ADVANCES IN IMMUNOASSAY TECHNOLOGY

Edited by **Norman H. L. Chiu**
and **Theodore K. Christopoulos**

Advances in Immunoassay Technology
Edited by Norman H. L. Chiu and Theodore K. Christopoulos

Published by InTech
Janeza Trdine 9, 51000 Rijeka, Croatia

Notice
Statements and opinions expressed in the chapters are these of the individual contributors and not necessarily those of the editors or publisher. No responsibility is accepted for the accuracy of information contained in the published chapters. The publisher assumes no responsibility for any damage or injury to persons or property arising out of the use of any materials, instructions, methods or ideas contained in the book.

Publishing Process Manager Maja Bozicevic

Technical Editor Teodora Smiljanic

Cover Designer InTech Design Team

Additional hard copies can be obtained from orders@intechopen.com

Advances in Immunoassay Technology,
Edited by Norman H. L. Chiu and Theodore K. Christopoulos
p. cm.
ISBN 978-953-51-0440-7

For EU product safety concerns:
IN TECH d.o.o., Prolaz Marije Krucifikse Kozulić 3, 51000 Rijeka, Croatia,
info@intechopen.com or visit our website at intechopen.com.

Meet the editors

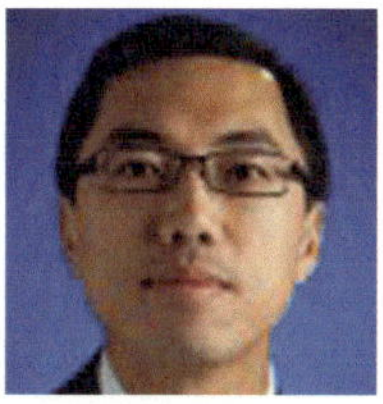

Dr Norman H. L. Chiu is an Associate Professor of Chemistry at the University of North Carolina at Greensboro, USA. He is also an affiliated member of the Joint School of Nanoscience and Nanoengineering in Greensboro, and the Comprehensive Cancer Center at the Wake Forest University. He received his B.Sc. in Chemistry from the University of Liverpool, UK, M.Sc. in Analytical Chemistry from the University of Bristol, UK, and Ph.D. in Biochemistry from the University of Windsor, Canada. He and Dr. Theodore Christopoulos were the first to develop an expressible enzyme-coding DNA label for immunoassays. As a Postdoctoral Research Fellow, he extended his research experience on method development with Dr. Charles R. Cantor at Boston University and Sequenom Inc, USA.

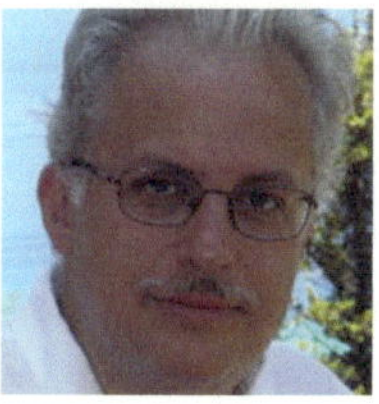

Dr Theodore K. Christopoulos is Professor and Chair, Department of Chemistry, University of Patras, Greece. He received a B.Sc. in Pharmacy (1982) and a Ph.D. in Analytical Chemistry (1987) from the University of Athens, Greece as well as a Postdoctoral Diploma in Clinical Chemistry (1991) from the University of Toronto, Canada. From 1989 to 1992 he was a Postdoctoral Research Associate at the Department of Clinical Biochemistry, University of Toronto. From 1992 to 1999 he worked as Assistant, Associate and Full Professor at the Department of Chemistry & Biochemistry, University of Windsor, Canada. He is the recipient of the 1997 Grannis award for "Excellence in Research and Scientific Publication" from the U.S. National Academy of Clinical Biochemistry.

Contents

Preface

Over the past decade, the development and applications of immunoassays have continued to grow exponentially. This book focuses on some of the latest advances in immunoassay technology, which include new materials and methods. The book contains nine invited chapters that are divided into three sections. In the first section, the basics for producing recombinant antibodies, the use of polyacrylonitrile fibre as a solid surface, and the nature of interference in immunoassays are summarized. The second section begins with a chapter on the basic concepts of different types of immunosensors, some of which allow label-free detection of specific analytes. This is followed by chapters on piezoelectric immunosensors and surface plasmon resonance biosensors. A chapter on using nanopores as a label-free biosensing platform and its potential for immunosensing is also included in the second section. The third section starts with a chapter that describes different platforms for carrying out multiplexed immunoassays. This is followed by a chapter on the advantages and limitations of multiplexed bead immunoassays.

The Editors express their thanks and appreciation to the authors for their contributions to this book project. Moreover, they are thankful to the Editorial Office at InTech for their support. They are also grateful to the *love* and support from their families, and acknowledge the assistance from their co-workers. Last but not least, they wish to thank all their former teachers and mentors for sharing their knowledge and experience with them.

Dr. Norman H. L. Chiu
Department of Chemistry and Biochemistry,
The University of North Carolina at Greensboro,
USA

Dr. Theodore K. Christopoulos
Department of Chemistry,
University of Patras,
Greece

Part 1

New Materials and Assay Interference

1

Recombinant Antibodies and Non-Antibody Scaffolds for Immunoassays

Bhupal Ban and Diane A. Blake
Department of Biochemistry and Molecular Biology, Tulane University School of Medicine, New Orleans, Louisiana, USA

1. Introduction

The measurement of trace amounts of physiologically active small molecules (for example, lipids, drugs, other synthetic chemicals and metals) is critical for both clinical and environmental analyses. Most small molecules can be analyzed using highly sophisticated analytical techniques, including high pressure liquid chromatography (HPLC), gas chromatography (GC), and inductively coupled plasma atomic emission spectroscopy (ICPAES). However, these methods require extensive purification, experienced technicians, and expensive instruments and reagents. Immunoassays offer an alternative to these instrument-intensive methods. Immunoassays rely on an antibody (Ab), or mixture of antibodies, for recognition of the molecule being analyzed (the analyte). Immunoassays are frequently applied to the analysis of both low molecular ligands and macromolecular drugs, and are also applied in such important areas as the quantitation of biomarkers that indicate disease progression and immunogenicity of therapeutic drug candidates. The performance of immunoassays is critically dependent on the binding properties of the antibody used in the analysis, and identification of suitable antibodies is often a major hurdle in assay development. Recombinant antibodies will play a major role in future immunoassay development.

2. Natural and recombinant antibody fragments

The antibody is the key reagent of an immunoassay and it can be produced by animal immunization, hybridoma technology, and/or recombinant techniques. Most, but not all, production methods require immunization of an animal with an antigen. An antigen is a molecule that can be recognized by the immune system (immunogenicity) and that can be bound specifically to an antibody (reactogenicity). Molecules with both immunogenicity and reactogenicity are called "complete antigens" and molecules that possess only reactogenicity are called "incomplete antigens". Incomplete antigens, also called haptens, encompass a wide variety of molecules, including drugs, explosives, pesticides, herbicides, polycyclic aromatic hydrocarbons, and metal ions. These haptens can induce the immune system to produce antibodies only when they are covalently conjugated to a larger carrier molecule such as a protein.

Although polyclonal antibodies hold their place as the reagents of choice for general-purpose applications in the biological sciences, the volume of serum that can be obtained from immunized animals and batch-to-batch differences in affinity and cross-reactivity make them less attractive for quantitative immunoassays. The first milestone for the generalized the use of immunoassays was the development of hybridoma technology, which overcame problems of heterogeneity and supply (Kohler & Milstein, 1975). While traditional monoclonal antibodies are used throughout biological research, many potential applications remain unfulfilled. The production of monoclonal antibodies requires considerable time, expense and expertise, as well as specialized cell culture facilities. The use of animal immunization means that the selection for relevant binding specificities occurs in the uncontrolled serum environment. This technology is adequate for stable antigens but not for molecules that are highly toxic, not immunogenic in mammals or not stable enough to withstand the immune processing steps required for the *in vivo* immune response. Most importantly, when working with monoclonal antibodies, it is not possible to alter or improve an antibody's binding properties without cumbersome procedures that convert the molecules to recombinant forms that can be engineered. All these reasons urged the development of strategies aimed at the production of recombinant antibodies (rAbs) and alternative scaffolds (Gebauer & Skerra, 2009) of smaller dimensions that can be easily selected, manipulated and produced using standard molecular biology techniques.

There are several distinct classes of natural antibodies (IgG, IgM, IgA, and IgE) that provide animals with key defenses against pathogenic organisms and toxins. Most immunoassay systems rely upon IgG as the immunoglobulin of choice. IgG is bivalent, and its ability to bind to two antigenic sites greatly increases its functional affinity and confers high retention time on cell surface receptors. The basic structure of an IgG molecule is shown in figure 1. Most IgG molecules are composed of two heavy chains (HC) and two light chains (LC), which are stabilized and linked by inter- and intra-chain disulfide bonds. The HC and LC can be further subdivided into variable regions and constant regions. The antigen binding site is formed by the combination of the variable region of the HC and LC. Most IgG molecules have two identical antigen binding sites, which are usually flat and concave for protein antigens, but which may form a pocket when the antibody has been selected against a hapten. Within the HC and LC variable regions are 3 hypervariable regions, also called complementary determining regions (CDRs), and 4 frameworks regions (FRs). The greatest sequence variation among individual antibodies occurs within the CDRs, while the FRs are more conserved. In general, it is assumed that the CDR regions from the LC and HC associate to form the antigen binding site. The lower part of the IgG molecule contains the heavy chain domains (crystallizable fragment, Fc) that are responsible for important biological effector functions. In additional to these conventional antibodies, camelids and sharks produce unusual antibodies composed only of heavy chains, also shown in figure 1. These peculiar heavy chain antibodies lack light chains (and, in the case of camelid antibodies also CH1 domain). Therefore, the antigen binding site of heavy chain antibodies is formed only by a single domain that is linked directly via a hinge region to the Fc domain. Intact IgG molecules, the bivalent $(Fab')_2$, or the monovalent (Fab), all of which contain the antigen binding site(s), can be used in immunoassays.

Recombinant antibody forms have also been developed to facilitate antibody engineering. The single chain fragment variable (scFv) molecule is a small antibody fragment of 26-27 kDa. It contains the complete variable domain of the HC and LC, typically linked by a 15 aa long hydrophilic and flexible polypeptide linker. The scFv fragments can also include a His tag for purification, an immunodetection epitope and a protease-specific cleavage site. The

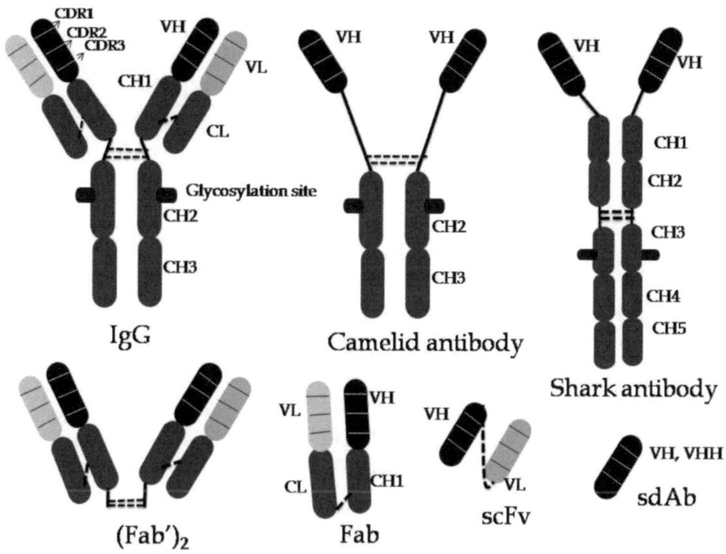

Fig. 1. Structure of conventional, camelid and shark antibodies and of antibody fragments.

orientation of the HC and LC domains is critical for binding activity, expression and proteolytic stability. Although a vast number of recombinant antibody (rAb) structures have been proposed (Holliger & Hudson, 2005), scFv fragments derived from mammalian IgGs and the single domain antibodies (sdAbs), which include the VHH from camelid and llama and the VH from shark, are the antibody fragments most widely used for both research and industrial applications (Kontermann, 2010; Wesolowski et al., 2009).

3. Principles and selection platforms of rAbs

Powerful combinatorial technologies have enabled the development of *in vitro* immune repertoires and selection methodologies that can be used to derive antibodies with or without the direct immunization of a living host (Hoogenboom, 2005; Marks & Bradbury, 2004). Recombinant antibody technology has provided an alternative method to engineer antibody fragments with the desired specificity and affinity within inexpensive and relatively simple host systems. Effective *in vitro* libraries have been constructed using either the entire antigen-binding fragment (Fab) or the single chain variable fragment (scFv), which represents the smallest domain capable of mediating antigen recognition. The simplest and most widely used antibody libraries utilize the scFv format, although single domain heavy chain libraries (VH and VHH) have also been constructed. The construction of *in vitro* libraries using different sources will be reviewed herein.

3.1 Antibodies from immune antibody libraries

The first rAbs were derived from pre-existing hybridomas; now, however, rAbs are mostly isolated from immune antibody libraries, i.e., antibody libraries generated from genetic material derived from immunized animals or naturally infected animals or humans. These libraries are biased for binding to the antigen. Thus, affinity maturation takes place *in vivo* and the chances of isolating the high-affinity antibodies are increased. Immune libraries are constructed using HC and LC variable domain gene pools amplified directly from immune sources; lymphoid sources include peripheral blood, bone marrow, spleen and tonsil (Huse et al., 1989; Schoonbroodt et al., 2005). In contrast to hybridoma technology, which can sample no more ~10% of the immune repertoire of an animal, a recombinant immune library, when prepared with the appropriate primers, can sample >80% of the immune repertoire and the diversity of antibodies that can be derived from a single immunized donor is much higher than what is possible using hybridomas. Selection is performed *in vitro,* which enhances the ability to select for rare antibody specificities. In addition, the immune repertoires of almost any species can be trapped, even those where hybridoma technology has not been described (chicken and llama), is not freely available (rabbit), or is not very robust (sheep). Immune libraries can provide higher-affinity binders than non-immune libraries. Immunizations are generally required for each targeted antigen, although multi-antigen immunizations have been performed successfully (Li et al., 2000). Advantages and disadvantages of immune libraries include: (1) the ease of preparation compared to naïve libraries; (2) the time requirement for animal immunization; (3) the unpredictability of the immune response of the animal to an antigen of interest; (4) lack of immune response to some antigens; and (5) the necessity of construction of new libraries for each new antigen.

3.2 Antibodies from nonimmune, synthetic, and semi- synthetic libraries

Non-immune (naïve) libraries are derived from normal, unimmunized, rearranged V gene from the IgM/IgG mRNA of B cells, peripheral blood lymphocytes, bone marrow, spleen or tonsil. These libraries are not explicitly biased to contain clones binding to antigens; as such they are useful for selecting antibodies against a wide variety of antigens. Using specific sets of primers and PCR, IgM and IgG variable regions are amplified and cloned into specific vectors designed for selection and screening (Bradbury & Marks, 2004; Marks et al., 1991, 2004). An ideal naïve library is expected to contain a representative sample of the primary repertoires of the immune system, although it will not contain a large proportion of antibodies with somatic hypermutations produced by natural immunization. The major advantages and disadvantages of using very large naïve libraries are: (1) the large antibody repertoire, which can be selected for binders for all antigens including non-immunogenic and toxic agents; (2) a shorter time period to binding proteins, because selection is performed on an already existing library; (3) low affinity antibodies are obtained from these libraries; and (4) it is technically demanding to construct these large non-immune repertoires. Many of these disadvantages may be bypassed by using synthetic antibody libraries.

Synthetic antibody libraries are created by introducing degenerate, synthetic DNA into the regions encoding CDRs of the defined variable-domain frameworks. Synthetic diversity bypasses the natural biases and redundancies of antibody repertoires created *in vivo* and allows control over the genetic makeup of V genes and the introduction of diversity (Hoogenboom & Winter, 1992). A synthetic library has been described that was constructed on the basis of existing information on the structure of the antigenic site of proteins and small molecules (Persson et al., 2006; Sidhu & Fellouse 2006).

Semi-synthetic libraries have been constructed by incorporating CDR loops with both natural and synthetic diversity into one or more of the antibody framework regions. High diversity semi-synthetic repertoires have been generated by introducing partially or completely randomized sequences mainly into the CDR3 region of the heavy chain. This process generates highly complex libraries and facilitates the selection of antibodies against self-antigens, which are normally removed by the negative selection of the immune system (Barbas et al.,1992). An efficient cloning system (*in vivo* Cre/loxP site specific recombination) combined with dual antibody cloning strategies allows construction of very large repertoires with about 10^{9-11} individual clones (Sblattero & Bradbury, 2000). Semi-synthetic libraries, however, have the disadvantage of always containing a certain number of non-functional clones, stemming from PCR errors, stop codons in the random sequence, or improperly folded protein products.

4. *In vitro* selection procedures for rAbs from combinatorial libraries

Recombinant antibody technologies provide the investigator with a great deal of control over selection and screening conditions and thus permit the generation of antibodies against highly specialized antigen conformations or epitopes. The most powerful methods, phage, yeast, and ribosomal display technologies, are complementary in their properties and can be used with naïve, immunized or synthetic antibody repertoires.

4.1 Phage display libraries for the isolation of antibodies

Phage display-based selections are now a relatively standard procedure in many molecular biology laboratories. The generation of antibody fragments with high specificity and affinity for virtually any antigen has been made possible using phage display. Phage display libraries are produced by cloning the pool of genes coding for antibody fragments into vectors that can be packed into the viral genome. The rAb is then expressed as an antibody fragment on the surface of mature phage particles. Selection of specific antibody fragments involves exposure to antigen, which allows the antigen-specific phage antibodies to bind their target during the bio-panning. The binding is followed by extensive wash steps and subsequent recovery of antigen-specific phage. The phage particles can then be used to infect *E. coli* bacteria. Different display systems can lead to monovalent (single copy) or to multivalent (multiple copy) display of the antibody fragment, depending on the type of anchor protein and display vector used (Sidhu et al., 2000). The most popular system uses a monovalent display vector system, which is convenient for selecting antibodies with higher affinity. Monovalent display is achieved by using a direct fusion to a minor viral coat protein (pIII). The vector into which most antibody libraries are cloned is a phagemid vector that requires a helper phage for the production of phage particles. Use of a phagemid vector makes propagation in bacteria much easier to accomplish than would be possible with a phage vector (Hust & Dubel, 2005). A general scheme for the isolation of antibody fragments by phage display is shown in figure 2. Libraries with 10^{6-11} individual clones can be made using recombinant-based protocols. Due to limitations of the *E. coli* folding machinery, complete IgG molecules are very difficult to express in *E. coil* and display on the surface of phage. Therefore, smaller antibody fragments such as Fab, scFv and sdAb are primarily used for antibody phage display.

4.2 Yeast surface display

Yeast surface display is a powerful method for isolating and engineering antibody fragments (Fab, scFv) from immune and non-immune libraries, and has been used to isolate recombinant antibodies with binding specificity to variety of proteins, peptides, and small molecules (Boder & Wittrup, 2000; Chao et al., 2006). In this system, antibodies are displayed on the surface of yeast *Saccharomyces cerevisiae* via fusion to an α-agglutinin yeast adhesion receptor, which is located in the yeast cell wall.

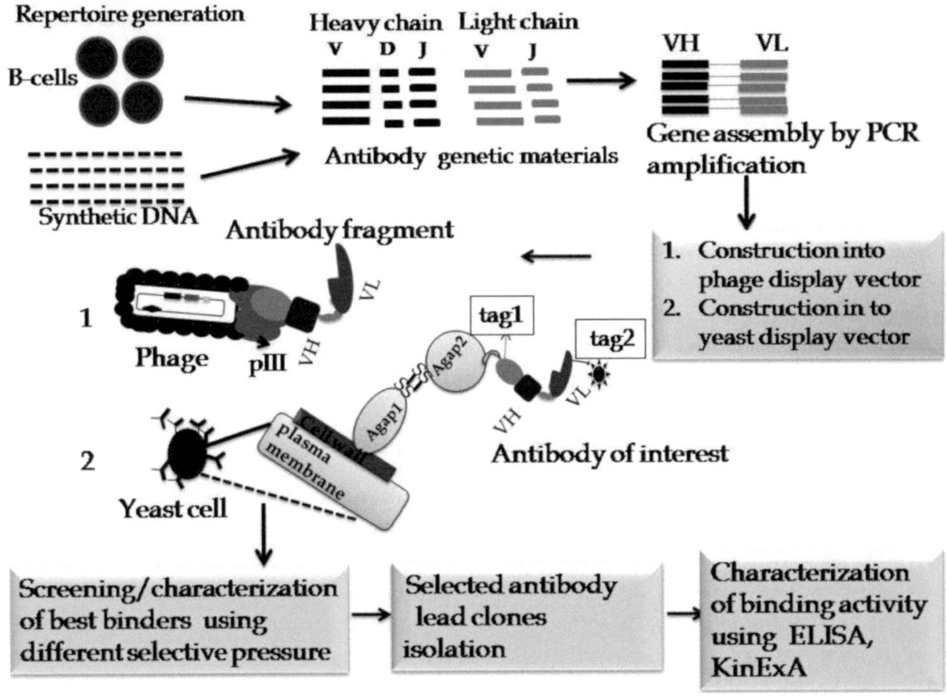

Fig. 2. Schematic diagram for construction of antibody libraries and *in vitro* display system; phage and yeast display.

Like phage display, yeast display provides a direct connection between genotype and phenotype; a plasmid containing the gene of interest is contained within yeast cells, while the encoded antibody is expressed on the surface. The display level of each yeast cell is variable, with each cell displaying $1x10^4$ to $1x10^5$ copies of the scFv. Variation of surface expression and avidity can be quantified using fluorescence activated cell sorting (FACS), which measures both antigen binding and antibody expression on the yeast cell surface (Feldhaus et al., 2003). The main advantage of yeast surface display over other display technologies is the eukaryotic expression bias of yeast, which contains post-translational modification and processing machinery similar to that of mammalian cells. Thus, yeast may be better suited for the expression of antibodies as compared to prokaryotes such as *E. coli*. Yeast display libraries have been used during the affinity maturation of scFvs from mutagenic libraries (Boder et al., 2000; Lou et al., 2010; Orcutt et al., 2011). Limiting factors of yeast display include a more limited transforming efficacy of yeast as compared to bacteria, which can lead to a smaller functional library size (about 10^7-10^9) than is possible with other display technologies.

4.3 Ribosomal display

Ribosomal display is an *in vitro* selection and evolution technology for proteins and peptides from large libraries (Dreier & Pluckthun, 2011; Hanes & Pluckthun, 1997). The general scheme of ribosomal display is shown in figure 3. This display system was developed from a peptide-display approach that was extended to screen scFv and scaffold proteins having very high affinity for antigen (K_ds as low as 10^{-11} M) from very large libraries (Binz et al., 2004; Zahnd et al., 2007). The DNA library coding for proteins such as antibodies and scaffolds are transcribed *in vitro*. The mRNA has been engineered without a stop codon; therefore, the translated protein remains attached to the peptidyl tRNA and occupies the ribosomal tunnel. This allows the protein of interest to protrude out of the ribosome and fold. Ribosomal display is performed entirely *in vitro*, and it has two advantages over other selection technologies. First, the diversity of the libraries is not limited by the transformation efficiency of bacterial cells (~1x10^{11} to 1x10^{13}), but only by the number of ribosomes and different mRNA molecules present in the test tube. Second, random mutations can be introduced easily after each selection round, as no cells must be transformed after any diversification step. In ribosomal display, the physical link between the genotype and the corresponding phenotype is accomplished by a complex consisting of mRNA, ribosome and protein.

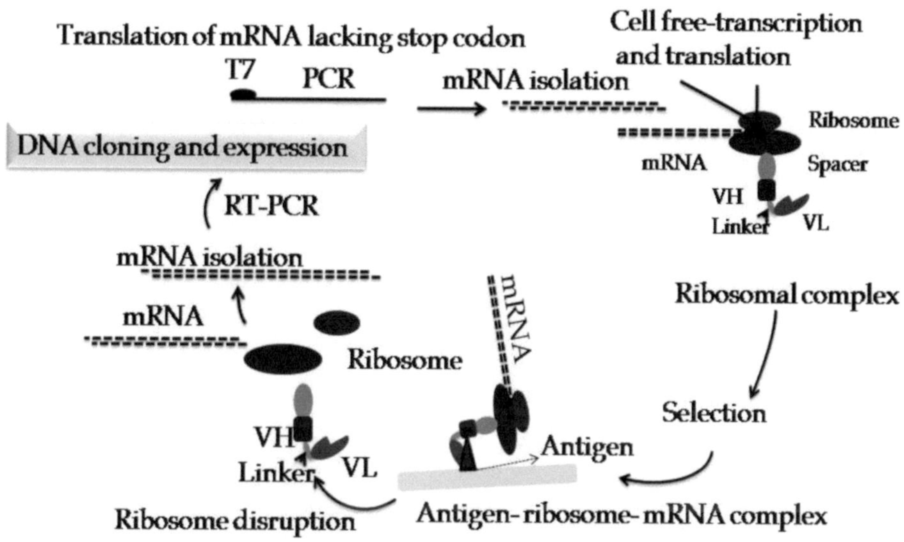

Fig. 3. Schematic diagram for isolation of specific antibody fragment from ribosomal display

Ribosomal display has been used to isolate antibodies that bind to haptens with nanomolar affinities (Yau et al., 2003). A summary of the *in vitro* display systems available to researchers is shown in table 1.

5. Applications of rAbs against low molecular ligands

A large number of rAbs have been used successfully to develop diagnostic kits, therapeutics and biosensors (Holliger et al., 2005; Huang et al., 2010; Kramer & Hock, 2003). The majority of the targets were large molecular weight analytes such as proteins and peptides. Prior to 1990, there were few reports of the isolation of rAbs against low molecular weight molecules (haptens) such as drugs of abuse, vitamins, hormones, metabolites, food toxins and environmental pollutants, including heavy metals and pesticides. Hapten-specific antibodies

Name	Display	Library size	Main applications	Advantages	Disadvantages
Phage display	Monovalent Multivalent	10^{10} to 10^{11}	Abs from natural & synthetic libraries; Affinity maturation & stability increase	Easy and versatile for large rAbs panels	Laborious to make large libraries; Not truly monovalent
Yeast surface display	Multivalent	10^7	Abs from natural & synthetic libraries; Affinity maturation & stability increase	Rapid when used in combination with random mutagenesis	Small rAb panels, FACS expertise required
Ribosome display	Monovalent	10^{12} to 10^{13}	Abs from natural & synthetic libraries; Affinity maturation & stability increase	Intrinsic mutagenesis, fastest of all systems	Small rAb panels, limited selection scope and technically sensitive

Table 1. Comparing the main *in vitro* selection platforms for isolation of rAbs

are necessary reagents for the development of immunoassays, immunosensor technologies (Charlton et al., 2001), and immunoaffinity chromatography purification columns (Sheedy & Hall, 2001). Commercial immunoassays for haptens such as small environmental contaminants still rely mostly on polyclonal antibodies rather than monoclonal or recombinant antibodies fragments (Sheedy et al., 2007). The complexity and costs associated with the production of anti-hapten antibodies by hybridoma technology and the preferential selection of antibodies that recognize the conjugated form of the haptens over antibodies that specifically recognize free haptens are two of the most important problems that have limited the development and application of antibodies that recognize haptens and other low molecules ligands. Moreover, some small molecular weight ligands will not trigger the animal immune system even when conjugated to a carrier protein, thereby making the production of antibodies against that such analytes very difficult.

In recent years, the production of recombinant antibodies to low molecular weight ligands has increased significantly, as shown in table 2. A single methyl or hydroxyl group can have a considerable effect on the biological properties of a steroid hormone. Similarly, protein phosphorylation, acetylation and sulfation, all of which are relatively simple post-translational modifications in chemical terms, can dramatically affect signal transduction (Bikker et al., 2007; Hoffhines et al., 2006; Kehoe et al., 2006). Antibodies capable of discerning such relatively simple chemical modification are of great values in studying these effects. The display methods to tailor both affinity and specificity have generated antibodies capable of discerning minor difference between related small molecules far better than those obtained by immunization.

6. Improving the specificity and affinity of rAbs to low molecular weight ligands

Although recombinant antibody technology has been able to open the bottleneck in the isolation of antibodies against virtually any antigen, it remains difficult to obtain high-affinity antibodies against small molecules using immune and naïve libraries. Various approaches have been utilized, including identifying the key binding residues, developing more effective procedures for selection of the most specific binders and avoiding interfacial effects that can compromise the yield and stability of rAbs.

Target Hapten	Ab format	Antibody library	*In vitro* display	Reference
Aflatoxin B1	scFv	Naïve	Phage	(Moghaddam et al., 2001)
Digoxigenin	scFv	Naïve	Phage	(Dorsam et al., 1997)
Doxorubicin	scFv	Naïve	Phage	(Vaughan et al., 1996)
Estradiol	scFv	Naïve	Phage	(Dorsam et al., 1997)
Indole-3-acetic acid	VHH	Naïve	Phage	(Sheedy et al., 2006)
Fluorescein	scFv	Naïve	Phage	(Vaughan et al., 1996)
Phenyloxazolone	scFv	Naïve	Phage	(de Haard et al., 1999)
Picloram	VHH	Naïve	Ribosome	(Yau et al., 2003)
Progesterone	scFv	Naïve	Ribosome	(He et al., 1999)
Fumosinin B1	scFv	Naïve	Phage	(Lauer et al., 2005)
Atrazine	scFv	Immune	Phage	(Li et al., 2000)
Azo-dye RR1	VHH	Immune	Phage	(Spinelli et al., 2000)
Cortisol	scFv	Immune	Phage	(Chames & Baty, 1998)
Digoxin & analogues	scFv	Immune	Phage	(Short et al., 1995)
Isoproturon	scFv	Immune	Phage	(Li et al., 2000)
Mecoprop	scFv	Immune	Phage	(Li et al., 2000)
Simazine	scFv	Immune	Phage	(Li et al., 2000)
Triazine	scFv	Immune	Phage	(Kramer, 2002)
4-Hydroxy-3-iodo-5-nitrophenol	scFv	Semi-synthetic	Phage	(van Wyngaardt et al., 2004)
Fluorescein	scFv	Semi-synthetic	Phage	(van Wyngaardt et al., 2004)
Microcystin LR	scFv	Semi-synthetic	Phage	(Strachan et al., 2002)
Phtalic acid	scFv	Semi-synthetic	Phage	(Strachan et al., 2002)
Trichlocarbon	VHH	Naïve	Phage	(Tabares-da Rosa et al., 2011)
6-Monoacetylmorphine but not morphine	scFv	Naïve	Phage	(Moghaddam et al., 2003)
Metallic gold	Fv	Naïve	Phage	(Watanabe et al.,, 2008)
Anti-Aluminum	VHH	Semi-synthetic	Phage	(Hattori et al., 2010)
Anti-Cobalt	VHH	Semi-synthetic	Phage	(Hattori et al., 2010)
Anti-Uranium	scFv	Immune	Phage	(Zhu et al., 2011)
Domoic acid	scFv	Immune	Phage	(Shaw et al., 2008)
Azoxystrobin	VHH	Immune	Phage	(Makvandi-Nejad et al., 2011)
Methamidophos	scFv	Immune	Phage	(Li et al., 2006)

Table 2. List of small molecule-specific recombinant antibodies

There are, however, unique challenges to the development of antibodies that will perform well in assays for low molecular weight ligands. Antigen binding sites are generated by the cooperation between the variable domains of the HC and LC (VH/VL). The amino acids of FRs compose rigid scaffolds that position the amino acids in the CDRs in loops that extend outward from scaffold. These loops play important roles in making contact with the antigen. Hapten antigens have remained a great challenge for immunodiagnostics, because the hapten portion of the antigen often ends up almost buried inside the concave-shaped antigen binding pocket. The extended shape of this binding pocket then facilitates additional interactions between amino acid residues in binding site and portions of the hapten-protein conjugate present in the bridge between the hapten and the protein carrier. These additional interactions mean that the antibody often binds to the much more tightly to the hapten-protein conjugate than to the soluble hapten. In our laboratory, we have studied this phenomenon with 10 different anti-hapten antibodies. In this study, the antibody always bound more tightly to the protein conjugate than to the soluble antigen. The differences in affinity ranged from 1.5 to 1600 fold, depending upon the antibody being analyzed (Blake et al., 1996, Melton, 2010). Thus, when given a choice, anti-hapten antibodies almost always prefer binding to the hapten-protein conjugate, and additional soluble hapten is required to inhibit this interaction, thus reducing assay sensitivity. Selective panning and affinity maturation are methods available in recombinant technology for reducing selective binding of hapten antibodies to the hapten-protein conjugate.

6.1 Panning optimization

A variety of selection strategies have been reported for the isolation of high affinity rAbs against chelated metals and other haptens (Sheedy et al., 2007; Zhu et al., 2011). The most successful strategies employed first loose and then increasingly stringent panning conditions to enrich the population of phage antibodies as follow: (i) the concentration of coating antigen was gradually decreased during successive rounds of panning (Strachan et al., 2002; Zhu et al., 2011); (ii) soluble hapten was used to elute ligand-specific antibodies in place of the triethylamine more commonly used for elution; (iii) during the panning of immune scFv libraries, the conjugate carrier protein and/or other linker peptides were included for several intermediate incubation steps at high concentration and subsequently decreased to remove phage antibodies that bound to the protein conjugate rather than the soluble hapten; (iv) the phage antibodies were incubated with structural analogues of the hapten prior to incubation with the immobilized target hapten to eliminate phage antibodies with unwanted cross reactivities (Charlton et al., 2001; Zhu et al., 2011). Such panning optimization strategies have led to the isolation of antibodies with higher affinity and specificity and lower levels of cross-reactivity. For an example from the isolation of antibodies to metal-chelate complexes, such subtractive panning strategies were employed to isolate an antibody that bound tightly to uranium in complex with 2,9-dicarboxyl-1,10-phenanthroline, (DCP), but weakly to metal-free DCP. In successive rounds of panning, the phage antibody population was incubated with a high concentration of carrier protein (BSA) and increasing concentrations of soluble DCP in immunotubes coated with decreasing concentrations of a UO_2^{2+}-DCP-BSA conjugate as shown in table 3.

Round of Selection	Percent of maximum conjugate coated onto immunotubes	Percent of maximum metal-free chelator added to the phage binding buffer	Percent of maximum carrier protein added to the phage binding buffer
1	100	10	100
2	100	10	100
3	10	20	100
4	10	20	100
5	1	100	100

Table 3. General selection strategy for the isolation of scFvs that bind to a metal-loaded but not a metal-free chelator (Zhu et al., 2011).

6.2 *In vitro* antibody affinity maturation

The affinity maturation procedure contains two stages: (a) making a modified antibody library with a larger diversity than the original library (b) selecting desired antibodies molecules from the library using the previously discussed *in vitro* display and panning methods. An antibody's affinity for its antigen is dependent on the identity and conformation of the amino acid sidechains in the CDRs of both the HC and LC. Improvement in the antigen-binding affinity can be attained using a number of strategies. The mostly common used are random mutagenesis, site-direct mutagenesis and chain shuffling. These processes are often referred to as *in vitro* affinity maturation, to distinguish the process from the affinity maturation that takes place in the animal. Although a considerable number of successful affinity maturation processes have been reported for antibodies against macromolecule antigens like proteins, affinity maturation for low weight molecules like haptens and metals is obviously more difficult, and consequently, only a limited number of successful studies have thus far been reported.

6.2.1 Random mutagenesis (Error Prone PCR; E-p PCR)

Random mutagenesis is the process that most closely mimics the *in vivo* process of somatic hypermutation. This process makes no assumptions as to which sites are the best to mutate in order to increase affinity, and it is also technically rather simple to execute. Error prone PCR uses low fidelity polymerization conditions to introduce a low level of point mutations randomly throughout a wide region of a target gene (e.g. , the entire VH and VL). Error prone PCR has been used to demonstrate the effect of mutation frequency on the affinity maturation of antibodies against both proteins and small ligands (Daugherty et al., 2000). When wild type antibodies to the hapten, diogoxin, were subjected to E-p PCR, the higher affinity clones isolated from libraries all contained aromatic residues substitutions in the antibody binding site. These resides were thought to be important for hydrophobic interaction with the planer aromatic structure of digoxin (Short et al., 1995). A disadvantage of E-p PCR is that surface-selection often enriches binders with increased tendency for dimerization, especially when using the scFv format. In addition, most of the mutants lacked detectable expression or lost antigen-binding affinity. A few mutants lost specificity and showed increased cross-reactivity to analogs (Fuji, 2004; Sheedy et al., 2007). Point mutation can cause profound effects on the binding affinity and specificity of an antibody for its small ligands. The affinity maturation processes reported for anti-hapten scFvs are listed in table 4.

6.2.2 Site-directed mutagenesis

In site-directed mutagenesis, the investigator changes specific amino acid residues. Site-directed mutagenesis is often used in combination with in silico modeling, crystallographic data, and ligand docking programs, which allow the investigator to hypothesize about the roles that individual binding site amino acid residues have in antigen binding. The CDRs of VH and VL are usually targeted for both haptens and protein antigens (Siegel, et al., 2008), and mutations in CDRs as opposed to within the framework residues generally contribute more to increases in affinity (Orcutt et al., 2011; Short et al., 2002). In one study, the most significant increase in affinity was correlated with mutations in the light chain CDR1 even though this CDR1 was not contacting the hapten directly (Valjakka et al., 2002). Hapten-specific antibodies whose affinity has been increased by site directed mutagenesis are listed in table 4.

Target hapten	Fold increase in affinity	Ab format/ *in vitro* display	Affinity maturation	Reference
phOx-GABA	290	scFv/Phage	Chain shuffling	(Marks et al., 1992)
Cortisol	7.9	scFv/Phage	Site-directed	(Chames et al., 1998)
Estradiol-17 β	12	Fab/Phage	Site-directed	(Kobayashi et al., 2010)
Fluorescein	2600	scFv/Yeast	Ep-PCR /DNA -shuffling	(Boder et al., 2000)
Testosterone	35	Fab /Phage	Site-directed	(Valjakka et al., 2002)
Tacrolimus	15	scFv/Yeast	Site-directed	(Siegel et al., 2008)
DOTA-chelate	1000	scFv/Yeast	Site-directed	(Orcutt et al., 2011)

Table 4. List of successful affinity maturations of anti-hapten antibodies

6.3 Shuffling of antibody genes

Shuffling of antibody genes to create new antibody libraries can be accomplished in several ways: chain shuffling, DNA shuffling, and staggered extension processes.

6.3.1 Chain shuffling

In this procedure, one of the two chains (VH of VL) is fixed and combined with a repertoire of partner chains to yield a secondary library that can be searched for superior pairings against antigens. This approach takes advantage of "random" mutations that have been introduced into VH and VL germline genes *in vivo*. Phage display and yeast display are often used to facilitate the selection of improved binders from these secondary libraries (Lou et al., 2010; Marks, 2004; Persson et al., 2006). This procedure has also been used to increase the affinity of anti-hapten antibodies and the results are reviewed in table 4. Chain shuffling is only a suitable mutagenesis strategy when VH and VL sequences are available from immune libraries. Chain shuffling is, therefore, not useful with naïve libraries since heavy and light chains available in these libraries have not been exposed to the antigen of interest.

6.3.2 DNA shuffling by random fragmentation and reassembly

DNA shuffling is based on repeated cycles of point mutagenesis, recombination and selection, which allows *in vitro* molecular evolution of protein (Stemmer, 1994). The process mimics somewhat the natural mechanism of molecular evolution (Ness et al., 1999). This shuffling technique involves the digestion of a large antibody gene with DNase I to create a pool of random DNA fragments. These fragments can then be reassembled into full-length genes by repeated cycles of annealing in the presence of DNA polymerase. DNA shuffling offers several advantages over more traditional mutagenesis strategies. It uses longer DNA sequences and also permits the selection of clones with mutations outside of the antibody binding site.

7. Modification of rAbs fused with signal enhancer proteins

Antibody engineering enables the preparation of fusion proteins combining scFvs and enzymes via the expression of a single scFv-enzyme fusion gene. Such recombinant scFv-fusion proteins have been reported for numerous applications, including the detection of a plant virus (Griep et al., 1999), the human pathogen hantaviruses (Velappan et al., 2007), other protein targets such as *Bacillus anthraces* (Wang et al., 2006), cholera and ricin toxins (Swain et al., 2011), and the haptens morphine (Brennan et al., 2003) and 11-deoxycortisol (11-DC) (Kobayashi et al., 2006). These fusion proteins provide a much higher signal/noise ratio in the ELISA format than conventional enzyme-labeled antibodies because the fusion proteins can be obtained as a single molecule species having a 1:1 rAb/enzyme ratio, and thus are uncontaminated by unconjugated enzyme and rAb molecules. As an example, the sensitivity of a competitive immunoassay for 11-deoxycortisol was 10,000-fold higher when an scFv-alkaline phosphatase fusion protein replaced the standard enzyme-labeled secondary antibody (Kobayashi et al., 2006; Martin et al., 2006).

8. Beyond antibody fragments (Scaffold protein)

Conventional diagnostic immunoassays are limited to the analysis of a few hundred assays per day, whereas with antibody microarrays using individually addressable electrodes, thousands of assays can be run in parallel (Dill et al., 2004). Antibody fragments are providing valuable alternatives to full length mAbs for new biosensing devices because they provide small, stable, highly specific reagents against the target antigens. In addition, because the recombinant antibody is smaller than the intact IgG, the density of binding sites that can be immobilized on the surface of these sensors can be increased. The stability of surface-immobilized ligands is also crucial in immunoassay format. Therefore, a great deal of interest has been focused on simplifying the antibody scaffold, and molecular engineering has pushed the concepts of antibody miniaturization to develop more stable binders that are less sterically hindered when immobilized on surfaces.

To overcome the limitation of antibodies, the several alternative protein frameworks have been developed. Design of these protein frameworks, collectively called "scaffolds" or "scaffold proteins", usually involves the adaptation of structurally well-defined polypeptide frameworks by the introduction of novel functionality. The new functionality is added to those parts of the protein surface that are not considered important for protein folding or stability. The recent development of non-biological alternatives to antibodies, including both scaffold proteins and plastibodies, may create distinct opportunities for future improvements in immunoassay technology. This could be particularly relevant in applications where compatibility of the binding probe with organic solvents and the ability to withstand thermal and mechanical stress are required. Currently, there are more than 60 non-antibody scaffolds suggested as affinity ligands, primarily for therapeutic and diagnostic purposes (Binz et al., 2005a; Caravella & Lugovskoy, 2010; Lofblom et al., 2010; Skerra, 2007). One of the current problems with bacterial expression of antibody fragments is that of disulfide bond formation, which occurs primarily in the periplasm of bacterial cells. Because of the intradomain disulfide bonds required for proper immunoglobulin folding, neither scFvs nor Fabs are compatible with intracellular expression and only very stable scFv fragments have been expressed in the cytoplasm of *E. coli* (Martineau & Betton, 1999; Ohage et al., 1999). The ideal scaffold therefore should be stable without disulfide bonds, expressed in high amounts in *E. coli* and compatible with current display techniques. The scaffold should contain loops or other structures on its surface that can be modified to form the binding site. This can be a natural binding site or created *de novo*. Randomizations made to the binding region should be able to generate binders with high specificity and affinity (Binz & Pluckthun, 2005b; Gebauer et al., 2009; Gronwall & Stahl, 2009; Kim et al., 2009; Lofblom et al., 2010). All of the scaffolds reported to date, including affibodies, anticalins, and designed ankyrin repeats (DARPin), can be engineered for interaction with analytes by mimicking the way the immune system shuffles sequences to create diversity in loop structures. The goal is to randomize the loops without affecting the overall structure and stability of protein. Thus, it is possible to engineer binding properties that are totally independent of their original biological function. An example of this strategy is the recently developed anticalin with picomolar affinity for DTPA-chelated lanthanides, especially Y^{III} (Kim et al., 2009). This anticalin forms a tight non-covalent complex (with slow dissociation kinetics) under physiological conditions in the presence of the chelated metal ion and, after fusion with an appropriate targeting domain; it may provide an ideal tool for applications in 'pretargeting' radioimmunotherapy. Notably, the only established non-Ig scaffold that intrinsically provides pockets and thus allows tight and specific complexation of small molecules is the one of the lipocalins.

9. Conclusion

Immunoassay techniques provide simple, powerful and inexpensive methods for the measurement of small ligands. However, the progress of the development of new immunoassays and related immunotechnologies is still limited by the availability of antibodies with the desired affinities and specificities for given applications. Advances in molecular biology have led to the ability to synthesize antibodies *in vitro*, completely without the use of animals. Recombinant molecular technology that can generate variability, combined with high-throughput screening methodologies, can be used to produce engineered antibody-like molecules and novel antibody-mimic domains on scaffold proteins. The rAbs fused with other functional proteins can enhance the sensitivity of antibody-based assays and reduce the cost and labor involved in chemically synthesizing conjugates. Antibody engineering had already matured into a technology available to the general scientific community. Further advances will lead to better binding proteins that will permit the development of novel, high-throughput sensing systems for low molecular weight ligands.

10. Acknowledgments

The authors acknowledge funding from the Office of Science, Department of Energy (DE-SC0004959) and from the USPHS, NIEHS (U19-ES020677).

11. References

Barbas, C. F., 3rd, Bain, J. D., Hoekstra, D. M., & Lerner, R. A. (1992). Semisynthetic combinatorial antibody libraries: a chemical solution to the diversity problem. *Proc Natl Acad Sci U S A*, 89(10), 4457-4461.

Bikker, F. J., Mars-Groenendijk, R. H., Noort, D., Fidder, A., & van der Schans, G. P. (2007). Detection of sulfur mustard adducts in human callus by phage antibodies. *Chem Biol Drug Des*, 69(5), 314-320.

Binz, H. K., Amstutz, P., Kohl, A., Stumpp, M. T., Briand, C., Forrer, P., Grutter, M. G., & Pluckthun, A. (2004). High-affinity binders selected from designed ankyrin repeat protein libraries. *Nat Biotechnol*, 22(5), 575-582.

Binz, H. K., Amstutz, P., & Pluckthun, A. (2005a). Engineering novel binding proteins from nonimmunoglobulin domains. *Nat Biotechnol*, 23(10), 1257-1268.

Binz, H. K., & Pluckthun, A. (2005b). Engineered proteins as specific binding reagents. *Curr Opin Biotechnol*, 16(4), 459-469.

Blake, D. A., Chakrabarti, P., Khosraviani, M., Hatcher, F. M., Westhoff, C. M., Goebel, P., Wylie, D. E., & Blake, R. C., 2nd (1996). Metal binding properties of a monoclonal antibody directed toward metal-chelate complexes. *J Biol Chem*, 271(44), 27677-27685.

Boder, E. T., Midelfort, K. S., & Wittrup, K. D. (2000). Directed evolution of antibody fragments with monovalent femtomolar antigen-binding affinity. *Proc Natl Acad Sci U S A*, 97(20), 10701-10705.

Boder, E. T., & Wittrup, K. D. (2000). Yeast surface display for directed evolution of protein expression, affinity, and stability. *Methods Enzymol*, 328, 430-444.

Bradbury, A. R., & Marks, J. D. (2004). Antibodies from phage antibody libraries. *J Immunol Methods*, 290(1-2), 29-49.

Brennan, J., Dillon, P., & O'Kennedy, R. (2003). Production, purification and characterization of genetically derived scFv and bifunctional antibody fragments capable of detecting illicit drug residues. *J Chromatogr B Analyt Technol Biomed Life Sci*, 786(1-2), 327-342.

Caravella, J., & Lugovskoy, A. (2010). Design of next-generation protein therapeutics. *Curr Opin Chem Biol*, 14(4), 520-528.

Chames, P., & Baty, D. (1998). Engineering of an anti-steroid antibody: amino acid substitutions change antibody fine specificity from cortisol to estradiol. *Clin Chem Lab Med*, 36(6), 355-359.

Chames, P., Coulon, S., & Baty, D. (1998). Improving the affinity and the fine specificity of an anti-cortisol antibody by parsimonious mutagenesis and phage display. *J Immunol*, 161(10), 5421-5429.

Chao, G., Lau, W. L., Hackel, B. J., Sazinsky, S. L., Lippow, S. M., & Wittrup, K. D. (2006). Isolating and engineering human antibodies using yeast surface display. *Nat Protoc*, 1(2), 755-768.

Charlton, K., Harris, W. J., & Porter, A. J. (2001). The isolation of super-sensitive anti-hapten antibodies from combinatorial antibody libraries derived from sheep. *Biosens Bioelectron*, 16(9-12), 639-646.

Daugherty, P. S., Chen, G., Iverson, B. L., & Georgiou, G. (2000). Quantitative analysis of the effect of the mutation frequency on the affinity maturation of single chain Fv antibodies. *Proc Natl Acad Sci U S A*, 97(5), 2029-2034.

de Haard, H. J., van Neer, N., Reurs, A., Hufton, S. E., Roovers, R. C., Henderikx, P., de Bruine, A. P., Arends, J. W., & Hoogenboom, H. R. (1999). A large non-immunized human Fab fragment phage library that permits rapid isolation and kinetic analysis of high affinity antibodies. *J Biol Chem*, 274(26), 18218-18230.

Dill, K., Montgomery, D. D., Ghindilis, A. L., & Schwarzkopf, K. R. (2004). Immunoassays and sequence-specific DNA detection on a microchip using enzyme amplified electrochemical detection. *J Biochem Biophys Methods*, 59(2), 181-187.

Dorsam, H., Rohrbach, P., Kurschner, T., Kipriyanov, S., Renner, S., Braunagel, M., Welschof, M., & Little, M. (1997). Antibodies to steroids from a small human naive IgM library. *FEBS Lett*, 414(1), 7-13.

Dreier, B., & Pluckthun, A. (2011). Ribosome display: a technology for selecting and evolving proteins from large libraries. *Methods Mol Biol*, 687, 283-306.

Feldhaus, M. J., Siegel, R. W., Opresko, L. K., Coleman, J. R., Feldhaus, J. M., Yeung, Y. A., Cochran, J. R., Heinzelman, P., Colby, D., Swers, J., Graff, C., Wiley, H. S., & Wittrup, K. D. (2003). Flow-cytometric isolation of human antibodies from a nonimmune Saccharomyces cerevisiae surface display library. *Nat Biotechnol*, 21(2), 163-170.

Fujii, I. (2004). Antibody affinity maturation by random mutagenesis. *Methods Mol Biol*, 248, 345-359.

Gebauer, M., & Skerra, A. (2009). Engineered protein scaffolds as next-generation antibody therapeutics. *Curr Opin Chem Biol*, 13(3), 245-255.

Griep, R. A., van Twisk, C., van der Wolf, J. M., & Schots, A. (1999). Fluobodies: green fluorescent single-chain Fv fusion proteins. *J Immunol Methods*, 230(1-2), 121-130.

Gronwall, C., & Stahl, S. (2009). Engineered affinity proteins--generation and applications. *J Biotechnol*, 140(3-4), 254-269.

Hanes, J., & Pluckthun, A. (1997). In vitro selection and evolution of functional proteins by using ribosome display. *Proc Natl Acad Sci U S A*, 94(10), 4937-4942.

Hattori, T., Umetsu, M., Nakanishi, T., Togashi, T., Yokoo, N., Abe, H., Ohara, S., Adschiri, T., & Kumagai, I. (2010). High affinity anti-inorganic material antibody generation by integrating graft and evolution technologies: potential of antibodies as biointerface molecules. *J Biol Chem*, 285(10), 7784-7793.

He, M., Menges, M., Groves, M. A., Corps, E., Liu, H., Bruggemann, M., & Taussig, M. J. (1999). Selection of a human anti-progesterone antibody fragment from a transgenic mouse library by ARM ribosome display. *J Immunol Methods*, 231(1-2), 105-117.

Hoffhines, A. J., Damoc, E., Bridges, K. G., Leary, J. A., & Moore, K. L. (2006). Detection and purification of tyrosine-sulfated proteins using a novel anti-sulfotyrosine monoclonal antibody. *J Biol Chem*, 281(49), 37877-37887.

Holliger, P., & Hudson, P. J. (2005). Engineered antibody fragments and the rise of single domains. *Nat Biotechnol*, 23(9), 1126-1136.

Hoogenboom, H. R. (2005). Selecting and screening recombinant antibody libraries. *Nat Biotechnol*, 23(9), 1105-1116.

Hoogenboom, H. R., & Winter, G. (1992). By-passing immunisation. Human antibodies from synthetic repertoires of germline VH gene segments rearranged in vitro. *J Mol Biol*, 227(2), 381-388.

Huang, L., Muyldermans, S., & Saerens, D. (2010). Nanobodies(R): proficient tools in diagnostics. *Expert Rev Mol Diagn*, 10(6), 777-785.

Huse, W. D., Sastry, L., Iverson, S. A., Kang, A. S., Alting-Mees, M., Burton, D. R., Benkovic, S. J., & Lerner, R. A. (1989). Generation of a large combinatorial library of the immunoglobulin repertoire in phage lambda. *Science*, 246(4935), 1275-1281.

Hust, M., & Dubel, S. (2005). Phage display vectors for the in vitro generation of human antibody fragments. *Methods Mol Biol*, 295, 71-96.

Kehoe, J. W., Velappan, N., Walbolt, M., Rasmussen, J., King, D., Lou, J., Knopp, K., Pavlik, P., Marks, J. D., Bertozzi, C. R., & Bradbury, A. R. (2006). Using phage display to select antibodies recognizing post-translational modifications independently of sequence context. *Mol Cell Proteomics*, 5(12), 2350-2363.

Kim, H. J., Eichinger, A., & Skerra, A. (2009). High-affinity recognition of lanthanide(III) chelate complexes by a reprogrammed human lipocalin 2. *J Am Chem Soc*, 131(10) , 3565-3576.

Kobayashi, N., Iwakami, K., Kotoshiba, S., Niwa, T., Kato, Y., Mano, N., & Goto, J. (2006). Immunoenzymometric assay for a small molecule,11-deoxycortisol, with attomole-range sensitivity employing an scFv-enzyme fusion protein and anti-idiotype antibodies. *Anal Chem*, 78(7), 2244-2253.

Kobayashi, N., Oyama, H., Kato, Y., Goto, J., Soderlind, E., & Borrebaeck, C. A. (2010). Two-step in vitro antibody affinity maturation enables estradiol-17beta assays with more than 10-fold higher sensitivity. *Anal Chem*, 82(3), 1027-1038.

Kohler, G., & Milstein, C. (1975). Continuous cultures of fused cells secreting antibody of predefined specificity. *Nature*, 256(5517), 495-497.

Kontermann, R. E. (2010). Alternative antibody formats. *Curr Opin Mol Ther, 12*(2), 176-183.

Kramer, K. (2002). Synthesis of a group-selective antibody library against haptens. *J Immunol Methods*, 266(1-2), 209-220.

Kramer, K., & Hock, B. (2003). Recombinant antibodies for environmental analysis. *Anal Bioanal Chem*, 377(3), 417-426.

Lauer, B., Ottleben, I., Jacobsen, H. J., & Reinard, T. (2005). Production of a single-chain variable fragment antibody against fumonisin B1. *J Agric Food Chem*, 53(4), 899-904.

Li, T., Zhang, Q., Liu, Y., Chen, D., Hu, B., Blake, D.A., & Liu, F. (2006) Production of recombinant antibodies against methamidophos from a phage-display library of a hyperimmunized mouse. *J Agric Food Chem*, 54(24), 9085-9091.

Li, Y., Cockburn, W., Kilpatrick, J. B., & Whitelam, G. C. (2000). High affinity ScFvs from a single rabbit immunized with multiple haptens. *Biochem Biophys Res Commun*, 268(2), 398-404.

Lofblom, J., Feldwisch, J., Tolmachev, V., Carlsson, J., Stahl, S., & Frejd, F. Y. (2010). Affibody molecules: engineered proteins for therapeutic, diagnostic and biotechnological applications. *FEBS Lett*, 584(12), 2670-2680.

Lou, J., Geren, I., Garcia-Rodriguez, C., Forsyth, C. M., Wen, W., Knopp, K., Brown, J., Smith, T., Smith, L. A., & Marks, J. D. (2010). Affinity maturation of human botulinum neurotoxin antibodies by light chain shuffling via yeast mating. *Protein Eng Des Sel*, 23(4), 311-319.

Makvandi-Nejad, S., Fjallman, T., Arbabi-Ghahroudi, M., Mackenzie, C. R., & Hall, J. C. (2011). Selection and expression of recombinant single domain antibodies from a hyper-immunized library against the hapten azoxystrobin. *J Immunol Methods*. in press.

Marks, J. D. (2004). Antibody affinity maturation by chain shuffling. *Methods Mol Biol*, 248, 327-343.

Marks, J. D., & Bradbury, A. (2004). PCR cloning of human immunoglobulin genes. *Methods Mol Biol*, 248, 117-134.

Marks, J. D., Griffiths, A. D., Malmqvist, M., Clackson, T. P., Bye, J. M., & Winter, G. (1992). By-passing immunization: building high affinity human antibodies by chain shuffling. *Biotechnology (N Y)*, 10(7), 779-783.

Marks, J. D., Hoogenboom, H. R., Bonnert, T. P., McCafferty, J., Griffiths, A. D., & Winter, G. (1991). By-passing immunization. Human antibodies from V-gene libraries displayed on phage. *J Mol Biol*, 222(3), 581-597.

Martin, C. D., Rojas, G., Mitchell, J. N., Vincent, K. J., Wu, J., McCafferty, J., & Schofield, D. J. (2006). A simple vector system to improve performance and utilisation of recombinant antibodies. *BMC Biotechnol*, 6, 46.

Martineau, P., & Betton, J. M. (1999). In vitro folding and thermodynamic stability of an antibody fragment selected in vivo for high expression levels in Escherichia coli cytoplasm. *J Mol Biol*, 292(4), 921-929.

Melton, S. J. (2010) Ph.D. Thesis, Biomedical Sciences Graduate Program, Tulane University School of Medicine, New Orleans, LA, USA.

Moghaddam, A., Borgen, T., Stacy, J., Kausmally, L., Simonsen, B., Marvik, O. J., Brekke, O. H., & Braunagel, M. (2003). Identification of scFv antibody fragments that specifically recognise the heroin metabolite 6-monoacetylmorphine but not morphine. *J Immunol Methods*, 280(1-2), 139-155.

Moghaddam, A., Lobersli, I., Gebhardt, K., Braunagel, M., & Marvik, O. J. (2001). Selection and characterisation of recombinant single-chain antibodies to the hapten Aflatoxin-B1 from naive recombinant antibody libraries. *J Immunol Methods*, 254(1-2), 169-181.

Ness, J. E., Welch, M., Giver, L., Bueno, M., Cherry, J. R., Borchert, T. V., Stemmer, W. P., & Minshull, J. (1999). DNA shuffling of subgenomic sequences of subtilisin. *Nat Biotechnol*, 17(9), 893-896.

Ohage, E. C., Wirtz, P., Barnikow, J., & Steipe, B. (1999). Intrabody construction and expression. II. A synthetic catalytic Fv fragment. *J Mol Biol*, 291(5), 1129-1134.

Orcutt, K. D., Slusarczyk, A. L., Cieslewicz, M., Ruiz-Yi, B., Bhushan, K. R., Frangioni, J. V., & Wittrup, K. D. (2011). Engineering an antibody with picomolar affinity to DOTA chelates of multiple radionuclides for pretargeted radioimmunotherapy and imaging. *Nucl Med Biol*, 38(2), 223-233.

Persson, H., Lantto, J., & Ohlin, M. (2006). A focused antibody library for improved hapten recognition. *J Mol Biol*, 357(2), 607-620.

Sblattero, D., & Bradbury, A. (2000). Exploiting recombination in single bacteria to make large phage antibody libraries. *Nat Biotechnol*, 18(1), 75-80.

Schoonbroodt, S., Frans, N., DeSouza, M., Eren, R., Priel, S., Brosh, N., Ben-Porath, J., Zauberman, A., Ilan, E., Dagan, S., Cohen, E. H., Hoogenboom, H. R., Ladner, R. C., & Hoet, R. M. (2005). Oligonucleotide-assisted cleavage and ligation: a novel directional DNA cloning technology to capture cDNAs. Application in the construction of a human immune antibody phage-display library. *Nucleic Acids Res*, 33(9), e81.

Shaw, I., O'Reilly, A., Charleton, M., & Kane, M. (2008). Development of a high-affinity anti-domoic acid sheep scFv and its use in detection of the toxin in shellfish. *Anal Chem*, 80(9), 3205-3212.

Sheedy, C., & Hall, J. C. (2001). Immunoaffinity purification of chlorimuron-ethyl from soil extracts prior to quantitation by enzyme-linked immunosorbent assay. *J Agric Food Chem*, 49(3), 1151-1157.

Sheedy, C., MacKenzie, C. R., & Hall, J. C. (2007). Isolation and affinity maturation of hapten-specific antibodies. *Biotechnol Adv*, 25(4), 333-352.

Sheedy, C., Yau, K. Y., Hirama, T., MacKenzie, C. R., & Hall, J. C. (2006). Selection , characterization, and CDR shuffling of naive llama single-domain antibodies selected against auxin and their cross-reactivity with auxinic herbicides from four chemical families. *J Agric Food Chem*, 54(10), 3668-3678.

Short, M. K., Jeffrey, P. D., Kwong, R. F., & Margolies, M. N. (1995). Contribution of antibody heavy chain CDR1 to digoxin binding analyzed by random mutagenesis of phage-displayed Fab 26-10. *J Biol Chem*, 270(48), 28541-28550.

Short, M. K., Krykbaev, R. A., Jeffrey, P. D., & Margolies, M. N. (2002). Complementary combining site contact residue mutations of the anti-digoxin Fab 26-10 permit high affinity wild-type binding. *J Biol Chem*, 277(19), 16365-16370.

Sidhu, S. S., Weiss, G. A., & Wells, J. A. (2000). High copy display of large proteins on phage for functional selections. *J Mol Biol*, 296(2), 487-495.

Siegel, R. W., Baugher, W., Rahn, T., Drengler, S., & Tyner, J. (2008). Affinity maturation of tacrolimus antibody for improved immunoassay performance. *Clin Chem*, 54(6), 1008-1017.

Skerra, A. (2007). Alternative non-antibody scaffolds for molecular recognition. *Curr Opin Biotechnol*, 18(4), 295-304.

Spinelli, S., Frenken, L. G., Hermans, P., Verrips, T., Brown, K., Tegoni, M., & Cambillau, C. (2000). Camelid heavy-chain variable domains provide efficient combining sites to haptens. *Biochemistry*, 39(6), 1217-1222.

Stemmer, W. P. (1994). Rapid evolution of a protein in vitro by DNA shuffling. *Nature*, 370(6488), 389-391.

Strachan, G., McElhiney, J., Drever, M. R., McIntosh, F., Lawton, L. A., & Porter, A. J. (2002). Rapid selection of anti-hapten antibodies isolated from synthetic and semi-synthetic antibody phage display libraries expressed in Escherichia coli. *FEMS Microbiol Lett*, 210(2), 257-261.

Swain, M. D., Anderson, G. P., Serrano-Gonzalez, J., Liu, J. L., Zabetakis, D., & Goldman, E. R. (2011). Immunodiagnostic reagents using llama single domain antibody-alkaline phosphatase fusion proteins. *Anal Biochem*, 417(2), 188-194.

Tabares-da Rosa, S., Rossotti, M., Carleiza, C., Carrion, F., Pritsch, O., Ahn, K. C., Last, J. A., Hammock, B. D., & Gonzalez-Sapienza, G. (2011). Competitive selection from single domain antibody libraries allows isolation of high-affinity antihapten antibodies that are not favored in the llama immune response. *Anal Chem*, 83(18):7213-7220

Valjakka, J., Hemminki, A., Niemi, S., Soderlund, H., Takkinen, K., & Rouvinen, J. (2002). Crystal structure of an in vitro affinity- and specificity-matured anti-testosterone Fab in complex with testosterone. Improved affinity results from small structural changes within the variable domains. *J Biol Chem*, 277(46), 44021-44027.

van Wyngaardt, W., Malatji, T., Mashau, C., Fehrsen, J., Jordaan, F., Miltiadou, D., & du Plessis, D. H. (2004). A large semi-synthetic single-chain Fv phage display library based on chicken immunoglobulin genes. *BMC Biotechnol*, 4, 6.

Vaughan, T. J., Williams, A. J., Pritchard, K., Osbourn, J. K., Pope, A. R., Earnshaw, J. C., McCafferty, J., Hodits, R. A., Wilton, J., & Johnson, K. S. (1996). Human antibodies with sub-nanomolar affinities isolated from a large non-immunized phage display library. *Nat Biotechnol*, 14(3), 309-314.

Velappan, N., Martinez, J. S., Valero, R., Chasteen, L., Ponce, L., Bondu-Hawkins, V., Kelly, C., Pavlik, P., Hjelle, B., & Bradbury, A. R. (2007). Selection and characterization of scFv antibodies against the Sin Nombre hantavirus nucleocapsid protein. *J Immunol Methods*, 321(1-2), 60-69.

Wang, S. H., Zhang, J. B., Zhang, Z. P., Zhou, Y. F., Yang, R. F., Chen, J., Guo, Y. C., You, F., & Zhang, X. E. (2006). Construction of single chain variable fragment (ScFv) and BiscFv-alkaline phosphatase fusion protein for detection of Bacillus anthracis. *Anal Chem*,78(4), 997-1004.

Watanabe, H., Nakanishi, T., Umetsu, M., & Kumagai, I. (2008). Human anti-gold antibodies: biofunctionalization of gold nanoparticles and surfaces with anti-gold antibodies. *J Biol Chem*, 283(51), 36031-36038.

Wesolowski, J., Alzogaray, V., Reyelt, J., Unger, M., Juarez, K., Urrutia, M., Cauerhff, A., Danquah, W., Rissiek, B., Scheuplein, F., Schwarz, N., Adriouch, S., Boyer, O., Seman, M., Licea, A., Serreze, D. V., Goldbaum, F. A., Haag, F., & Koch-Nolte, F. (2009).Single domain antibodies: promising experimental and therapeutic tools in infection and immunity. *Med Microbiol Immunol*, 198(3), 157-174.

Yau, K. Y., Groves, M. A., Li, S., Sheedy, C., Lee, H., Tanha, J., MacKenzie, C. R., Jermutus, L., & Hall, J. C. (2003). Selection of hapten-specific single-domain antibodies from a non-immunized llama ribosome display library. *J Immunol Methods*, 281(1-2), 161-175.

Zahnd, C., Amstutz, P., & Pluckthun, A. (2007). Ribosome display: selecting and evolving proteins in vitro that specifically bind to a target. *Nat Methods*, 4(3), 269-279.

Zhu, X., Kriegel, A. M., Boustany, C. A., & Blake, D. A. (2011). Single-chain variable fragment (scFv) antibodies optimized for environmental analysis of uranium. *Anal Chem*, 83(10), 3717-3724.

2

Polyacrylonitrile Fiber as Matrix for Immunodiagnostics

Swati Jain, Sruti Chattopadhyay, Richa Jackeray, Zainul Abid and Harpal Singh
Indian Institute of Technology-Delhi, New Delhi, India

1. Introduction

Accurate assessment of various clinical, elemental, chemical antigenic substances from different sources is imperative for monitoring, preventive and treatment measures. Instrumental techniques, chromatographic analysis and immunological assays have progressed for the accurate measurement of various analytes over last decades [N. C. Van de Merbel, 2008; R. M. Lequin 2005; R. M. Twyman 2005; H. Richardson 1998; J. Garcia-de-Lomas 1997]. Immunoassays provide an easy, simple and sensitive route for the precise determination of analytical concentration. They utilize the concept of high specificity of antibodies to their analogues antigen forming a complex which can be detected using secondary antibody (Ab) coupled with certain labels. These markers or labeling agents can be radionuclides, chemiluminescent substrates, fluorophores or enzymes leading to measurable results. In the areas of safety regulations, instrumentation and convenience of protocol, enzyme immunoassays have easily surpassed others over the years. Enzyme catalyzed immunochemical test had caught the imagination of researchers leading to development of numerous immunoassays over the years. The future of enzyme immunoassays will bring more rapid test results with simplified procedures catering to wider audience for clinical applications. Extension of basic concept may also encompass a broader consumer-base consisting of increasing number of potential users which will transcend boundaries of technical disciplines [Maggio, E. T. 1979]. The following introduction descibes enzyme immunoassays in brief with emphasis on polymeric matrices as solid support in ELISA. This chapter describes the designing of solid phase immunoassay using surface functionalized polyacrylonitrile fibers for the sensitive and specific determination of various antibodies. Pendent nitrile groups on polyacrylonitrile fibres were successfully reduced to generate amino groups on the surface of the fibers. The newly formed amino groups of the fibers were activated by a bi-functional spacer-glutraldehyde for the covalent linking of antibodies. Sandwich immuno-complex was developed on these PAN fibers which provided high sensitivity, specificity and reproducibility for the detection of various small analytes.

1.1 Enzyme immunoassays

Enzyme immunoassays have become popular in clinical and medical fields. The concept first described by Landsteiner gained momentum in the late 1950s and 60s setting the stage for the pioneering work for the rapid development of immunological assays. Utilization of enzymes as isotopic label has greatly overshadowed fluorophores and radioactive substances. The broad range of application of enzyme immunoassay to determine the concentration of serum proteins & hormone levels, illicit & therapeutic drugs, cardiovascular ligands, carcinofetal proteins, immune status, chemotherapeutics and pathogenic microbes will attest to this. Enzyme Immunoassay is a prominent methodology based on selective recognition and high affinity of antigen and antibody coupling along with the sensitivity of simple enzyme assays. They utilize antibodies or antigen coupled to an easily assayed enzyme that posses a high turnover number to enhance assay signal as some chromogenic substrate is converted to coloured product whose intensity is directly proportional to antigenic concentration [Lequin, 2005].

These immunoassays can be broadly categorized into two major types depending on the assay formats. The first one being homogenous assay in which the immunological reaction occurs in solution phase. Homogeneous immunoassays do not require a separation and washing step, but the enzyme label must function within the sample matrix. As a result, assay interference caused by the matrix may be problematic for samples of environmental origins (i.e., soil, water, etc.). For samples of clinical origin (human or veterinary applications), high target analyte concentrations and relatively consistent matrices are often present. Thus for clinical or field applications, the homogeneous immunoassay format is popular, whereas the heterogeneous format predominates for environmental matrices [Rubestein et al., 1972; Pulli, et al., 2005; Voller, 1979]. Heterogeneous assays such as Enzyme Linked Immuno-Sorbent Assays (ELISAs) are most widely used detection method which utilizes the concept of immobilization of biomolecules on solid support. These have atleast one separation step allowing the differentiation of reacted from un-reacted materials. The enzymatic activity is quantified either in bound state or free fraction by an enzyme catalyzed process of a relatively nonchromatic substrate to highly chromatic product.

1.1.1 Solid-phase immunoassays

Solid phase enzyme immunoassays, which include Enzyme Linked Immunosorbent Assay-ELISA and Western blot, have become popular as qualitative and semi-quantitative sample screening methods for the laboratory diagnosis of infectious diseases, auto-immune disorders, immune allergies and neoplastic diseases [Condorelli & Zeigler, 1993; Derer, et al., 1984; Gosling, 1990; Rordorf, et al., 1983; Voller, et al.,1976]. In ELISA, antibody immobilized on the solid support detects the specific antigen present in the sample and this immune complex is detected by a high turn-over enzyme conjugated antibody. The excess of reagents are washed off in each step and the subsequent substrate interaction yields a coloured product either for the direct visualization or for measuring the optical density. Thus, the ELISAs are among the most specific analytical techniques providing a low detection limit and are economical, versatile, robust, achieve easy separation of free and bound moieties and be automated on demand [Engvall 1977; Peruski A. H. & Peruski L.F., 2003; Wilson & Walker, 1994]. Within the past decade, immunochemical methods have proven to be an alternative or a supplement to the established chromatographic methods.

Sandwich ELISA is a dominant format where a "sandwich" type complex is formed with immobilized antibody, target molecule and secondary antibody labeled with enzyme. Immobilization anchors the first antibody which recognizes the specific antigen from the sample which is detected by enzyme conjugate. Excess of reagents are washed off in each step and the subsequent substrate reaction yields coloured signal for direct visual or spectrometric assessment. The amount of enzyme activity is measured under standard conditions is directly proportional to the antigen present in sample. The immobilization however, should not lead to loss of activity of biomolecule due to change in the orientation and steric hindrance [Moulima, et al., 1998].

1.1.2 Immobilization techniques

1.1.2.1 Physical adsorption

Commonly used immobilization methods include physical absorption or adsorption of biomolecules on the solid support. This involves immobilization of biomolecules through weak forces such as vander waal, electrostatic, hydrophobic interaction and hydrogen bonding. However, non-specific interaction may lead to desorption of the biomolecule during the integral intensive washing steps of assay ensuing erroneous results [Honda, et al., 1995; Rejeb, et al., 1998; Palma, et al., 2004; Palmer, et al., 2004; Tedeschi, et al., 2003]. A controlled covalent attachment of Abs is more preferred to random adsorption so as to achieve better homogeneity in antibody coating.

1.1.2.2 Covalent attachment

Covalent attachment involves the chemical interaction of counter functionalities present on solid matrix and biological entity. The covalent bond induces flexibility to the bond relieving it from steric hindrance and crowding of biomolecules leading to conformational stability. Tethering analytical compound to solid support via functional groups leads to its reduced non-specific absorption, greater stability and better biological activity and enhanced signal output. Lehtonen and Vilijen [Lehtonen & Viljanen, 1980] have studied the antigen attachment in ELISA for the detection of chicken anti-bovine serum albumin antibodies and compared the non-covalent and covalent coupling of biomolecules. They have used polystyrene (PS), nylon and cynogen bromide (CNBr) activated paper and have reported the substantial leakage of antigen from both PS (30%) and nylon (60%) while less desorption was observed for the CNBr activated paper during washing steps. Covalent immobilization is difficult with the non-functionalized surfaces including PS. Eckert et al [Eckert, et al., 2000] have grafted glycidal methacrylate on PS microtiter plate for immobilizing proteins and have reported poor reproducibility of the results. Hence, modified and synthesized functional groups containing solid surfaces are being employed for ELISA.

1.1.3 Polymeric matrices as solid support for immobilization

Efficient tailoring of physico-chemical properties of polymers like molecular weight, shape, size, and easy functionalization render them amenable for the covalent attachment of biomolecules in ELISA. A covalent linkage of antibodies to solid support is preferred which gives more sensitive assays as negligible desorption occurs during extensive washing steps and imparts very low extent of non-specific interaction of biomolecules. Hence, surface and interface chemistry of lots of polymeric materials is currently manipulated to make them amenable for covalent immobilization. The conglomeration of material science and molecular biology has lead to the development of new technologies which benefit from the exquisite specificity of biomolecules and controllable surface properties of polymeric materials. Polymeric materials are surface modified for the generation of an array of functional groups improving hydrophilicity, hydrophobicity, biocompatibility, conductivity apart from providing active groups for the covalent immobilization of biomolecules. Many polymeric materials such as polyethylene, nitrocellulose (NC), Dacron, polyvinyl chloride (PVC), nylon, polyacrylonitrile (PAN) etc. have been widely studied as bioassay's matrix over the years as a reliable interface between materials and biological moieties [Charles, et al., 2006; Jackeray, et al., 2010; Jain, et al., 2008; Venditti, et al.,2008].

1.1.4 Polyacrylonitrile fibers

Polyacrylonitrile in various forms like membranes, fibers and nano-fibers have been exploited in different fields of composites, protective clothing, pervoporation, water treatment, gas separation technology, nanosensors, enzyme immobilization, haemodialysis, biochemical product purification and other biomedical applications [Che, et al., 2005; Nouzaki, et al., 2002; Shinde, et al., 1995; Sreekumar, et al., 2009]. This wide popularity is due to their excellent thermal & mechanical properties, chemical stability, abrasion resistance, high tensile strength and tolerance to most solvents, bacteria & photo-irradiation [Frahn, et al., 2004; Iwata, et al., 2003; Kim, et al., 2001; Musale & Kulkarni, 1997]. Polyacrylonitrile (PAN) is the most important fiber and film/membrane forming polymer. PAN hollow fiber membranes such as AN 69 (produced by HOSPAL, fabricated from an acrylonitrile/methallyl sulphonate copolymer) have already been used as dialyzers and high flux dialysis therapy [Valette, et al., 1999; Thomas, et al., 2000]. PAN hollow fibers are already used as dialysers that remove low molecular weight compounds and proteins. PAN fibers have high surface area, very high mechanical strength, abrasion resistance & posses' insect resistance. Though PAN has many superior properties, it has few demerits of moderate hydrophilicity, low moisture absorption and lack of active functionality limiting its usages. However, the presence of nitrile groups along with the fiber backbone offers multidirectional approaches to modify fibers for specific applications unlike synthetic membranes which can be damaged during the modification [Wen & Shen, 2002, 41].

There is a lot of interest in modifying PAN by changing its surface structure by plasma and photo-induced graft co-polymerization [Deng et al., 2003; Hartwig, et al., 1994; Ulbricht, et al., 1995; Zhao, et al., 2005; Zhao, et al., 2004] enzymatic [E. Battistel, et al., 2001] and chemical modifications including hydrolysis and reduction of PAN fibers. Haiquing Liu *et al* [Liu & Hsieh, 2006 48] have hydrolysed PAN nanofibers to improve its water absorbing capacity. A PAN derivative of poly (acrylonitrile-maleic acid) containing reactive carboxy functionality were synthesized and fabricated to nanofiber and used to immobilize lipase by Sheng-Feng Li [Li et al., 2007]. Ezeo Battistel et al have used nitrile hydratase to enzymatically modify PAN fibers to introduce amide groups. Zhao Jia et al [Jia & Du, 2006] have hydrolyzed and chlorinated PAN fibers and then grafted natural polymer casein to improve moisture absorption and water retention properties. Fumihiro Ishimura [Ishimura & Seijo, 1991] has reduced the PAN fiber and immobilized penicillin acylase to study the activity of the enzyme after the attachment on the fibers in terms of specific activity and immobilization yields.

Nitrile groups of PAN fibers have been partially & completely hydrolyzed and reduced to generate amide, carboxy and amine functionality respectively by researchers using chemical, irradiation and enzymatic techniques [Li et al., 2007; Matsumoto, et al., 1980]. Zhao Jia et al have grafted casein directly on PAN fibers to improve their antistatic and water retention properties [Leirião, et al., 2003]. Fumihiro Ishimura has reduced the PAN fiber and immobilized penicillin acylase to study the activity of the enzyme after the attachment on the fibers in terms of specific activity and immobilization yields [Ishimura & Seijo, 1991].

2. PAN fibers-surface modification and their evaluation for the colorimetric detection of analytes

2.1 Reduction of PAN fibers

In a 250 mL RB flask equipped with water condenser, equivalent quantities of lithium aluminium hydride (LAH) (1.5 g) and polyacrylonitrile PAN fibers (1.5 g) were reacted in excess of pre-dried diethyl ether, AR grade (120 mL) [Matsumoto, et al., 1980]. The reaction mixture was stirred continuously in a moisture free environment under the nitrogen blanket at room temperature (27±2^{0}C) for different time periods (0.5 h, 1 h, 6 h, 12 h and 24 h). The fibers were thoroughly washed to remove the excess of LAH and dried in vacuum oven for 4 h. They were then stored in the desiccator for further use.

2.2 Activation of the aminated fibers and immobilization of antibodies

10 mg aminated PAN fibers (PAN-NH_2) were activated using 12.5% glutaraldehyde/borate buffer (pH 8.5) in a micro-centrifuge tube at 4 ^{o}C for 3 h. The fibers were thoroughly washed with borate buffer (pH 8.5) and Tween/PBS (pH 7.2) to remove excess of glutaraldehyde [Leirião, et al., 2003; Matsumoto, et al., 1984]. Glutaraldehyde activated PAN fibers (PAN-NH_2-Glu) were used for the immobilization of enzyme conjugated antibodies. 10 mg of differently aminated PAN-NH_2-Glu were incubated with GAR-HRP (1 mL) of various dilutions ranging from 1:1000-1:64000 for 16 h at 4 ^{o}C with occasional shaking. The fibers were washed with Tween/PBS (pH 7.4). After the removal of unbound antibodies, peroxidase activity of the bound antibody on the fiber was measured by the means of conversion of colorless substrate 3, 3′, 5, 5′ tetramethyl benzidine (TMB) to a colored product immediately after 10 min. 100 μL of this solution was transferred to the 96-well microtiter plate and the color development was quenched by adding equal volume of conc. sulphuric acid (0.5 M). The optical density was measured at 450 nm with Biorad ELISA plate reader.

2.3 Evaluation of the modified fibers for the detection of analyte (RAG) by performing checkerboard ELISA

A checkerboard or 2-Dimensional serial dilution method was carried out to optimize the concentration and dilution of the analyte and enzyme-label respectively. A checkerboard titration is single experimental set in which the concentration of two components is varied that will result in a pattern. 10 mg of activated PAN fibers (PAN-NH_2-Glu) were immobilized with 1 mL of GAR-IgG antibody (1 μg/mL to 5 μg/mL) for 16 h at 4 ^{o}C. Unbound antibodies were removed and the fibers were washed with Tween/PBS. The unbound sites of the fibers were blocked with 12% skimmed milk (1 mL). These primary antibody immobilized fibers were incubated with a fixed concentration (1 mL) of complimentary antibody RAG-IgG (60 ng/mL) for 1.5 h at 37 ^{o}C. After washing with Tween/PBS, the fibers were again incubated with 1 mL of enzyme conjugate of the first antibody - GAR-HRP, conjugate dilutions ranging from 1:2000-1:32000 for 1.5 h at 37 ^{o}C. Subsequently, the conjugate was decanted and the fibers were washed with Tween/PBS buffer. After the removal of unbound conjugate, the activity of HRP was evaluated, using its substrate TMB as mentioned earlier and the optical density was recorded. Non-specific binding (NSB) of the modified fibers was also evaluated. 10 mg of modified PAN fibers were immobilized with 1 mL of 60 ng/mL of the analyte RAG-IgG. They were blocked with 1 mL of 12% skimmed milk and were incubated with the subsequent GAR-HRP conjugate dilutions (1:2000- 1:32000) after the washing steps. A complimentary set of experiments were performed to determine the sensitivity of the assay i.e. to measure the minimal detectable concentration of the analyte RAG. The activated PAN fiber with optimized primary antibody GAR-IgG concentration, (determine by previous experiment) was incubated with serial dilutions (120 ng/mL-1 ng/mL) of RAG-IgG antibody taken as analyte for 1.5 h at 37 ^{0}C. After washing, fibers were incubated with GAR-HRP of 1:8000 dilutions (as optimized previously) for 1.5 h at 37 ^{0}C and then the fibers were washed again with Tween/PBS. The activity of peroxidase was measured using its substrate TMB and optical density was recorded with the ELISA plate reader.

The developed ELISA system was compared with conventional ELISA using polystyrene (PS) 96-well microtiter plates. Same experimental procedure was followed as that with the activated PAN fibers. The fibers were also compared with the ELISA system where the PS 96-well microtiter plates were pre-treated with 12.5% glutaraldehyde for 3 h at 4 ^{0}C.

2.4 Detection of human blood IgG's using the developed assay of modified PAN fibers

Human blood was taken and 10 µL was spotted on a wattman filter paper no. 1, the blood dots were air dried at 37 ^{0}C for 1 h and then stored at 4 ^{0}C for further use. When required, the filter paper with the dotted blood was punched from a standard puncing machine and discs of 5 mm diameter were obtained. All the blood spotted samples discs were eluted in 100 µL of PBS of pH 7.4 for 1 h at room temperature. After this, serial dilutions of the eluted samples were performed to obtain 1:10, 1:100, 1:1000 and 1:10000 dilutions. These were stored at 4 ^{0}C for further use.

10 mg of the reduced PAN fibers were taken after the activation with glutaraldehyde in a microcentrifuge tube and incubated with 1 mL of 3 µg/mL of GAH-IgG for 16 h at 4 ^{0}C. Antibody immobilized fibers were washed with Tween/PBS and incubated with 1 mL of the human blood elute (undiluted) for 1 h at 37 ^{0}C. After washing, the non-specific binding sites were blocked with 12% skimmed milk at 4 ^{0}C. Blocking solution was removed and fibers were washed and incubated with 1:8000 enzyme conjugate of anti-species of human antibody RAH-HRP for 1 h at 4 ^{0}C. The fibers were washed and the activity of the peroxidase was measured by adding the substrate TMB. The OD was recorded in ELISA plate reader. To determine the sensitivity of the developed assay for human blood, the eluted and serially diluted human blood samples were incubated with the GAH-IgG antibody immobilized PAN fibers followed by the aforementioned ELISA steps. The specificity of the developed assay was further checked using rabbit blood.

3. Results and discussion

3.1 Amine content

The pendent nitrile groups present on the surface of polyacrylonitrile fibers were successfully reduced to primary amino groups with LAH as schematically diagrammed in

Scheme 1. The amine content determined by performing acid-base titrations revealed that with the increasing reduction time, the primary amine content increased and was found to be highest for 12 h reduction time after that amination decreased. As the reduction time increased, prolonged action of the reducing agent LAH ensures the conversion of more number of nitrile groups to amino groups. However, it was also observed that with very high reduction time e.g. 24 h the content of amino groups reduced. The explanation to the decreased amine value is not clear but similar pattern was also reported in US Patent No 4486549 [Matsumoto, et al., 1984]. Physical changes also indicated reduction of fibers such as change of colour from shinning white to pale yellow which increased with the advancement of reaction. Extent of the reduction also influenced and increased the brittleness (noted by ease of tearing of fibers) and roughness (gauzed by touching) in the fibers.

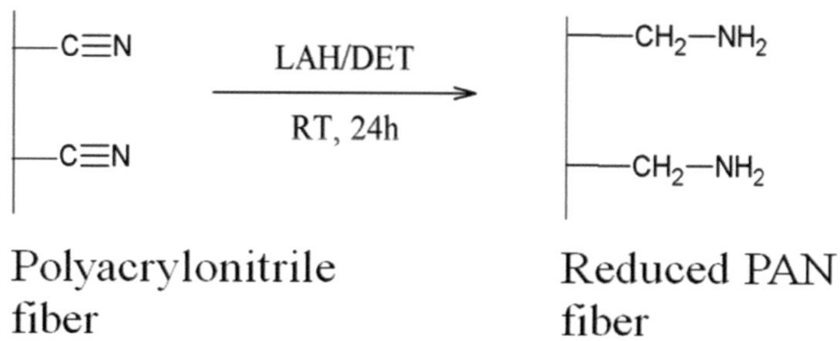

Scheme 1. Reduction of pendent nitrile groups of polyacrylonitrile fibers to amino groups

SI No.	Time of reduction (h)	Content of Amino groups (μM/g)
1.	0.5	28.75
2.	1	36.29
3.	6	78.5
4.	12	126.1
5.	24	108.75

Table 1. Content of amino groups of PAN fibers as measured by acid–base titration method

3.2 ATR-FTIR spectroscopy

FTIR spectroscopic studies showed an appearance of broad band from 3400-3500 cm^{-1} after reduction, which is attributed to the N-H stretching vibration, demonstrating the formation of the primary amine groups. IR spectra were also used to monitor the relationship between surface amination and the reduction time. It was observed that as the reduction time increased from 0.5 h to 12 h, the band corresponding to amino groups increased, but decreased for fiber reduced for 24 h. Relatively, as the reduction time increased, the peak 2241 cm^{-1}, corresponding to the C N stretching vibration of nitrile group decreased in magnitude and completely vanished in the spectra of the fiber reduced for higher time periods. Also as the reduction progresses, the peaks corresponding to C-N stretching and bending vibration diminished and vanished for the fibers reduced for higher time periods. A peak at 1730 cm^{-1} corresponding to C-O stretching of C=O is observed probably due to the addition of small percentage of methyl methacrylate/vinyl acetate added during the polymerization.

After glutaraldehyde treatment absorption peak of stretching vibration of imines group (N=C) comes at 1655 cm^{-1} (Fig. 2 A). However, the peak of free carbonyl group of glutaraldehyde at 1720 cm^{-1} was not visible as it is merged with the peak of methacrylate/acetate groups. The spectra of GAR-IgG antibody immobilized PAN fibers showed absorption band at 2506 cm^{-1} different from that of glutaraldehyde activated PAN fibers (Fig. 2 C), which also correspond to the spectrum of antibody (given in the Fig.2 B for comparison). The band around 2506 cm^{-1} may be attributed to the O-H stretching of carboxyl group present in the *Fc* region of Ab [Allmer, et al., 1989].

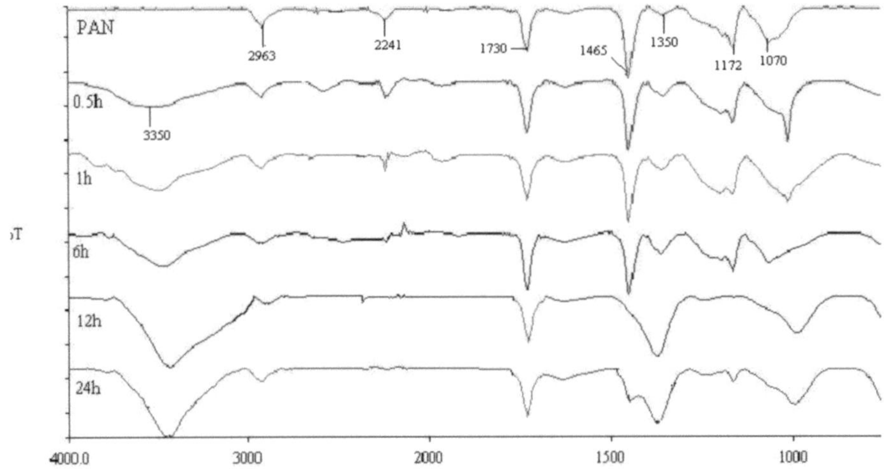

Fig. 1. ATR-FTIR spectra of unmodified and aminated PAN fibers

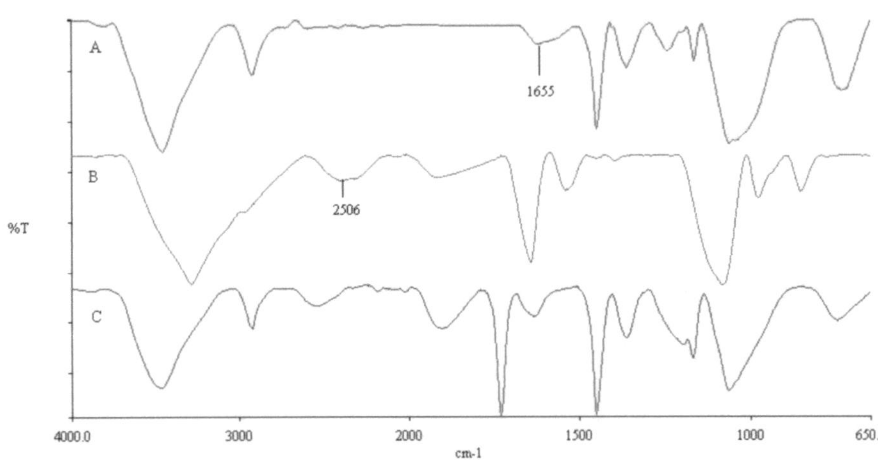

Fig. 2. ATR-FTIR spectra of (A) glutaraldehyde treated reduced PAN fibers (B) Antibody GAR-IgG (C) GAR-IgG immobilized PAN fiber

3.3 Differential scanning calorimetry

Thermal properties of unmodified and reduced PAN fibers were studied in DSC and are given in Fig. 3, 4 and Table 2. It was observed that two thermal transitions occurred for dry PAN fibers in the first cycle of heating and only one in the second cycle. On first cycle of heating a transition is observed at 96 ^{0}C. A sharp peak also appears at 150 ^{0}C which is attributed to the cyclization of PAN (Fig. 3a) involving the pendent nitrile groups present on its surface as given in Scheme II [S. Hajir, et al., 2003]. It was observed that for the fibers reduced for 0.5 h and 1 h, the peak cyclization temperature shifted to 162 ^{0}C and 166 ^{0}C respectively (Table 2). However, fibers reduced for 6 h, 12 h and 24 h (Fig. 3c) did not show any second transition. This altered cyclization behavior of modified PAN indicates that negligible nitrile groups were available to facilitate the cyclization process on heating as majority of them were converted to amino groups on reduction.

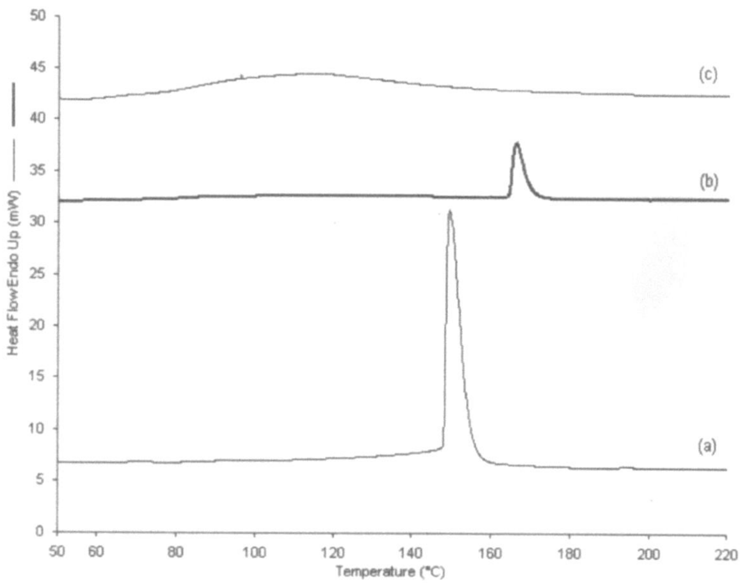

Fig. 3. Cyclization temperature of (a) unmodified PAN fibers and (b) 1 h reduced fibers (c) 6 h reduced fibers

Glass transition temperature (T_g) of PAN and reduced fibers as recorded during second cycle of heating is given in Table 2 and is graphically presented in Fig. 4. T_g of PAN was observed at 96 ^{0}C as a result of chain mobility caused by the weakening of vander waals forces in the amorphous region of the polymer [Zhang & Li, 2005]. However, no significant change in the glass transition temperature was observed in reduced fibers. No change in T_g indicate that polymeric backbone was not affected by the reduction of pendent nitrile groups.

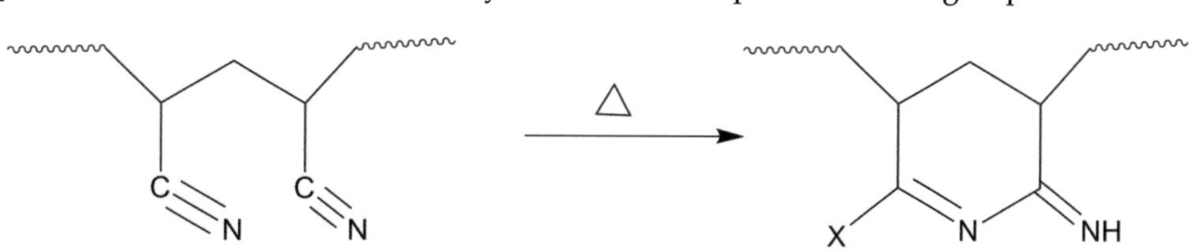

Scheme 2. Cyclization of nitrile groups of PAN upon heating in DSC

Fiber type	Initial exothermic temp. (^{0}C)	End exotherm ic temp. (^{0}C)	Cyclization temp. (^{0}C)	Heat energy (mJg^{-1})	Glass transition temperature T_g (^{0}C)
PAN	146	160	150	0.374	96.351
PAN-NH_2 (0.5h)	157	180	162	0.348	110.7
PAN-NH_2 (1h)	164	174	166	0.352	98.294
PAN-NH_2 (6h)	-	-	-	0.356	101.327
PAN-NH_2 (12h)	-	-	-	0.388	98.921
PAN-NH_2 (24h)	-	-	-	0.604	102.350

Table 2. Thermal behavior of the unmodified and fibers reduced for different time periods

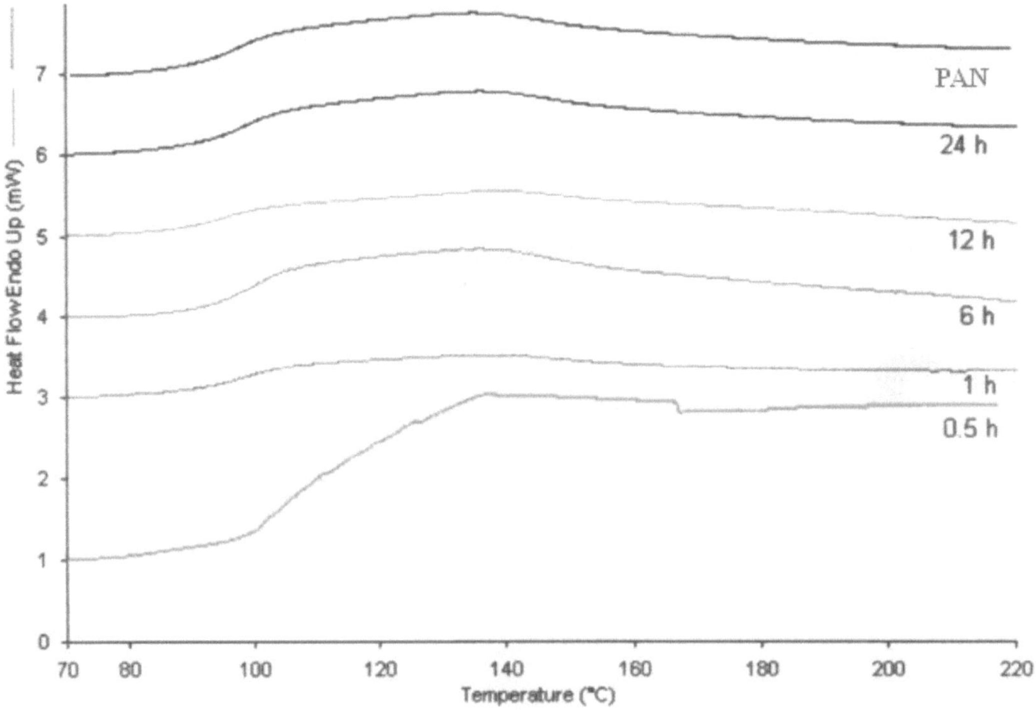

Fig. 4. Thermal studies of reduced fibers using DSC

3.4 Scanning electron microscopy

Scanning electron micrographs of unmodified and reduced PAN fibers are depicted in Fig 5 a-f. Unmodified fibers were found to be smooth and untangled with fiber diameter of 50-70 µm. No significant morphological changes were observed for 0.5 h and 1 h reduced fibers (Fig. 5 b-c). However, as the reduction time increased fibers gradually become rough, rugged and the extent of entanglement also increased, indicating conversion of a large number of nitrile to amino groups. Similar observations are also reported by other authors [Liu and Heish, 2006]. 24 h reduced fibers were further used for immobilization and development of the assay due to its consistent and reproducible immobilization results. Hence, its morphology was also studied after glutaraldehyde activation and antibody immobilization. The micrographs of activated and GAR-IgG antibody immobilized fibers are presented in Fig. 6. No major morphological changes were observed on activation of the fibers with glutaraldehyde. After immobilization of antibodies, topography of the fiber changed (Fig 6 b & c). Deposition of the antibody can be seen on the modified fibers after immobilization on higher magnification.

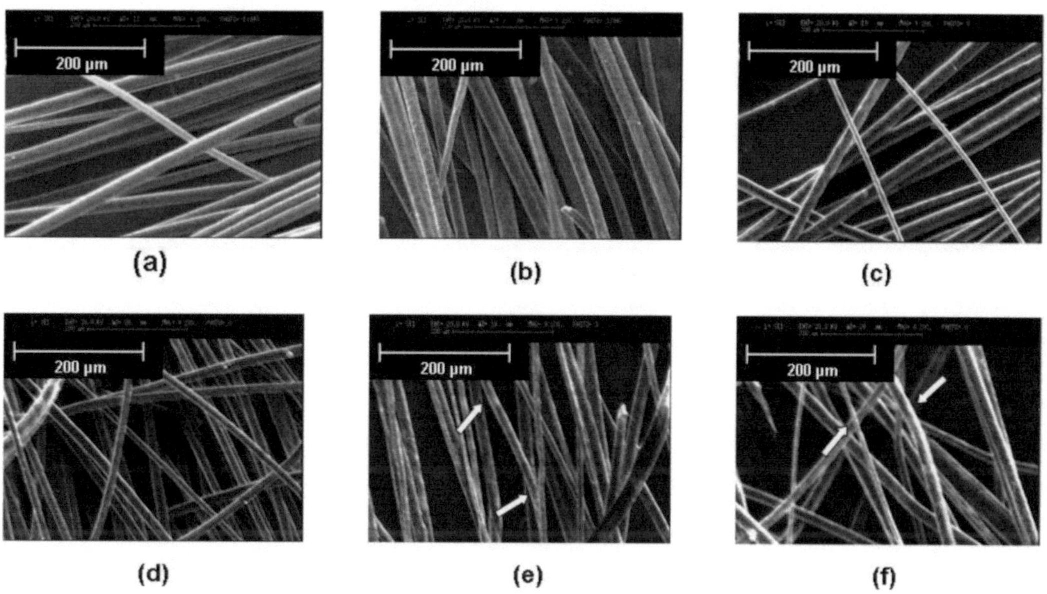

Fig. 5. Scanning electron micrographs of unmodified and reduced fibers (a) Unmodified PAN fibers (b) 0.5 h (c) 1 h (d) 6 h (e) 12 h and (f) 24 h reduced fibers

3.5 Antibody immobilization

Reduced PAN fibers were activated with excess of glutaraldehyde. The primary amine groups of the reduced fibers reacted with one of the aldehydic groups of the bi-functional glutaraldehyde to form the imine linkage (Scheme III). The free aldehyde group of glutaraldehyde covalently binds to the amino groups of residues/units (generally lysine) in the antibodies and the antibodies coupled with enzymes, providing a stable linkage. Thus, antibodies were covalently immobilized on the glutaraldehyde activated PAN fibers.

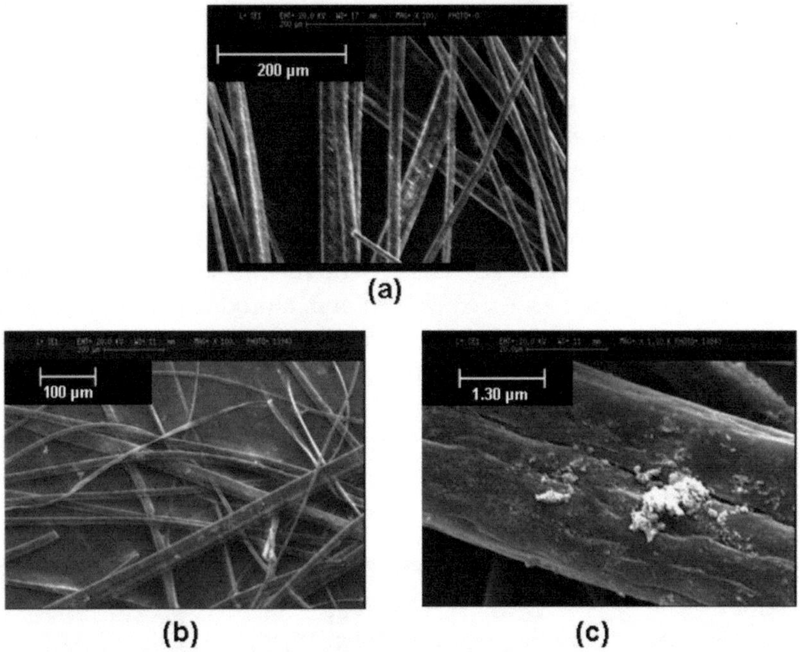

Fig. 6. Scanning electron micrographs of (a) glutaraldehyde activated fibers (b) antibody immobilized PAN fibers (c) Immobilized fibers at higher magnification

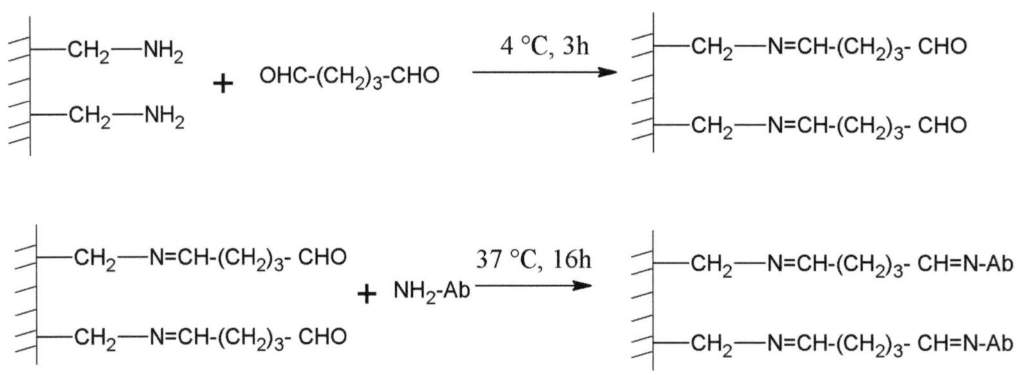

Scheme 3. Activation of the reduced fibers with glutaraldehyde and immobilization of antibody on the activated fibers

The attachment of the Ab on the fibers was visualized through confocal laser scanning microscope using fluorophore tagged antibody Goat anti-Rabbit-Fluorescien isothiocyanate (GAR-FITC) (Fig. 7 b). Glutaraldehyde activated fibers were coupled with 1:400 dilution of GAR-FITC for 16 h at 4 °C. They were washed with Tween/PBS and studied under the microscope in dark. The null method was applied to deduce the autofluorescence [Jang, et al., 2006] of the polyacrylonitrile (Fig. 7 a) from the fluorescence of dye FITC attached on fiber as GAR-FITC.

A range of HRP conjugated antibodies were prepared in 1X-PBS buffer to evaluate the efficiency of immobilization on aminated PAN fibers. Effect of conjugate dilution shows a

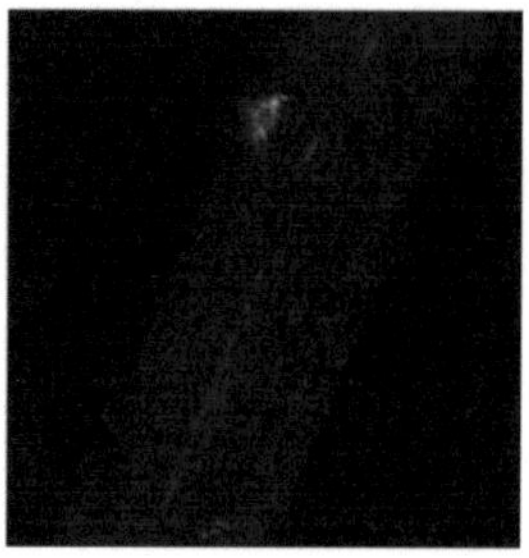

(a) (b)

Fig. 7. Confocal laser scanning electron microscope image of (a) unmodified PAN (b) modified PAN-NH_2-Glu-GAR-FITC at 512 HV voltage

typical sigmoidal curve (Fig. 8). With an increase in the conjugate GAR-HRP dilution from 1:2000 to 1:64000 in the immobilization system, there was a decrease in the optical density (O.D.) recorded. A sigmoidal pattern may be attributed to the saturation of PAN fibers with the Ab at the higher concentration/lower dilutions. Competitive Ab-Ab interaction of GAR-HRP molecule for binding to aldehydic groups and steric hindrance are the principal factor leading to the plateau of O.D. values for the immobilization at higher concentrations of conjugate. Very low optical density was observed at lower dilutions as negligible binding occurs, since less conjugate was present for binding. Similar pattern was observed for the time varied reduced fibers (0.5 h to 24 h) as given in Fig. 9. Efficacy of differently aminated PAN fibers for immobilization of Ab was studied. Various conjugate dilutions GAR-HRP, ranging from 1:2000-1:64000 were immobilized onto fibers reduced from 0.5 h to 24 h. The result showed that with increase in reduction time, the O.D. increased indicating greater immobilization of the antibody-HRP conjugate occurred on the modified fibers (Fig.9). It was also observed that the O.D. was highest for 12 h reduction time. However, the fibers, which were reduced for 24 h showed the most stabilized readings on repeated experimentation as against that of 12 h reduction time period. Therefore, 24 h reduced fibers were further used for the detection of the analyte.

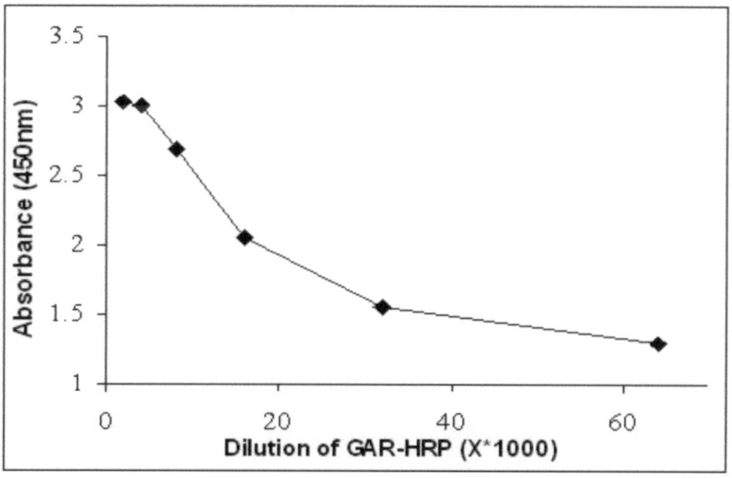

Fig. 8 Activity of GAR-HRP immobilized on modified PAN fiber

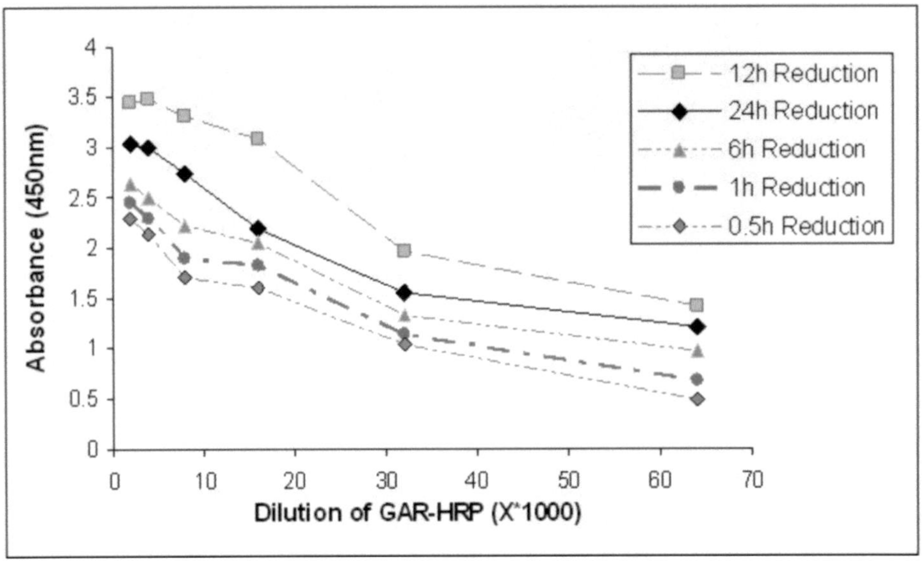

Fig. 9. Activity of GAR-HRP immobilized on PAN fibers reduced for different time periods (0.5 h to 24 h)

3.6 Evaluation of the modified fibers for the detection of analyte (RAG) by performing checkerboard ELISA

A checkerboard is a typical sandwich ELISA technique, where the antibody immobilized to the solid support binds with the complimentary Ab or antigen in the solution. This complex is incubated with the secondary Ab conjugated with an enzyme which provides a colorimetric reaction for the detection of antigen/analyte spectrophotometerically. Reduced PAN fibers were studied to develop a reproducible assay for the detection of analyte over a biologically relevant assay range. Therefore, optimum concentration of each assay reagent has to be standardized empirically. In the first experiment, a varied concentration of primary antibody GAR-IgG was immobilized on to reduced fibers activated by glutaraldehyde. Analyte RAG-IgG was immobilized with a fixed conc. of 60 ng/mL and then serially diluted secondary Ab conjugate GAR-HRP was incubated with the fibers. The assay was carried out in triplicate and the averages of the results are presented in Fig 10 and 11. The result showed that with the increase in primary antibody GAR-IgG concentration from 1 µg/mL to 5 µg/mL and secondary Ab dilution from 1:2000-1:32000, an antibody saturation pattern in optical density (Fig.10) was observed. This curve showed maximum O.D. for 3 µg/mLGAR-IgG conc. at 1:8000 conjugate dilutions, thus, these values were established as the optimized concentration and dilution. This indicated that at higher concentration saturation of primary Ab occurred due to Ab-Ab interactions and steric hindrance. The NSB of Ab on modified PAN fibers was observed from 0.85 to 0.23 for the dilutions 1:2000 to 1:32000 of the conjugate GAR-HRP.

Sensitivity is an important parameter while developing any immunogenic assay. The sensitivity of the assay was determined for the modified PAN fibers by varying the concentration of the analyte RAG-IgG. In the second experimental set up, primary antibody

GAR-IgG (3 µg/mL) and conjugate GAR-HRP (1:8000) were fixed for 10 mg of PAN-NH_2-Glu and the analyte RAG-IgG was varied over a range from 0.9 ng/mL to 120 ng/mL. Over this range of analyte concetration, it was observed that the lowest detectable concentration hence sensitivity of the assay was 3.75 ng/mL (Fig.11).

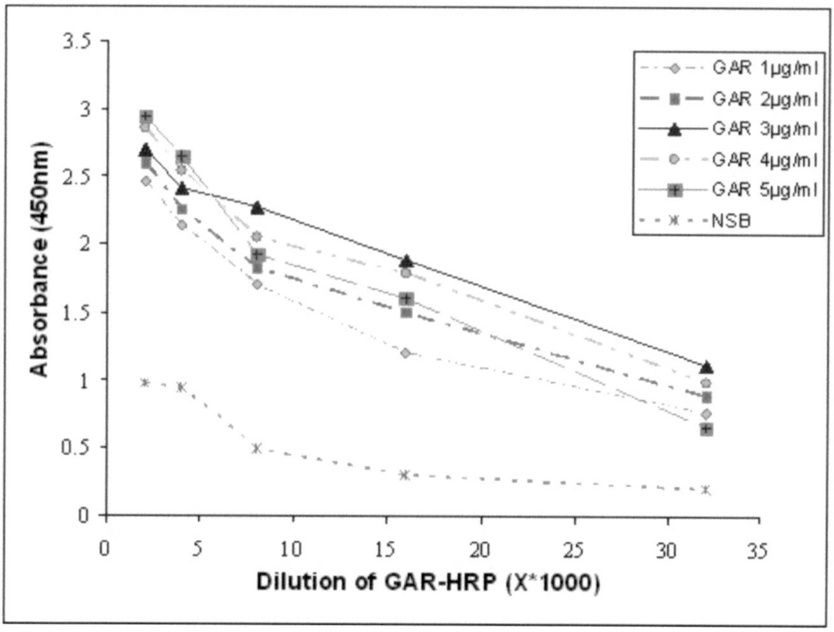

Fig. 10. PAN-NH_2-Glu fiber - ELISA at different primary antibody (GAR-IgG) and conjugate dilution (GAR-HRP)

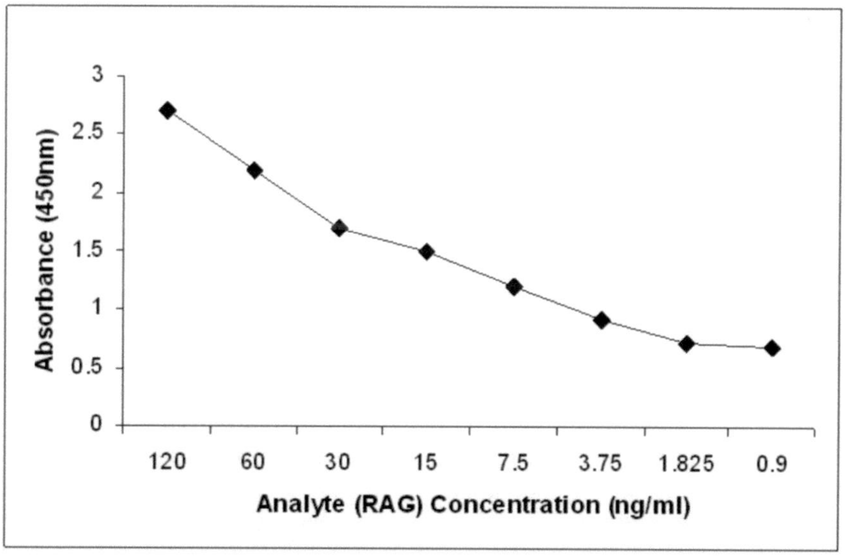

Fig. 11. PAN-NH_2-Glu fiber - ELISA at different analyte concentrations with the 3µg/ml primary antibody GAR concentration and 1:8000 antibody enzyme conjugate GAR-HRP

The results were compared with the conventional ELISA method where the assay was performed on 96-well PS microtiter plate as well as glutaraldehyde pretreated plate and are presented in Fig. 12. It was observed that with the increase in analyte concentration the O.D. increased for all the three solid supports. But the O.D. of modified PAN fibers was always higher than both of the plates. Glutaraldehyde pre-treated and non-treated plates showed decreased activity due to loss of reagents during extensive washing. This confirms, simply adsorbed antibodies bind to solid support get detached while washing, leading to less sensitive assays. Thus, covalent binding on modified PAN fibers leads to high sensitivity and specificity. The advantages of covalent binding are also reported by other authors [Palma, et al., 2004; Tedeschi, et al. 2003; Tyagi, et al., 2009]. From these studies it can be concluded that modified PAN fibers as a solid support are more sensitive, specific and cost effective as compared to PS 96-well microtiter plates.

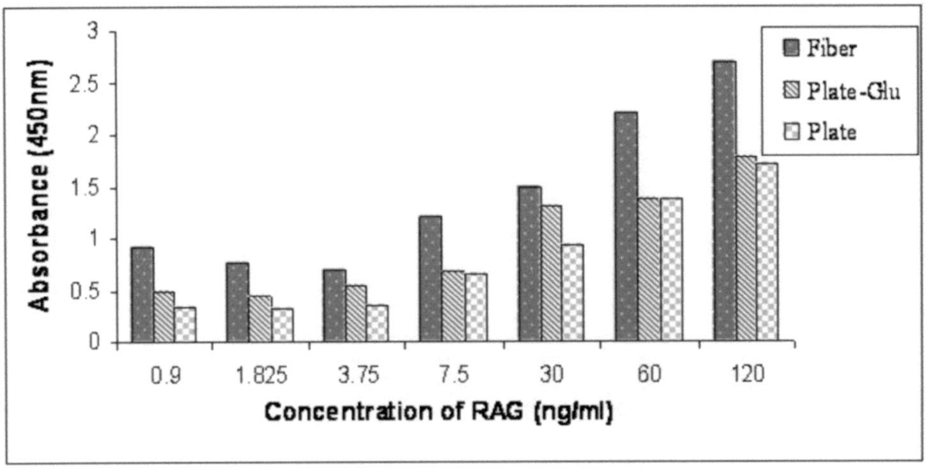

Fig. 12. Comparison of antibody immobilized PAN-NH_2-Glu fiber with the conventional PS microtiter plate and PS plate pre-treated with 12.5% glutaraldehyde

3.7 Detection of human blood IgG's

Modified PAN fibers were used for the detection of antibodies present in human blood. Antispecies of human blood IgG were covalently immobilized on the fibers, which specifically binds with the IgG's of the human blood. This complex was detected with the antispecies-HRP antibody conjugate as visualized by the development of the coloured product on addition of substrate. Sensitivity of the developed assay on modified PAN fibers coated for human blood was also checked and is given in Fig. 13. The human blood elute of 10 fold and 100 fold dilution gave high O.D. values. With further dilutions, the absorbance decreased and negligible intensity was recorded for 1:10000 dilutions. It was also observed that the O.D. of neat elute was lesser than that of 1:10 diluted sample, indicating lesser immobilization of human IgG's with the neat eluate. This can be attributed to the overpopulation of IgG, resulting in their deformed orientation and led to non-homogeneity during immobilization [Endo, et al., 1987, 60]. These results thus established that blood sample as low as 0.1 µL can be easily detected through the developed assay. GAH-IgG immobilized modified PAN fibers were also used for specificity test against human and rabbit blood elutes. Negligible readings were recorded for rabbit blood elute where the O.D.

of neat human blood elute was substantial. The GAH and RAH-HRP used in the assay specifically binds with the antispecies of human blood IgG's. This confirms the non-specificity of the assay with respect to blood of any other organism.

These results were compared with the conventional PS 96-well microtitre plates (Fig. 13). A slightly higher absorbance was recorded for modified PAN fibers in comparison to PS microtiter plate and the glutaraldehyde activated plate. This relates to better sensitivity of the assay due to covalent binding of Ab's to fibers. Modified fibers also showed lesser extent of non-specific binding caused due to physical adsorption and were more specific towards the detection of human blood.

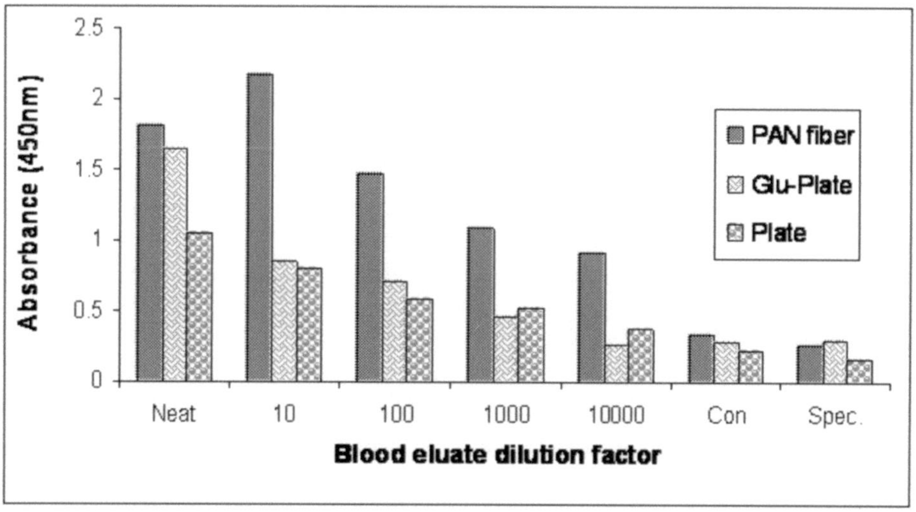

Fig. 13. Human antibody detection by modified PAN fibers-ELISA and comparison with conventional PS microtiter plate and PS plate pre-treated with 12.5% glutaraldehyde

4. Conclusions and prospects

In our work pendent nitrile groups of multifilamentous polyacrylonitrile (PAN) fibers were reduced to amino groups using lithium aluminum hydride for different time of reduction and amine content was estimated by performing acid-base titrations. Modified fibers were characterized by spectroscopic and analytical techniques for the generation of amino groups. The newly formed amino groups of the fibers were activated by using glutaraldehyde for the covalent immobilization of biomolecules. Modified PAN fibers were evaluated as a matrix for sandwich ELISA by using Goat anti-Rabbit antibody (GAR-IgG), Rabbit anti-Goat (RAG-IgG) as analyte and enzyme conjugate GAR-HRP. The fibers reduced for 24 h were able to detect the analyte RAG-IgG at a concentration as low as 3.75 ng/mL. PAN-ELISA gave more promising results when compared with the conventional polystyrene (PS) 96-well microtitre plate-ELISA. The sensitivity, specificity and reproducibility of the developed immunoassay was further established with antibodies present in human blood using Goat anti-Human (GAH-IgG) antibody and the corresponding anti-species HRP enzyme conjugate. These standardized modified PAN fibers when applied for human blood antibody identification showed that 0.1 μL blood elute was sufficient for ELISA. These immunoassays demonstrate that Modified PAN-ELISA can be exploited as a solid matrix for the detection of variety of biomolecules. Immunoassay developed on modified PAN fibers provides a low detection limit, is versatile, robust and achieve easy separation of free and bound moieties. The sensitivity, specificity and the reproducibility of the developed immunoassay indicate the potential application of modified PAN fibers in the field of immunodiagnostics.

5. Acknowledgment

Authors of this chapter are thankful towards Department of Biotechnology (DBT), Council for Scientific and Industrial Research (CSIR) India, University Grant Commission (UGC), Govt. of India and Lockheed Martin Corporation, USA, for their generous financial and technical support.

6. References

A. H. Peruski and L. F. Peruski Jr. (2003). Immunological methods for Detection and Identification of Infectious Disease and Biological Warfare Agents. Clinical and Diagnostic lab Immunology, Vol. 10, No. 4, (July 2003), pp.506-513

Allmer, K., Huly, A. and Runby, B. (1989). Surface modification of polymers. III. Grafting of stabilizers onto polymer films. *Journal of Polymer Science Part A: Polymer Chemistry,* Vol. 27, No. 10, (March 2003), pp. 3405-3417

Battistel, E., Morrea, M. and Marinetti, M. (2001). Enzymatic surface modification of acrylonitrile fibers. *Applied Surface Science*, Vol. 177, pp. 32-41

Charles, P. T., Velez, F., Soto, C. M., Goldman, E. R., Martin, B. D., Rav, R. I. and Taitt, C. R. (2006). A galactose polyacrylate-based hydrogel scaffold for the detection of cholera toxin and staphylococcal enterotoxin B in a sandwich immunoassay format. *Analytica Chimica Acta*, Vol.578, No. 1, (18 September 2006), pp. 2-10

Che, A. F., Nie, F. Q., Uang, X. D., Xu, Z. K. and Yao, K. (2005). Acrylonitrile-based copolymer membranes containing reactive groups: Surface modification by the immobilization of bimolecules. *Polymer,* Vol. 46, pp. 11060-11065

Condorelli, F. and Ziegler, T. J. (1993). Clinical Microbiology, Vol. 31, pp.717-719

Deng, S., Bai R., and Paul J. Chen. (2003). Aminated Polyacrylonitrile Fibers for Lead and Copper Removal. *Langmuir*, Vol.19 No. 12, (May, 2003) pp.5058–5064

Derer, M. M., Miescher, S., Johansson, B., Frost, H. and Gordon J. (1984). Application of the dot immunobinding assay to allergy diagnosis. *Journal of Allergy and Clinical Immunology*, Vol. 74 No. 1, (July 1984) pp. 85-92

Eckert, A.W., Gröbe, D. and Rothe, U. (2000). Surface-modification of polystyrene-microtitre plates via grafting of glycidylmethacrylate and coating of poly-glycidylmethacrylate. *Biomaterials*, Vol. 21 No. 5, (March 2000) pp. 441-447

Endo, N., Kato, Y. and Hara, T., (1987). A novel covalent modification of antibodies at their amino groups with retention of antigen-binding activity. *Journal of Immunological Methods*, Vol.104, No. 1-2 (*23 November 1987)*, pp 253-258

Engvall, E. (1977). Quantitative enzyme immunoassay (ELISA) in microbiology. *Medical Biology*, Vol. 55 No. 4, (August 1977), pp. 193

Frahn, J., Malsch, G, Matuschewski, H., Schedler, U. and Schwarz, H. (2004). Separation of aromatic/aliphatic hydrocarbons by photo-modified poly(acrylonitrile) membranes. *Journal of Membrane Science*, Vol. 234, No. 1-2, (1 May 2004), pp. 55-65

Garcia-de-Lomas J. and Navarro D. (1997). New Directions in Diagnosis. *Journal of Pediatric Infectious Diseases*, Vol.16, No. 3, (March 1997), pp. S43-S48

Gosling, J. P. (1990). A decade of development in immunoassay methodology. Clinical Chemistry, Vol. 36, No. 8, pp.1408–1427

Hajir, S., Bajaj, P. and Sen, K. (2003). Thermal behavior of acrylonitrile carboxylic acid copolymers. *Journal of Applied Polymer Science*, Vol.88, No. 3, (18, April), pp. 685-698

Hartwig, A., Mulder, M. and Smolders, C. (1994). Surface amination of poly(acrylonitrile). *Advances in Colloid and Interface Science*, Vol. 52, (19 September 1994), pp. 65-78

Honda, T., Miwatani, T., Yabushita, Y., Koike, N., and Okada, K. I. (1995). A novel method to chemically immobilize antibody on nylon and its application to the rapid and differential detection of two Vibrio parahaemolyticus toxins in a modified enzyme-linked immunosorbent assay. *Clinical and Diagnostics Lab Immunonology,* Vol. 2 No. 2, (March 1995) pp.177–181

Ishimura, F. and Seijo H. (1991) Immobilization of penicillin acylase using porous polyacrylonitrile fibers. *Journal of Fermentation Bioenggineering,* Vol. 71, No. 2 pp. 140-143

Iwata, M., Adachi, T., Tomidokoro, M., Ohta, M., Kobayashi T. (2003). Hybrid sol–gel membranes of polyacrylonitrile–tetraethoxysilane composites for gas permselectivity. *Journal of Applied Polymer Science,* Vol. 88, No. 7, (16 May 2003), pp. 1752-1759

Jackeray, R., Jain, S., Chattopadhyay, S., Yadav, M., Shrivastav, T. G. and Singh, H. (2010). Surface Modification of Nylon Membrane by Glycidyl Methacrylate Graft Copolymerization for Antibody Immobilization. *Journal of Applied Polymer Science,* Vol.116, No. 3, (May 2010) pp. 1700–1709

Jain, S., Jackeray, R., Chattopadhyay, S., Abid, Z., Kumar, M. and Singh, H. (2010), Detection of anti-tetanus toxoid antibodies on modified polyacrylonitrile fibers. *Talanta,* Vol.82, No. 5, pp.1876–1883

Jang, J., Bae, J. and Park, E., (2006). Polyacrylonitrile Nanofibers: Formation Mechanism and Applications as a Photoluminescent Material and Carbon-Nanofiber Precursor. *Advanced Functional Materials,* Vol.16, No. 11 pp. 1400-1406

Jia, Z. and Du, S. (2006). Grafting of casein onto polyacrylonitrile fiber for surface modification. *Fibers and Polymers,* Vol. 7, No.3, pp. 235-240

Kim, J. H., Ha, S. Y., Nam, S. Y., Rhim, J. W., Baek, K. H. and Lee Y. M. (2001). Selective permeation of CO_2 through pore-filled polyacrylonitrile membrane with poly(ethylene glycol). *Journal of Membrane Science,* Vol. 186, No. 1 (15 May 2001), pp. 97-107

Lehtonen, O. P. and Viljanen, M. K. J., Journal of Immunological Methods (1980) Antigen attachment in ELISA. *Journal of Immunological Methods,* Vol. 34, No. 1, (12 May 1980), pp. 61-70

Leirião, P. R. S., Fonseca, L. J. P., Taipa, M. A., Cabral, J. M. S. and Mateus, M. (2003). Horseradish peroxidase immobilized through its carboxylic groups onto a polyacrylonitrile membrane: Comparison of enzyme performances with inorganic beaded supports, *Applied Biochemistry Biotechnology,* Vol. 110, No.1, pp. 1-10

Lequin, R. M. (2005). Historical note on Enzyme immunoassay (EIA)/Enzyme linked immunosorbent Assay (ELISA). *Clinical Chemistry,* Vol.51, No. 12, pp. 2415–2418

Li, S. F., Chen, J. P., Wen, W. T. (2007). Electrospun polyacrylonitrile nanofibrous membranes for lipase immobilization. *Journal of Molecular Catalysis B: Enzymatic* Vol.47, pp. 117-124

Liu, H., Hsieh, You-L. (2006). Preparation of water-absorbing polyacrylonitrile nanofibrous membrane. *Macromolecular Rapid Communication*, Vol.27, pp. 142-145

Maggio, E. T. (1979). Introduction, In: *Enzyme Immunoassays*, Maggio E. T. (1-3), CRC, Inc., Boston

Matsumoto, K., Izumi, R., Seijo, H., Mizuquchi, H. (1984). U.S. Patent: 4486549 Dec. 4

Matsumoto, K., Seijo, H., Karube, I. and Suzuki, S. (1980). Amperometric determination of choline with use of immobilized choline oxidase. *Biotechnology and Bioengineering*, Vol. 31, No. 5, (May 1980), pp. 1071-1086

Moulima, B. J., Galisteo, G. F., Hidelgo, A. R. (1998) *Journal of Biomaterial Science: Polymer Edition*, Vol.9, pp. 1103-1110

Musale, D. A. and Kulkarni, S. S., (1997). Relative rates of protein transmission through poly(acrylonitrile) based ultrafiltration membranes. *Journal of Membrane Science*, Vol.136, No.1-2, (10 December 1997), pp.13-23

Nouzaki, K., Nagata, M., Araib, J., Idemotob, Y., Kourab, N. and Yanagishita H. (2002). Preparation of polyacrylonitrile ultrafiltration membranes for wastewater treatment. *Desalination*, Vol. 144, No.1-3, (10 September 2002), pp. 53-59

Palma, R. J., Manso, M., Rigueiro, J. P., Garcia-Ruiz, J. P., Martinez-Duarte, J. M. (2004). Surface biofunctionalization of materials by amine groups. *Journal of Material Research*, Vol. 19 No. 8, pp. 2415-2420

Palmer, T., Enzymes: Biochemistry, Biotechnology and Clinical Chemistry, East-west Press, 2004, New Delhi

Pulli, T., Höyhtyä, M., Söderlund, H., Takkinen, K. (2005). One step homogenous immunoassays for small analytes. *Analytical Chemistry*, Vol. 77, No. 7, pp. 2637-2642

Rejeb, S. B., Tatulian, M., Khonsari, F. A. and Durand, N. F. (1998). Functionalization of nitrocellulose membranes using ammonia plasma for the covalent attachment of antibodies for use in membrane-based immunoassays. *Analytica Chimica Acta*, Vol. 376, No. 1, (4 December 1998), pp. 133-138

Richardson, H., Smaill F. (1998). Recent Advances: Medical microbiology. *Clinical Reviews BMJ*, Vol. 317, No. 7165, (October 1998), pp. 159-162

Rordorf, C., Gambke, C. and Gordon J. (1983). A multidot immunobinding assay for autoimmunity and the demonstration of novel antibodies against retroviral antigens in the sera of MRL mice. *Journal of Immunological Methods*, Vol. 59, No.1, pp. 105-112

Rubestein, K. E., Schneider, R. S. and Ullman, E. F. (1972). Homogeneous enzyme immunoassay: A new immunochemical technique. *Biochemical and Biophysical Research Communication*, Vol.47 *, No. 4, (26 May 1972), pp. 846-851*

Shinde, M. H., Kulkarni, S. S., Musale, D. A., Joshi S.G. (1999). Improvement of the water purification capability of poly(acrylonitrile) ultrafiltration membranes. *Journal of Membrane Science*, Vol. 162, No. 1-2, (1 September 1999), pp. 9-22

Sreekumar, T. V., Das, A., Chandra, L., Srivastava, A. and Rao, K. U. (2009). Inherently Colored Antimicrobial Fibers Employing Silver Nanoparticles. *Journal of Biomedical Nanotechnology*, Vol. 5, No.6, pp. 115-120

Tedeschi, L., Domenici, C., Ahluwalia, A., Baldini, F. and Mencaglia, A. (2003). Antibody immobilisation on fibre optic TIRF sensors. *Biosensors and Bioelectronics,* Vol. 19, No. 2, (15 November 2003), pp. 85-93

Thomas, M., Valette, P., Mausset, A.L. and Dejardin, P. (2000). High molecular weight kininogen adsorption on hemodialysis membranes: influence of pH and relationship with contact phase activation of blood plasma influence of pre-treatment with poly(ethyleneimine). *International Journal of Artificial Organs,* Vol.23 No. 1, pp. 20-26

Twyman, R. M. (2005). Immunoassay Applications/Clinical pp. 317-324

Tyagi, C., Tomar, L., and Singh, H. (2009). Glycidyl methacrylate-co-N-vinyl-2-pyrrolidone coated polypropylene strips: Synthesis, characterization and standardization for dot-enzyme linked immunosorbent assay. *Analytica Chimica Acta,* Vol. 632, No. 2, (November 2008) pp.256-265

Ulbricht, M., Oechel A., Lehmann, C., Tomaschewski, G. and Hicke, H.G. (1995). Gas-phase photoinduced graft polymerization of acrylic acid onto polyacrylonitrile ultrafiletration membranes. *Journal of Applied Polymer Science,* Vol. 55, pp. 1707-1723

Valette, P., Thomas, M. and Dejardin, P. (1999). Adsorption of low molecular weight proteins to hemodialysis membranes: experimental results and simulations. *Biomaterials,* Vol. 20, No. 17, (September 1999), pp. 1621-163,

Van de Merbel N. C. (2008). Quantitative determination of endogenous compounds in biological samples using chromatographic techniques. *Trends in Analytical Chemistry,* Vol.27, No.10, (November 2008), pp.924-933

Venditti, I., Fratoddi, I., Russo, M., Bellucci, S., Iozzino, L., Staiano, M., Aurilia, V., Varriale, A., Rossi, M., Auria, S., (2008). Nanobeads-based assays: The case of gluten detection. *Journal of Physics: Condensed Matter,* Vol. 20, pp. 474202-474205

Voller, A. (1979). Heterogeneous enzyme-immunoassays and their applications In: *Enzyme Immunoassays,* Maggio E. T. (181-196) CRC, Inc., Boston

Voller, A., Bidwell, D. E. and Bartlett, A. (1976). Enzyme immunoassays in diagnostic medicine: Theory and practice. *Bulletin of World Health Organization,* Vol. 53, pp. 55-65

Wen, B. and Shan, X. Q. (2002). Improved immobilization of 8-hydroxyquinoline on polyacrylonitrile fiber and application of the material to the determination of trace metals in seawater by inductively coupled plasma mass spectroscopy. *Analytical and Bioanalytical Chemistry,* Vol. 374 No. 5, (November 2002) pp.948–954

Wilson, K. and Walker, J., Practical Biochemistry: Principles and Techniques, Cambridge University Press 1994, UK

Zhang, W. and Li, M. (2005). DSC Study on the Polyacrylonitrile Precursors for Carbon Fibers. *Journal of Material Science and Technology,* Vol. 21, No. 4, pp.581-584

Zhao, Z. P., Li, J. D., Wang, D. and Chen C. X. (2005). Nanofiltration membrane prepared from polyacrylonitrile ultrafiltration membrane by low-temperature plasma:4. Grafting of N-vinylpyrrolidone in aqueous solution. *Desalination,* Vol. 184, pp. 37-44

Zhao, Z. P., Li, J. D., Wang, D. and Chen, C. X. (2004). Nanofiltration membrane prepared from polyacrylonitrile ultrafiltration membrane by low-temperature plasma: I Graft of acrylic acid in gas. *Journal of Membrane Science*, Vol. 232, pp. 1-8

3

Interferences in Immunoassays

Johan Schiettecatte, Ellen Anckaert and Johan Smitz
UZ Brussel, Laboratory Clinical Chemistry and Radioimmunology, Belgium

1. Introduction

Interference in immunoassays is a serious but underestimated problem (Ismail et al, 2002a). Interference is defined as "the effect of a substance present in the sample that alters the correct value of the result, usually expressed as concentration or activity, for an analyte" (Kroll & Elin, 1994). Immunoassays are analytically sensitive and measurements can frequently performed without prior extraction. However, immunoassays may lack adequate specificity and accuracy. Specificity of an immunoassay does not only depend on the binding property of the antibody but also the composition of the antigen and its matrix is important. Specificity can also be influenced by reagent composition and immunoassay format. Substances that alter the measurable concentration of the analyte in the sample or alter antibody binding can potentially result in assay interference (Tate & Ward, 2004).

Interference can be analyte-dependent or analyte–independent and it may increase (positive interference) or decrease (negative interference) the measured result. The common interferences of hemolysis, icterus, lipemia, effects of anticoagulants and sample storage are independent of the analyte concentration. Analyte-dependent interferences in immunoassays are caused by interaction between components in the sample with one or more reagent antibodies. They include heterophilic antibodies, human anti-animal antibodies, auto-analyte antibodies, rheumatoid factor and other proteins. Interferences may lead to falsely elevated or falsely depressed analyte concentration depending on the nature of the interfering antibody or the assay design (reagent limited versus reagent excess assays). The magnitude of the effect depends on the concentration of the interferant, but it is not necessarily directly proportional. It can also lead to discordant results between assay systems (Selby, 1999; Tate & Ward, 2004).

Interference can have important clinical consequences and may lead to unnecessary clinical investigation as well as inappropriate treatment with potentially unfavorable outcome for the patient (Ismail & Barth, 2001). It is important to recognize interference in immunoassays and put procedures in place to identify them wherever possible (Kricka, 2000).

2. Nature of Interference

Endogenous interfering substances can occur in both healthy and pathological patient samples. Sample properties are unique for each patient. Interference is caused by interaction with one or more steps in the immunoassay procedure and the analyte concentration or the antibody binding is influenced (Davies, 2005). Unsuspected binding protein(s) in the individual can interfere with the reaction between analyte and assay antibodies. In reagent-excess assays, like the common two-site immunometric assay (IMA), there is an increased chance of a cross-reactant forming a bridge between the two antibodies. Conformational changes to antigens can be induced by antibodies which may alter the specificity of antibodies. For these reasons there may be a higher prevalence of unpredictable cross-reaction in IMAs than in the single-site antigen-antibody reaction in reagent-limited assays (Boscato & Stuart, 1986). Exogenous antibodies given to a patient for therapy may also compete with the assay antibody for the analyte and disturb the antigen-antibody reaction resulting in immunoassay interference, e.g., administration of Fab fragments derived from anti-digoxin antibodies (Digibind) (Hursting et al., 1997).

Exogenous interferences are any interference caused by the introduction of external factors or conditions, in vivo or in vitro, not normally present in native, properly collected and stored samples. For example, hemolysis, lipemia, icterus, blood collection tube additives,

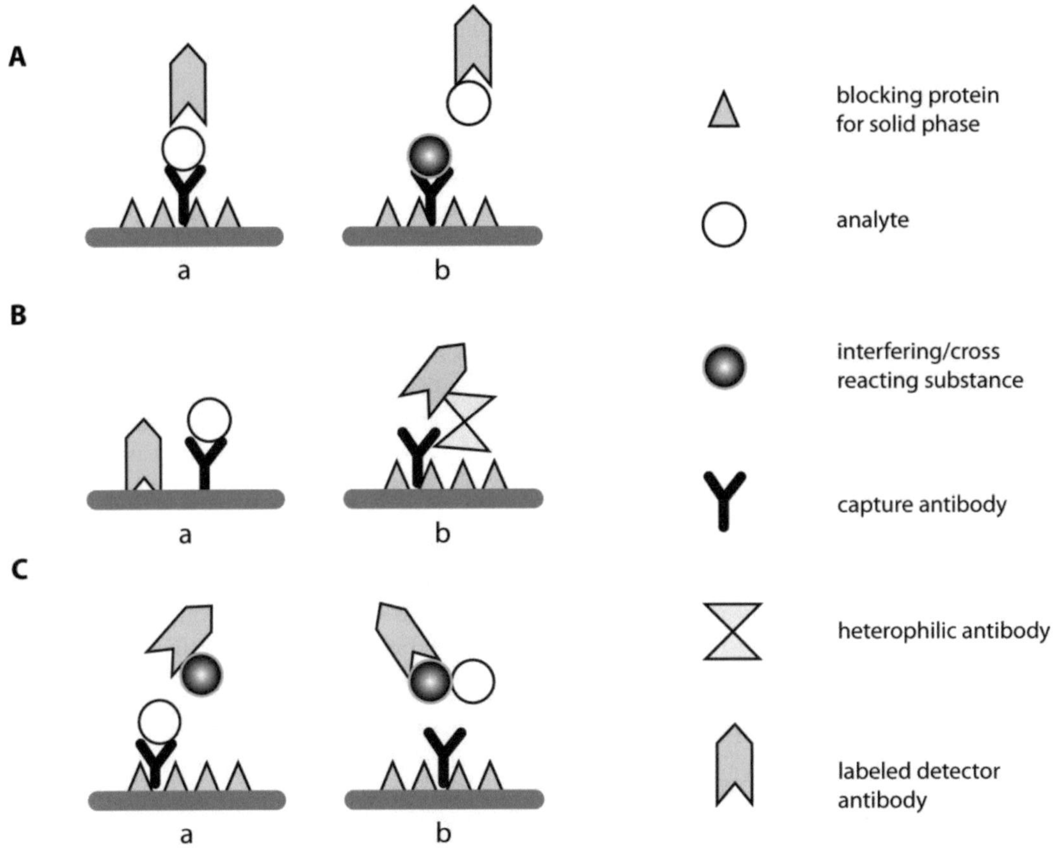

Fig. 1. Different interferences in immunometric immunoassays: Aa - assay without any interference; Ab - cross-reactivity of an interfering substance with capture antibody, resulting in false negative result; B - positive interference: Ba - unspecific binding of labelled detector antibody to a not blocked solid phase; Bb - "bridge" binding by heterophilic antibodies or HAMA, respectively; C - negative interference: Ca - change of sterical conformation after binding of interfering protein to Fc fragment of detector antibody Cb - masking of the epitope on analyte surface by a protein of the sample (Dodig, 2009).

administration of radioactive or fluorescent compounds, drugs, herbal medicines, nutritional supplements, sample storage and transport are all exogenous interferences that can adversely affect immunoassays (Selby, 1999).

Figure 1 summaries the possible interference mechanisms in IMAs.

3. Cross-reactivity

Cross-reactivity is the most common interference in immunoassays, but mostly in competitive assays. It is a non-specific influence of substances in a sample that structurally resemble the analyte (carry similar or the same epitopes as the analyte) and compete for binding site on antibody, resulting in over- or underestimation of analyte concentration. Cross-reaction is a problem in diagnostic immunoassays where endogenous molecules with a similar structure to the measured analyte exist or where metabolites of the analyte have common cross-reacting epitopes, and where there is administration of structurally similar medications (Kroll & Elin, 1994). The most common examples can be seen during determinations of hormone concentration, drugs and allergen-specific IgE. Hormones TSH (thyroid-stimulating hormone), LH (luteinising hormone) and hCG (human chorionic gonadotrophin) carry an analogue α-chain, and the β-chain determines the specificity of the respective hormone. Early hCG immunoassays cross-react with LH, but the development of more specific antibodies has led to most of today's assays for hCG having little or no cross-reaction with LH (Thomas & Segers, 1985). However, cross-reactivity with drugs and their metabolites is still a problem for the measurements of steroids which have an identical structure. For example, cortisol assays can show significant cross-reactivity with fludrocortisone derivates and result in falsely elevated cortisol levels in patients using these drugs (Berthod et al., 1988). The problem of cross-reactivity in active vitamin D ($1,25(OH)_2D$) determination due to possible positive interference of 25(OH) D is well known (Lai et al., 2010).

In competitive immunoassays for drugs of abuse screening, positive interference may result from medications or their metabolites that have similar chemical structures (Lewis et al., 1998).

In the regular monitoring of the transplant anti-rejection drug cyclosporine A in whole blood for dosage adjustment in patients after heart or liver transplantation, only the concentration of the parent drug should be used. Immunoassays for cyclosporine A show cross-reactivity for cyclosporine metabolites with levels up to 174% higher in individual patients compared with the HPLC reference method (Steimer, 1999).

In digoxin immunoassays, the presence of digoxin-like immunoreactive factors that are commonly found in renal failure, liver disease and hypertension, cause interference by cross-reaction (Dasqupta, 2006). Falsely suppression of results can also occur when a cross-reacting substance is present in the sample and during the wash or separation step the dissociation rate for the cross-reactant is greater than that for the analyte (Valdes & Jortani, 2002).

Interference due to cross-reactivity is highly dependent on assay specificity, which is not the focus of this chapter.

4. Alteration of the measurable concentration in the sample

4.1 Pre-analytical factors

All factors associated with the constituents of the sample are termed pre-analytical factors (Selby, 1999).

4.1.1 Blood collection

Blood collection tubes are not inert containers but have several constituents, including substances in and/or applied to rubber stoppers, tube wall material, surfactants, anticoagulants, separator gels and clot activators that can potentially interfere with immunoassays (Weber, 1990). Many laboratories have converted from glass to plastic collection tubes for convenience. Plastic blood collection tubes have been shown to be suitable for routine clinical chemistry analytes, hormone analysis and therapeutic drug monitoring (Wilde, 2005). But some low-molecular weight organic substances released by plastic tubes could interfere in some assays. The physical masking of the antibody by lipids and silicone oils present in some blood collection devices or tubes can physically interfere with Ag-Ab binding. The water-soluble silicone polymer coating the interior of serum separator tubes can interfere negatively with avidin-biotin binding in an IRMA for thyrotropin, prolactin, and hCG (Wickus et al, 1992). Conversely, silicone formed a complex with C-reactive protein (CRP) that enhanced the Ag-Ab reaction in the Vitros CRP assay resulting in falsely elevated results (Chang et al., 2003).

4.1.2 Sample type

For many immunoassays, serum is the matrix of choice; however, plasma can be a very useful alternative, as it eliminates the extra time needed for clotting, thereby reducing the overall pre-analytical time (Selby, 1999). Tubes containing anticoagulants must be filled to the mark, otherwise the concentration of the anticoagulants will be too high and this may affect the assay system, particularly the Ag-Ab characteristics. If several specimens are to be drawn at the same time the plain tube should always be first filled. The recommended order to fill being plain tube, citrate, lithium heparin, EDTA and finally fluoride/potassium oxalate. Care must still be taken to avoid cross-contamination between different additive tubes (Wilde, 2005). Sample type can affect analyte concentration with different results for samples collected in lithium heparin, EDTA, and sodium fluoride/potassium oxalate or tubes without anticoagulant reported for some analytes, e.g., cardiac troponin, hormones (Evans et al., 2001). If plasma is used for immunoassay, care must be taken to select the appropriate anticoagulant. Anticoagulants added to specimens in appropriate concentrations to preserve certain analytes, may cause problems with the assay of other analytes. Heparin may interfere with some antibody-antigen reactions.

4.1.3 Hemolysis, lipemia and icterus

Immunoassays are mostly unaffected by hemolysis and icterus unlike other analytes measured by spectral or chemical means (Tate & Ward, 2004). However, hemolysis may be unacceptable for immunoassays of relatively labile analytes like insulin, glucagon, calcitonin, parathyroid hormone, ACTH and gastrin, due to the release of proteolytic enzymes from erythrocytes that degrade these analytes. Samples with any sign of hemolysis are not acceptable for such assays. Because hemolysis may also interfere with some signal generation steps of different types of immunoassays, grossly hemolysed specimens should not be used. Lipemia can interfere in some immunoassays especially those using nephelometry and turbidimetry. Lipemia of serum or high levels of triglycerides, cholesterol or both may produce erroneous results in some assays by interfering with antigen binding, even when antibodies are linked to a solid support. Interferences by non-esterified fatty acids have been well documented for free thyroxine assays. Non-esterified fatty acids compete with thyroxine and its derivatives used as labels for endogenous protein binding sites and, depending on the assay format, may cause either falsely high or falsely low free thyroxine values. Binding of steroids may also be inhibited by non-esterified fatty acids. Hypertriglyceridaemia has been shown to cause falsely elevated results in some endocrine assays, using second antibody and polyethylene glycol separation techniques. Ideally, specimens should be collected from individuals following an overnight fast to reduce the immunoassay interference from lipids. Alternatively, ultracentrifugation but not dilution could be used to remove any excess lipids, or enzymatic cleavage by lipase may be used to treat samples before analysis. Excess bilirubin can also affect many different types of assays, including immunoassays (Wilde, 2005).

4.1.4 Stability and storage

Inappropriate specimen processing or storage can change the properties of a sample over time and affect immunoassay results. Most analytes are more stable when the sample is maintained in a cool or frozen condition. For some, especially the small peptide hormones, storage at -20°C and transportation in frozen state is necessary for reliable results. Such hormones include insulin, c peptide, gastrin, glucagon, ACTH and vitamin D (Wilde, 2005). For example, ACTH is reported to be stable in EDTA plasma at 4°C for only 18 hours compared with many other hormones that are stable for >120 hours (Ellis et al., 2003). Repeated freeze/thaw cycles can lead to denaturation, aggregation and loss of antigenicity of some proteins. Because EDTA chelates calcium and magnesium ions, which function as coenzymes for some proteases, blood specimens collected in EDTA are often more stable than serum or heparinised plasma. But elevated EDTA levels in the sample-reagent mixture, due to insufficient sample volume, can affect the activity of the alkaline phosphatase enzyme label used in chemiluminescence assays. Filling EDTA tubes to <50% affects intact parathyroid hormone and ACTH measurements by the Immulite assays (Glendenning et al., 2002). Some of the low mass polypeptide hormones such as ACTH, glucagon, gastrin and the gastrointestinal hormones are rapidly destroyed by enzymes present in blood and may require protection by addition of protease inhibitors (e.g., aprotonin) to the tube into which the blood sample is taken (Wilde, 2005).

4.1.5 Carryover

Integrated systems that combine clinical chemistry and immunoassay analysers are more and more used routinely. Sample to sample carryover is an inherent risk and can cause erroneously high test results for immunoassays (Armbruster & Alexander, 2006). Potential sample carryover due to inadequate washing or failure to detect a sample clot can also results in over- or under-estimation of values. If a sample to be assayed is preceded by a sample with a very high concentration of an analyte e.g. hCG, tumour markers, some of the analyte from the first sample on the instrument probe may significantly increase the concentration of the analyte in the second sample.

4.2 Hormone binding proteins

Hormone binding globulins can alter the measurable analyte concentration in the sample either by removal or blocking of the analyte (Tate & Ward, 2004). Important endogenous binding globulins are albumin (because of its large concentration), sex hormone binding globulin (SHBG), thyroid binding globulin (TBG) and cortisol binding globulin (CBG). For total hormone measurement, it is essential to displace all bound hormone from endogenous binding sites and to prevent the binding of labelled hormone to the endogenous binding site. This can be done by solvent extraction, denaturation of the binding proteins, by adding blocking agents or by immunoaffinity extraction. For example, increased or decreased SHBG concentrations can interfere in direct assays for steroids testosterone (Slaats et al., 1987) and estradiol (Masters & Hähnel, 1989) and binding of cortisol to CBG can be minimized by denaturation of the binding protein or by addition of blocking agent. In free hormone measurement, displacement of analyte from endogenous hormone binding proteins, e.g., free thyroxin (FT4) displaced from thyroid binding globulin (TBG) by non-esterified free fatty acids (NEFA), can alter assay equilibrium and either increase or decrease the free analyte concentration (Nelson & Wilcox, 1996). These NEFAs can be generated in-vitro in non-frozen samples from patients receiving heparin, secondary to the induction of heparin-induced lipase activity. Increased serum triglyceride levels can accentuate this problem (Mendel et al., 1987).

4.3 Autoanalyte antibodies

Autoantibodies have been described that can cause interference for a number of analytes including thyroid hormones in both free and total forms (Symons, 1989), thyroglobulin (Spencer et al., 1998), insulin (Sapin, 1997), prolactin (Fahie-Wilson & Soule, 1997) and testosterone (Kuwahara, 1998). Positive or negative influence may occur, depending on whether the autoantibody-analyte complex partitions into the free or the bound analyte fraction. Interference from autoantibodies can occur in both immunoassay formats (Tate & Ward, 2004).

Autoantibodies against thyroid hormones, especially anti-T4 and anti-T3 antibodies, have been reported in patients with Hashimoto's thyroiditis, Graves' disease, hyperthyroidism after treatment, carcinoma, goitre and non-thyroid autoimmune conditions. These endogenous factors particularly interfere in total T4, free T4, total T3 and free T3 methods. Thyroid hormone antibody interferences are difficult to predict and can occur even with frequently used and well-characterised methods. Antibody prevalence depends on the detection method used: it is low in healthy subjects but may be as high as 10% in patients with autoimmune disease although only a minority of such samples demonstrate substantial thyroid assay interference (Després & Grant, 1998). Their presence should be suspected when FT4 and TSH results appear to be discordant to the clinical findings.

Interference is also a serious problem in Tg assays largely due to endogenous Tg antibodies (TgAb). Serum TgAbs are present in up to 25% of differentiated thyroid cancer (DTC) patients and in 10% of the general population. It is important to use a Tg method that provides measurements that are concordant with the tumour status in DTC patients. IMA methods are prone to underestimate serum Tg when TgAb is present, increasing the risk that persistent or metastatic DTC will be missed. Because falsely low Tg results can occur by IMA and falsely elevated results by RIA, anti-Tg antibodies should be measured in all samples analysed for Tg and a possible interference should be retained in all TgAb positive samples (Spencer et al., 1998).

Anti-prolactin autoantibodies can be present in serum in the form of macroprolactin (macro-PRL). The presence of macro-PRL can cause macroprolactinemia with normal prolactin (PRL) concentrations and may lead to unnecessary medical or surgical procedures (De Schepper et al., 2002; Fahie-Wilson & Ahlquist, 2003). Macro-PRL is a macro-molecular complex of prolactin (PRL) with an IgG antibody (Schiettecatte et al., 2001, 2005) directed against specific epitope(s) on the PRL molecule. Macro-PRL is considered biologically inactive in vivo because of its decreased bioavailability. Macro-PRL is cleared more slowly than monomeric PRL and hence accumulates in the sera of affected subjects. The incidence of macro-PRL is up to 26% of all reported cases of hyperprolactinemia depending on the immunoassay system. Macro-PRL is detected in various degrees by different immunoassays (Smith et al., 2002). Laboratories should know the reactivity of the PRL assay with macro-PRL and ideally test for the presence of macro-PRL in all patients with hyperprolactinemia by gel filtration chromatography or pre-treatment with polyethylene glycol (PEG 6000). It is important to both recognize the presence of macro-PRL and provide an estimate of the monomeric PRL concentration because some patients with macroprolactinemia may have clinically significant, elevated monomeric PRL levels also (Van Besien et al., 2002; Fahie-Wilson, 2003).

5. Alteration of antibody binding

5.1 Heterophilic antibodies

Heterophilic antibodies are antibodies produced against poorly defined antigens. They are multi-specific antibodies of the early immune response and generally show low affinity and weak binding (Levinson & Miller, 2002). These antibodies react with many antigens and the variable region of other antibodies (anti-idiotypic antibodies). IgM antibodies play a key role in interfering sera from rheumatic patients as they can bind Fc fragments of human antibodies (Ismail et al., 2002b).

Interfering, endogenous antibodies should be called heterophilic when there is no history or medical treatment with animal immunoglobulins or other well-defined immunogens, and the interfering antibodies are multi-specific (reacts with immunoglobulin from two or more species) or exhibit rheumatoid activity (Kaplan & Levinson, 1999). In case of rheumatoid factor (RF), false elevated results arise from the binding of RF to the Fc constant domain of antigen-antibody complexes. The presences of RF in serum can cause falsely elevated analyte levels in troponin assays (Fitzmaurice et al., 1998), thyroid function tests (Martel et al., 2000), tumour marker assays (Berth et al., 2006) and falsely detected HCV-specific IgM (Stevenson et al., 1996).

In two-site IMA's, heterophilic antibodies can bridge two assay antibodies together and falsely elevates the patient value by producing an assay signal (Boscato & Stuart, 1986). Assays using either polyclonal or monoclonal antibodies can be affected. The same heterophilic may react differently for different antibody combinations hence causing rise in one assay but a lower result in another assay. The presence of excess non-human immunoglobulin in the assay buffers reduces the possibility of the interfering substances binding to the capture and detection antibody by binding instead to the interfering immunoglobulin. Although manufacturers routinely add blocking agents to their assay formulations, not all heterophilic interference can be blocked by non-immune globulin, including pooled globulin from several species as heterophilic antibodies may show reactivity to idiotypes that are not present in the blocking reagent. Both IgG and IgM heterophilic antibodies are reported to occur (Covinsky et al., 2000).

5.2 Human anti-animal antibodies

Human anti-animal antibodies (HAAA) are high-affinity, specific polyclonal antibodies generated after contact with animal immunoglobulin. They show strong binding and are produced in a high titer. HAAAs can be of the IgG, IgA, IgM, or rarely, the IgE class (Kricka, 1999). They compete with the test antigen by cross-reacting with reagent antibody of the same species to produce a false signal. The most common HAAAs are human anti-mouse antibodies (HAMA), but also antibodies to rat, rabbit, goat, sheep, cow, pig, horse may occur (Selby, 1999). HAMA is especially prevalent in serum of animal workers and in patients on mouse monoclonal antibody for therapy or imaging.

Interfering, endogenous antibodies should be called specific HAAAs when there is a history of medical treatment with animal immunoglobulin and immunoglobulin from the same species used in the immunoassay (Kaplan & Levinson, 1999). The nomenclature becomes confusing where the immunogen is not known and a heterophilic antibody is recognized in mouse or other animal-specific immunoassays.

HAMA interference has been reported for numerous analytes including cardiac markers assays (White & Tideman, 2002), thyroid function tests (Frost et al, 1998), drugs and tumour markers (Boerman et al., 1990). Two-site (sandwich) immunoassays are more prone to interference from antibodies to animal IgG in serum and may cross-react with reagent antibodies especially from the same species. HAMAs interfere by bridging between the immunoglobulin capture and the immunoglobulin detection antibodies resulting in false-positive results. False negative results due to HAMA interference are also possible in two-site assays, when the HAMA reacts with one of the antibodies preventing reaction with the analyte (Kricka, 1999). Methods that use only one mouse monoclonal in IMA assays are less prone to interference from HAMA.

5.3 High-dose hook effect

The hook effect is based on the saturation curve of antibody with antigen (Figure 2). It is caused by excessively high concentrations of analyte simultaneously saturating both capture and detector antibodies. The high-dose hook effect occurs mostly (but not exclusively) in one-step immunometric (sandwich) assays, giving a decrease in signal at very high concentration of analyte (Fernando & Wilson, 1992). In immunoassays with very large analyte concentration ranges (ferritin, growth hormone, hCG, PRL, Tg, tumor markers PSA, CA19.9, CA125); antigen-antibody reactions can go into antigen excess and result in falsely decreased results and potential misdiagnosis. In one step two-site immunoassays where capture and detection antibody are added simultaneously, free analyte and analyte bound to the labeled antibody compete for the limited number of antibody-binding sites of the detector and in the presence of very high analyte concentration will decrease in stead of increase label bound to the solid phase. High-dose hook effect can be avoided by increasing the quantity of the reagent antibodies and by reducing the amount sample required for analysis or by sample dilution (Cole, 2001). Careful assay design is necessary to ensure that the concentrations of both capture and detector antibodies are sufficiently high to cope with levels of analytes over the entire pathological range. It is common practice to re-assay samples at several dilutions as a check on the validity of the result (Davies, 2005).

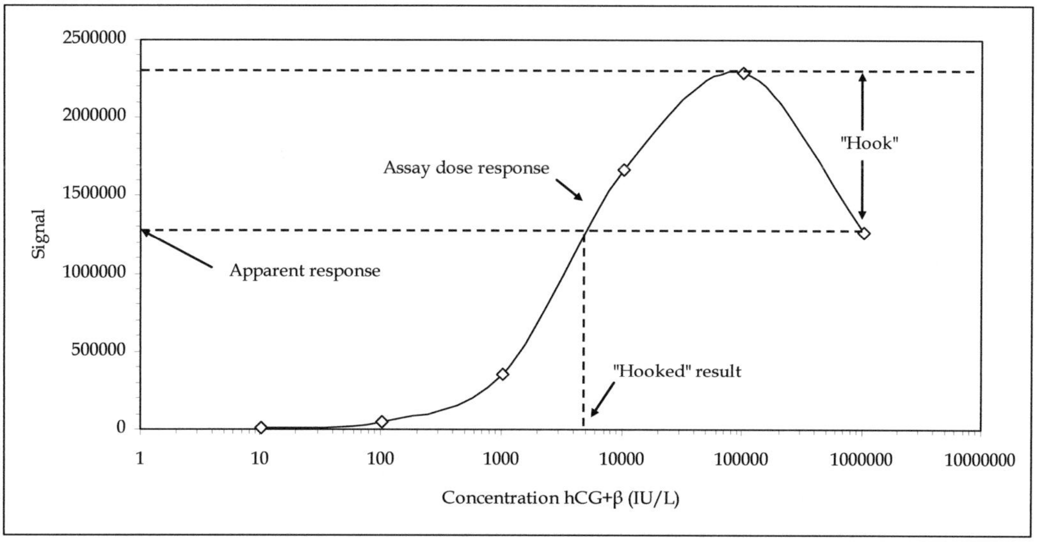

Fig. 2. High-dose hook effect in Elecsys hCG+β assay - an excessive amount of hCG overwhelms the binding capacity of the capture antibody. This results in an inappropriately low signal that causes an erroneous "hooked" result (6200 IU/L) for a patient with an excessively elevated serum hCG+ β concentration of 1 030 000 IU/L.

5.4 Other proteins

Interfering proteins of general relevance include albumin, complement, lysozyme, fibrinogen and paraprotein (Tate & Ward, 2004). They can affect antibody binding and can cause interference in immunoassays. Albumin may interfere as a result of its high concentration and its ability to bind or release large proportions of ligand. Complement binds to the Fc fragment of immunoglobulins and can block the analyte-specific binding sites of antibodies (Weber et al., 1990). Lysozyme can form a bridge between the solid-phase IgG and the detector antibody (Selby, 1999). IgG kappa paraprotein can bind to a TSH assay antibody and sterically block the binding of TSH and lead to falsely lowered TSH values (Luzzi et al., 2003).

6. Interference with detection systems

Occasionally, some samples contain compounds that artificially increase or decrease the magnitude of the response, without affecting antigen-antibody binding.

6.1 Endogenous signal-generating substances

The presence of endogenous signal-generating substances can interfere in the signal detection of an immunoassay. Diagnostic or therapeutic administration of radioisotopes can be carried over to the final counting tube, altering radioimmunoassay results. Endogenous europium can interfere in time-resolved fluorescence. With fluorescent immunoassays, interference can result from endogenous fluorescent substances, fluorescent drugs or fluorescein administration for the performance of retinal angiography (Davies, 2005).

6.2 Enzyme inhibitors/activators

In enzyme-labelled immunoassays, the presence of inhibitors or activators of the detection enzyme in the sample may alter the signal and thereby the immunoassay results. Enzyme inhibitors can be chemical or immunological. Antibodies that cross react with horse-radish peroxidase or alkaline phosphatase have been described. Azide present as preservative in some control sera may lead to suppression of enzyme activity in assays using peroxidase as label. Samples collected into tubes containing sodium fluoride may be unsuitable for some enzymatic immunoassay methods due to inhibition of the enzyme activity by fluoride (Davies, 2005).

6.3 Enzyme catalysts or cofactors

Enzyme-immunoassays can be affected by enzyme catalysts or cofactors, for example Cu^{2+} contamination promoting luminol chemiluminescence in the presence of H_2O_2.

Some label interferences can be resolved by utilising a heterogeneous assay format, a pre-treatment step, screening specimens for endogenous radioactivity before assay, use of non-isotopic labels/methods or diluting the sample so that the interfering substance is also diluted. These interferences can also selectively be depressed by adding suitable blocking agents (Davies, 2005).

7. Incidence of immunoassay interference

The prevalence of interference in modern immunoassays is low, but variable and dependent on the type of antibody interference. Heterophilic antibody and HAMA interference can vary from 0.05% to 6% depending upon the method of detection (Bjerner et al., 2002). Non-analyte antibody binding substances have been detected in proximally 40% of serum samples using a modified immunometric assay, termed an "interference assay" and they caused 15% interference in non-blocked assays (Boscato & Stuart, 1986). Ward et al. identified 7 out of 21,000 samples from a hospital population with heterophilic interference and HAMA, the interference being as low as 0.03% in blocked IMAs. However, the addition of blocking reagent does not guarantee the complete elimination of interference (Ward et al., 1997).

The extent of affected immunoassays was highlighted in a multicenter survey of erroneous immunoassay results from assays of 74 analytes in 10 donors conducted by 66 laboratories in seven countries (Marks, 2002). Approximately 6% of analytes gave falsely elevated results with the potential for incorrect clinical interpretation. Of these analytes, 1.8% (n=65) of results involving 13 analytes were determined to be heterophilic false-positive while another 4.2% (n=146) of results involving 17 analytes gave false-positives of uncertain etiology that were not restored to within the reference interval by addition of heterophilic blocking reagent. The blood was obtained from donors with RF-positive illnesses, multiple sclerosis, or lupus, and had detectable RF (31 to >1000 kIU/L) and/or HAMA (3-589 μg/L). Blood from nine of the ten donors resulted in false-positive results of uncertain etiology for six of seven estradiol assay systems (58% of analyses performed) and for two of eight cortisol systems (20% of analyses). For blood from one donor, eight of eleven FSH and LH assay systems reported false-lowered results. The highest percentage of heterophilic false-positive results in this survey occurred for myoglobin (48% of analyses performed in two of seven tested assay systems). From the available evidence, Levinson & Miller assumed that the amount of interference identified with modern blocked two-site immunoassays is very low, in the order of 10 per 20000 samples assayed (Levinson & Miller, 2002).

8. Techniques to minimise antibody interferences in immunoassay

Methods for the reduction of heterophilic and anti-animal interference in immunoassays are summarized in Table 1 (Selby, 1999; Tate & Wald, 2004). These include ways to remove or block the interfering antibody (Kricka, 1999). Prior extraction of the analyte from the sample can remove the interference. Gel chromatography can be effective to remove interferants. Immunoextraction using murine monoclonal antibody or protein G immobilized on Sepharose beads has been effectively used to remove HAMA interferences. Anti-animal interference can also be removed by precipitation with polyethylene (PEG) 6000 (Ismail, 2005). Heat treatment (70-90°C) of samples is of limited utility because few analytes are heat-stable and thus do not survive these antibody-denaturing conditions.

Addition of low concentrations of serum or immunoglobulin from the same species as the antibody reagents in the reaction mixture can prevent interference in some samples by neutralizing or inhibiting the interference. The blocking agent can be included in the assay diluent or the sample can be pre-treated before assay. Non-immune serum, polyclonal IgG, polymerized IgG, non-immune mouse monoclonal, or fragments of IgG (Fc, Fab, $F(ab')_2$) from the same species used to raise the reagent antibodies, are commonly used as blocking agents. However, in some cases addition of one or more of these blocking agents in immunoassay reagents is either insufficient or not successful in preventing interference. Determination of the exact amount of blocker sufficient to eliminate interference in all patient samples is difficult to determine in practice as the immune response to interfering antibodies is highly variable between individuals. The effectiveness of the added blocking agent depends on the species and subclass of the blocker (Selby,1999; Kricka, 1999; Tate & Ward, 2004). Several blocking reagents are available commercially: Heterophilic Blocking Reagent (HBR; Scantibodies), Immunoglobulin Inhibiting Reagent (IIR; Bioreclamation), Heteroblock (Omega Biologicals), MAB33 and Poly MAB 33 (Roche Diagnostics).

Another solution for the problem of human-animal antibody interferences is the use of Fab or $F(ab')_2$ fragments instead of the intact immunoglobulin as capture or detector antibodies in two-site assay, eliminating the interference of HAAAs with specificity for the Fc portion of an IgG antibody. Another strategy is to use chimeric antibodies. These chimeric antibodies are human antibodies where the variable regions are replaced with the corresponding part of a non-human antibody (mouse or rat). Interferences by anti-mouse or other animal antibodies are eliminated (Kricka, 1999). The latter are now used in some Roche immunoassays (Elecsys TSH, CEA, Troponin T) either as capture or detector antibody.

Removal of interfering antibody
• Extraction of analyte from sample
• Immunoextraction by addition of murine or other animal species serum immobilized onto Sepharose beads or immobilized Protein A suspension
• Polyethyleen glycol precipitation (PEG 6000)
• Heating to 70-90°C for heat-stable analytes
Addition of blocking agent from the same species as the antibody reagents
• The inclusion of one or more blocking agents in manufacturers' immunoassay reagent may be insufficient to overcome the interference
• Non-immune serum, species-specific polyclonal IgG, anti-human IgG or polymerized mouse IgG
• Non-immune mouse monoclonals
• Species-specific fragments of IgG (Fc, Fab)
• Heterophilic blocking reagents (HBR), immunoglobulin inhibiting reagent (IIR), and antibody blocking tubes
Assay redesign
• Use of Fab or F(ab')2 fragments
• Use of chimeric monoclonal antibodies

Table 1. Methods for reduction of interference from heterophilic antibodies and human anti-animal antibodies (Selby, 1999; Tate & Wald, 2004)

9. Testing for interferences in samples suspected of interference

Immunoassay results on samples suspected of interference can be checked by different procedures (Table 2). These include repeat analysis of the sample using a different immunoassay platform that, if possible, employs antibodies that are raised to a different species and normally gives agreement between methods. If HAMA interference is suspected, the alternate assays should not use monoclonal mouse antibodies because the assay may also be inaccurate. If a significantly different result is detected between methods there is a likelihood of interference. However, agreement between methods does not necessarily exclude interference nor does disagreement, if methods lack standardization and clinical decision limits differ (Tate & Wald, 2004). The false assumption that a result is correct because a majority of immunoassay methods give similar results was shown in the multicentre study by Marks in which nine of eleven LH and FSH methods were in agreement but gave falsely low results for a 72-year old postmenopausal woman who was positive for RF (Marks, 2002). Reanalysis using alternative technology such as liquid chromatography or tandem mass spectrometry should be considered if available (Ismael, 2009; Hoofnagle & Wener, 2009).

Another procedure for detecting and identifying a suspected interfering antibody is the use of commercially available blocking antibodies (Emerson et al., 2003). Statistically discrepant results before and after incubation with blocking agent would be indicative of interference. A difference between initial and treated value of 3 to 5 standard deviation (SD) suggest possible heterophilic interference, >5 SD indicates definite heterophilic interference (Preissner et al., 2005). However, 20-30% of samples with interfering antibodies may yield similar results after treatment with the blocking antibodies (Ismael, 2009).

Another test is making serial dilutions of the sample using manufacturer's diluent, provided that it contains non-immune globulin (Ismail, 2007). This could identify about 60% of samples with interference in which linearity and parallelism are lacking.

Using these three tests could identify interference in almost 90% of suspected samples (Ismail, 2009).

Repeat analysis with an alternate immunoassay that preferably uses antibody raised to a different species or using alternative technology such as liquid chromatography or tandem mass spectrometry
Measurement before and after addition of a blocking reagent
Measurement of dilutions of the sample with the manufacturer's diluent containing non-immune globulins
Sample pre-treatment e.g. PEG precipitation in Prolactin measurement

Table 2. Methods for testing of interference in suspected samples (Tate & Wald, 2004)

10. Conclusions

Interference in immunoassays from endogenous antibodies is still a major unresolved and underestimated analytical problem, which can have important clinical consequences. There is no single procedure that can rule out all interferences. It is important to recognize the potential for interference in immunoassay and to put procedures in place to identify them wherever possible. Most important is a consideration of the clinical picture. If there is any suspicion of discordance between the clinical and the laboratory data an attempt should be made to reconcile the difference. The detection of interference may require the use of another method, or measurement before and after treatment with additional blocking agent, or following dilution of the sample in non-immune serum. If testing is inconclusive and the interference cannot be identified, the analyte concentration should not be reported and laboratory report should indicate there is a discrepancy for that analyte due to some technical inaccuracy and suggest the test to be repeated using another sample.

Interference in immunoassay is one factor that contributes to the uncertainty of medical testing. Laboratories should be aware of the potential for interference in all immunoassays and how artefactual results may cause misinterpretation and a subsequent erroneous diagnosis and unwarranted treatment. The recognition of such aberrant test results requires constant surveillance of both laboratory and clinician. Since these interferences are relative uncommon, clinicians need to be aware of them and alert to the mismatch of clinical and biological data. Dialogue between the clinician and the clinical laboratory over unexpected immunoassay test results can avoid inappropriate clinical intervention based on abnormal test results.

11. References

Armbruster, D.A. & Alexander, D.B. (2006). Sample to sample carryover: a source of analytical laboratory error and its relevance to integrated clinical chemistry/immunoassay systems. *Clin Chim Acta*, Vol.373, pp. 37-43

Berth, M.; Bosmans, E.; Everaert, J.; Dierick, J.; Schiettecatte, J.; Anckaert, E. & Delanghe, J. (2006). Rheumatoid factor interference in the determination of carbohydrate antigen 19-9 (CA19-9). *Clin Chem Lab Med,* Vol.44, pp. 1137-1139

Berthod, C.; Rey, F. (1988). Enormous cross-reactivity of hydrocortisone hemisuccinate in the RIANEN RIA kit for cortisol determination. *Clin Chem*, Vol.34, pp. 1358

Bjerner, J.; Nustad, K.; Norum, L.F.; Hauge Olsen, K.; Børmer, O.P. (2002). Immunometric assay interference: incidence and prevention. *Clin Chem*, 2002, Vol.48, pp. 613–621

Boerman, O.C.; Segers, M.F.G.; Poels, L.G.; Kenemans, P.; Thomas, C.M.G. (1990). Heterophilic antibodies in human sera causing falsely increased results in the CA 125 immunofluorometric assay. *Clin Chem*, Vol.36,pp. 888–891

Boscato, L.M.; Stuart, M.C. (1986). Incidence and specificity of interference in two-site immunoassays. *Clin Chem*, Vol.32, pp. 1491–1495

Chang, C.Y. ; Lu, J.Y. ; Chien, T.I. ; Kao, J.T. ; Lin, M.C. ; Shih, P.C. & Yan, S.N. (2003). Interference caused by the contents of serum separator tubes in the Vitros CRP assay. *Ann Clin Biochem*, Vol.40, pp. 249–251

Cole, L.A.; Rinne, K.M.; Shahabi, S. & Omrani, A. (1999). False-positive hCG assay results leading to unnecessary surgery and chemotherapy and needless occurrences of diabetes and coma. *Clin Chem*, Vol.45, pp. 313–314

Cole, L.A.; Shahabi, S.; Butler, S.A.; Mitchell, H.; Newlands, E.S.; Behrman, H.R. & Verrill, H.L. (2001). Utility of commonly used commercial human chorionic gonadotropin immunoassays in the diagnosis and management of trophoblastic diseases. *Clin Chem*, Vol.47, pp. 308–315

Covinsky, M.; Laterza, O.; Pfeifer, J.D.; Farkas-Szallasi; T. & Scott M.G. (2000). An IgM λ antibody to Escherichia coli produces false-positive results in multiple immunometric assays. *Clin Chem*, Vol.46, pp. 1157–1161

Dasgupta, A. (2006). Therapeutic drug monitoring of digoxin: impact of endogenous and exogenous digoxin-like immunoreactive substances. *Toxicol Rev*, Vol.25, pp. 273–281

Davies, C. (2005). Concepts in *The Immunoassay Handbook*. 3nd edition, Elsevier Ltd., ISBN 0 08 044526 8, United Kingdom

De Schepper, J.; Schiettecatte, J.; Velkeniers; B.; Blumenfeld, Z.; Steinberg; M.; Devroey, P.; Anckaert, E.; Smitz, J.; Verdood, P.; Hooghe, R. & Hooghe-Peters, E. (2003). Clinical and biological characterization of macroprolactinemia with and without prolactin-IgG complexes. *Eur J Endocrinol*, Vol.149, pp. 201-207

Després, N. & Grant, A.M. (1998). Antibody interference in thyroid assays: a potential for clinical misinformation. *Clin Chem*, Vol.44, pp. 440–454

Dodig, S. (2009). Interferences in quantitative immunochemical methods. *Biochemia Medica*, Vol.19, pp. 50-62

Emerson, J.F.; Ngo, G. & Emerson, S.S. (2003). Screening for interference in immunoassays. *Clin Chem* , Vol.49, pp. 1163–1169

Evans, M.J.; Livesey, J.H.; Ellis, M.J. & Yandle, T.G. (2001) Effect of anticoagulants and storage temperatures on stability of plasma and serum hormones. *Clin Biochem.* , Vol.34, pp. 107–112

Ellis, M.J.; Livesey, J.H. & Evans, M.J. (2003). Hormone stability in human whole blood. *Clin Biochem.*, Vol.36, pp. 109–12

Fahie-Wilson, M.N. & Soule, S.G. (1997). Macroprolactinaemia: contribution to hyperprolactinaemia in a district general hospital and evaluation of a screening test based on precipitation with polyethylene glycol. *Ann Clin Biochem*, Vol.34:252–258

Fahie-Wilson, M.N. & Ahlquist, J.A. (2003). Hyperprolactinaemia due to macroprolactins: some progress but still a problem. *Clin Endocrinol.*, Vol.58:683–685

Fernando, S.A. & Wilson, G.S. (1992). Studies on the hook effect in the one-step immunoassay. *J Immunol Methods*, Vol.151, pp 47-66

Fitzmaurice, T.F.; Brown, C.; Rifai, N.; Wu, A.H.B. & Yeo, K.T.J. (1998). False increase of cardiac Tropinin I with heterophilic antibodies. *Clin Chem*, Vol.44, pp. 2212–2213

Frost, S.J.; Hine, K.R.; Firth, G.B. & Wheatley, T. (1998). Falsely lowered FT4 and raised TSH concentrations in a patient with hyperthyroidism and human anti-mouse monoclonal antibodies. *Ann Clin Biochem*, Vol.35, pp. 317–320

Glendenning, P.; Musk, A.A.; Taranto, M. & Vasikaran, S.D. (2002). Preanalytical factors in the measurement of intact parathyroid hormone with the DPC IMMULITE assay. *Clin Chem*, Vol.48, pp. 566–567

Hoofnagle, A.N. & Wener M.H. (2009) The fundamental Flaws of Immunoassays and the Potential solutions Using Tandem Mass spectrometry. *J Immunol Methods*, Vol.347, pp. 3-11

Hursting, M.J.; Raisys, V.A. & Opheim, K.E. (1987) Drug-specific Fab therapy in drug overdose. *Arch Pathol Lab Med*, Vol.111, pp. 693–697

Ismail, A.A.A. & Barth, J.H. (2001). Wrong biochemistry results. *Br Med J*, Vol 323, pp. 705–706

Ismail A.A.A.; Walker, P.L.; Cawood, M.L. & Barth, JH. (2002). Interference in immunoassay is an underestimated problem. *Ann Clin Biochem*, Vol.39, pp. 366-373

Ismail A.A.A.; Walker, P.L.; Barth, J.H.; Lewandowski, K.C.; Jones, R. & Burr, W.A. (2002) Wrong biochemistry Results: Two Case Reports and Observational Study in 5310 Patients on Potentially Misleading Thyroid-stimulating Hormone and Gonadotropin Immunoassay Results. *Clin Chem*, Vol.48, pp. 2023-2029

Ismail, A.A.A. (2005). A radical approach is needed to eliminate interference from endogenous antibodies in immunoassays. *Clin Chem*, Vol.51, pp. 25–26

Ismail, A.A.A. (2007). On detecting interference from endogenous antibodies in immunoassays by doubling dilutions test. *Clin Chem Lab Med*, Vol.45, pp. 851–854

Ismail, A.A.A. (2009). Interference from endogenous antibodies in automated immunoassays: what laboratorians need to know. *J Clin Pathol*, Vol.62, pp. 673–679

Kaplan, I.V. & Levinson, S.S. (1999). When is a heterophile antibody not a heterophile antibody? When it is an antibody against a specific immunogen. *Clin Chem*, Vol.45, pp. 616–618

Kricka, L.J. (1999). Human anti-animal antibody interferences in immunological assays. *Clin Chem*, Vol.45, pp. 942–956

Kricka, L.J. (2000) Interferences in immunoassays - still a threat. *Clin Chem*, Vol.46, pp 1037-1038

Kroll, M.H. & Elin, R.J. (1994). Interference with clinical laboratory analyses. *Clin Chem*, Vol.40, pp. 1996-2005

Kuwahara, A.; Kamada, M.; Irahara, M., Naka, O.; Yamashita, T. & Aono, T. (1998). Autoantibody against testosterone in a woman with hypergonadotropic hypogonadism. *J Clin Endocrinol Metab*, Vol.83, pp. 14–16

Lai, J.K.; Lucas, R.M.; Clements, M.S.; Harrison, S.L. & Banks E. (2010). Assessing vitamin D status: pitfalls for the unwary. *Mol Nutr Food Res*, Vol.54, pp. 1062–1071

Levinson, S.S. & Miller, J.J. (2002). Towards a better understanding of heterophile (and the like) antibody interference with modern immunoassays. *Clin Chim Acta*, Vol.325, pp. 1–15

Lewis J.H.; Dusci L.; Hackett P.; Potter J.M. (1998). Drugs of abuse: analytical and clinical perspective in the 1990s. *Clin Biochem Rev*, Vol. 19, pp. 18-52

Luzzi, V.I.; Scott, M.G. & Gronowski A.M. (2003). Negative thyrotropin assay interference associated with an IgGk paraprotein. *Clin Chem*, Vol.49, pp.709–710

Marks, V. (2002). False-positive immunoassay results: a multicenter survey of erroneous immunoassay results from assays of 74 analytes in 10 donors from 66 laboratories in seven countries. *Clin Chem*, Vol.48, pp. 2008–2016

Martel, J. ; Després, N. ; Ahnadi, C.E. ; Lachance, J.F. ; Monticello, J.E. ; Fink, G. ; Ardemagni, A. ; Banfi, G. ; Tovey, J. ; Dykes, P. ; John, R. ; Jeffery, J. & Grant, A.M. (2000). Comparative multicentre study of a panel of thyroid tests using different automated immunoassay platforms and specimens at high risk of antibody interference. *Clin Chem Lab Med*, Vol.38, pp. 785–793

Masters, A.M. & Hähnel, R. (1989). Investigation of sex-hormone binding globulin interference in direct radioimmunoassays for testosterone and estradiol. *Clin Chem*, Vol.35, pp. 979–984

Mendel, C.M.; Frost, P.H.; Kunitake, S.T. & Cavalieri, R.R. (1987). Mechanism of the heparin-induced increase in the concentration of free thyroxine in plasma. *J Clin Endocrinol Metab.*, Vol.65, pp. 1259–1264

Nelson, J.C. & Wilcox, R.B. (1996). Analytical performance of free and total thyroxine assays. Clin Chem, Vol.42, pp. 146–154

Preissner, C.M.; O'Kane, D.J.; Singh, R.J.; Morris, J.C. & Grebe, S.K.G. (2003). Phantoms in the assay tube: heterophile antibody interferences in serum thyroglobulin assays. *J Clin Endocrinol Metab*, Vol.88, pp. 3069–3074

Rotmensch, S. & Cole, L.A. (2000). False diagnosis and needless therapy of presumed malignant disease in women with false-positive human chorionic gonadotropin concentrations. *Lancet*, Vol.355, pp. 712–715

Sapin, R. (1997). Anti-insulin antibodies in insulin immunometric assays: a still possible pitfall. *Eur J Clin Chem Clin Biochem*, Vol.35, pp. 365–367

Schiettecatte, J.; De Schepper, J.; Velkeniers, B.; Smitz, J. & Van Steirteghem A. (2001). A rapid detection of macroprolactin in the form of prolactin-immunoglobulin G complexes by immunoprecipitation with anti-human IgG-agarose. *Clin Chem Lab Med*, Vol.39, pp. 1244-1248

Schiettecatte, J.; Van Opdenbosch, A.; Anckaert, E.; De Schepper, J.; Poppe, K.; Velkeniers, B. & Smitz, J. (2005). Immunoprecipitation for rapid detection of macroprolactin in the form of prolactin-immunoglobulin complexes. *Clin Chem*, Vol.51, pp. 1746-1748.

Selby, C. (1999). Interference in immunoassay. *Ann Clin Biochem*, Vol.36, pp. 704-721

Slaats, E.H.; Kennedy, J.C. & Kruijswijk, H. (1987). Interference of sex-hormone binding globulin in the "Coat-A-Count" testosterone no-extraction radioimmunoassay. *Clin Chem*, Vol.33, pp. 300–302

Smith, T.P.; Suliman, A.M.; Fahie-Wilson, M.N. & McKenna, T.J. (2002). Gross variability in the detection of prolactin in sera containing big big prolactin (macroprolactin) by commercial immunoassays. *J Clin Endocrinol Metab*, Vol.87, pp. 5410–5425

Spencer, C.A.; Takeuchi, M.; Kazarosyan, M.; Kazarosyan, M.; Wang, C.C.; Guttler, B.; Singer, P.A.; Fatemi, S.; LoPresti, J.S. & Nicoloff J.T. (1998). Serum thyroglobulin autoantibodies: prevalence, influence on serum thyroglobulin measurement, and prognostic significance in patients with differentiated thyroid carcinoma. *J Clin Endocrinol Metab*, Vol.83, pp. 1121–1127

Steimer, W. (1999). Performance and specificity of monoclonal immunoassays for cyclosporine monitoring: how specific is specific? *Clin Chem.*, Vol.45, pp. 371–381

Stevenson, D.L.; Harris, A.G.; Neal, K.R., Irving, W.L. (1996). on behalf of Trent HCV Study Group. The presence of rheumatoid factor in sera from anti-HCV positive blood donors interferes with the detection of HCV-specific IgM. *J Hepatol,* Vol XX, pp. 621–626

Symons R.G. (1989).Interference with the laboratory assessment of thyroid function. *Clin Biochem Rev*, Vol. 10, pp. 44-49

Tate, J. & Ward, G. (2004). Interferences in Immunoassay. *Clin Biochem Rev*, Vol.25, pp. 105-120

Thomas, C.M.G.; Segers M.F.G. (1985). Discordant results for goriogonadotropin: a problem caused by lutropin β-subunit interference? *Clin Chem*, Vol.31:159

Vanbesien, J.; Schiettecatte, J.; Anckaert, E.; Smitz, J.; Velkeniers, B. & De Schepper, J. (2002). Circulating anti-prolactin auto-antibodies must be considered in the differential diagnosis of hyperprolactinaemia in adolescents. *Eur J Pediatr*, Vol.161, pp 373-376

Valdes Jr, R. & Jortani, S.A. (2002). Unexpected suppression of immunoassay results by cross-reactivity: now a demonstrated cause for concern. *Clin Chem*, Vol.48, pp. 405–406

Ward, G.; McKinnon, L.; Badrick, T. & Hickman, P.E. (1997). Heterophilic antibodies remain a problem for the immunoassay laboratory. *Am J Clin Pathol*, Vol.108, pp. 417–21

Weber, T.H.; Käpyaho, K.I. & Tanner, P. (1990). Endogenous interference in immunoassays in clinical chemistry. A review. *Scand J Clin Lab Invest*, Vol.50 (Suppl 201), pp. 77–82

Wickus, G.G.; Mordan, R.J. & Mathews, E.A. (1992). Interference in the Allégro immunoassay system when blood is collected in silicone-coated tubes. *Clin Chem*, Vol.38, pp. 2347–2348

Wilde, C. (2005). Subject preparation, sample collection and handling in *The Immunoassay Handbook*. 3nd edition, Elsevier Ltd., ISBN 0 08 044526 8, United Kingdom

White, G.H. & Tideman, P.A. (2002). Heterophilic antibody interference with CARDIAC T quantitative rapid assay. *Clin Chem*, Vol.48, pp. 201–203

Part 2

Label-Free Technologies

4

Fundamentals and Applications of Immunosensors

Carlos Moina and Gabriel Ybarra
Instituto Nacional de Tecnología Industrial, Argentine Republic

1. Introduction

Immunosensors are compact analytical devices in which the event of formation of antigen-antibody complexes is detected and converted, by means of a transducer, to an electrical signal, which can be processed, recorded and displayed. Different transducing mechanisms are employed in immunological biosensors, based on signal generation (such as an electrochemical or optical signal) or properties changes (such as mass changes) following the formation of antigen-antibody complexes. In this chapter, the basics of immunosensors are presented focused on the different transduction techniques used in immunosensing.

2. The concept of biosensor: a convergence of biology, physical chemistry, and electronics

Most clinical analysis are carried out by specialized staff in laboratories employing desk-top instruments, thus assuring the highest possible confidence in the obtained results. However, there are many cases in which a critical clinical analysis cannot be performed in those optimal conditions because of the lack of trained analysts or the required facilities, as is often the case in underdeveloped or isolated areas. In those cases, biosensors, which are compact analytical devices for the detection of specific analytes, can be the only option to make a trustworthy medical diagnosis. Especially immunosensors, a type of biosensors aimed at the detection of the presence of specific antibodies or antigens, are particularly important for the diagnosis of diseases in remote environments, where carrying out immunoassays such as ELISA (Enzyme-Linked Immunosorbent Assay) is not an option. The advantages of point of care (POC) testing versus laboratory testing can be summarized in the diagram introduced by von Lode (Fig. 1).

Although the possibility of carrying out in situ or point of care diagnosis with a minimum required training is a major reason for the development of biosensors in general and immunosensors in particular, there are many other reasons. For instance, fast, non-expensive, multiple assays can ideally be performed with immunosensors and could be of help in epidemics to make proper diagnosis and follow the epidemic spreading.

In the rest of the chapter, we will present the basics of different types of immunosensors. We will begin considering the general outline of biosensors, which compromise three main components: a sensitive biological element, a transducer, and a signal processor. These three

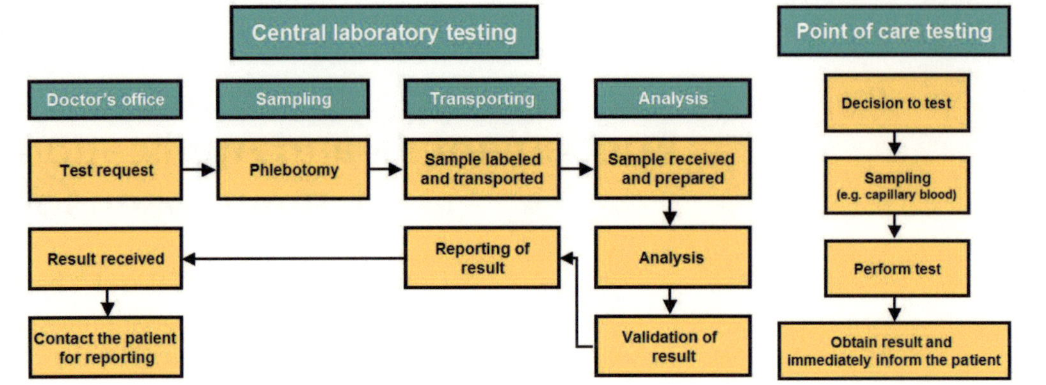

Fig. 1. Process of clinical testing in outpatient situations using central laboratory versus POC testing methods. The processes are shown in a simplified format and may sometimes contain additional steps (adapted from von Lode, 2005).

elements work together in integrated fashion as schematically shown in Fig. 2. The sensitive biological elements are usually biological materials such as enzymes, antibodies, cell receptors, nucleic acids, or microorganisms, although artificial biomimetic materials can also be employed. The sensitive biological element in the biosensors specifically recognizes the analyte in the sample generally via the formation of lock-and-key complexes: enzyme-substrate, antigen-antibody, and so on. The formed complex generates chemical signals or produces property changes, which are converted into an electrical signal by means of a transducer. There are several types of transducers and will be discussed with some detail in the rest of the chapter, the main ones being optical, electrochemical, and piezoelectric.

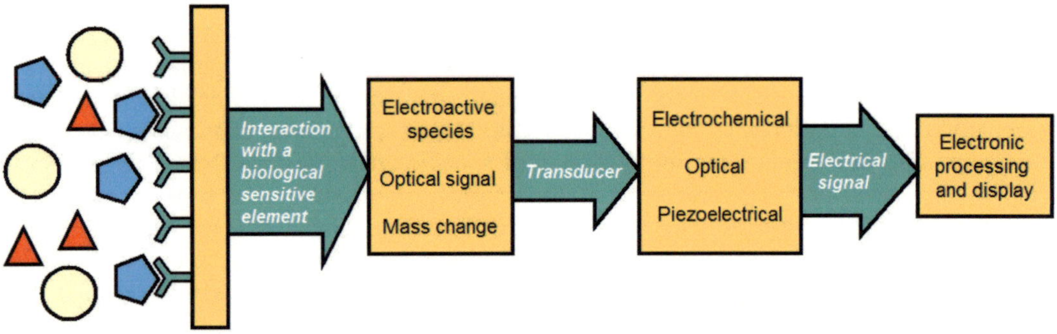

Fig. 2. Scheme of the basic integrated units that conform a biosensor.

Immunosensors make use of specific interactions between an antibody and an antigen. Antibodies are proteins generated by the immune system to identify bacteria, viruses, and parasites. The affinity between antibodies and antigens is very strong but of non-covalent nature. The development of sensitive and stable biological recognition elements is a key task in biosensors (Hock, 1997). However, biosensors, as a consequence of being highly integrated compact devices, are at a crossroad of different fields of knowledge. Biology and biotechnology are behind the key component of biosensors, as the sensitive biological elements provide the necessary specificity for the test. The generation of an electrical signal following the event of biological recognition involves the mastering of the transducing components, a field associated with chemical physics. Additionally, all these processes must be carried out at a small scale, with samples volumes in the order of microlitres, which requires the use of microfabricated structures and microelectronic circuits. Finally, biosensors can profit from the benefits of nanomaterials and nanostructures, such as large area to volume ratio, superparamagnetism, and surface enhanced resonance spectroscopy among many others, so nanotechnology has an increasing participation in the development of biosensors. Therefore, the biosensors field is by no means an exclusively biological field, but a truly multidisciplinary one.

3. Recognition and transducing in immunological biosensors

While biosensors can be used to detect many different analytes (not necessarily of biological nature as long as they interact specifically with the sensitive biological element), immunosensors are aimed mainly to the detection of the presence of certain antibodies or antigens in body fluids, especially in serum, although there is also a significant concern in the development of immunosensors employing antibodies for the detection of different analytes in diverse media, e.g. the quantification of TNT in groundwater via the formation of antibody-TNT complexes (Bromage et al., 2007). Therefore, the sensitive biological elements in immunosensors are antigens and antibodies (although in this chapter we will also include aptamers, which are single-stranded DNA molecules that work in fact as artificial antibodies forming aptamer-analyte complexes). Immunosensors can be designed for the detection of either antibodies or antigens; however, the detection of antibodies is preferred because the use of antibodies as sensitive biological elements may lead to a loss of affinity as a consequence of the immobilization of the antibodies onto a surface. Due to the high stability of the antigen-antibody complex once it is formed and the fact that the biological sensitive element is usually immobilized onto the surface of the transducer, most immunosensors are single use. Because some transducers are costly, there is a great concern in the regeneration of immunosensors, mainly by washing with an appropriate solution of high ionic strength or low pH.

Signal transducing in immunosensors can be carried out by different means, taking advantage of different properties changes or signal generation, which occurs following the formation of antigen-antibody complex. Although there are many kinds of transducers, this chapter is concerned with biosensors where the transducing mechanisms are related to the measurement of electrons, photons, and masses. Other mechanisms of transduction include thermal changes and pH variation. Therefore, the main transducers employed in immunosensors that this chapter will deal can be summarized as follows:

- *Electrochemical transducers.* In this case, an electrical signal is measured, which shows significant differences in magnitude if antigen-antibody complex are formed. The main electrochemical transducers are amperometric (measuring of current), potentiometric (measuring of electrode potential or voltage differences) and conductimetric (measuring of conductivity or resistance).
- *Optical transducers.* In this case, either an optical signal is generated (e.g. color or fluorescence) or a change in the optical properties of the surroundings following the antigen-antibody complex formation is measured.

- *Piezoelectric transducers.* The formation of antigen-antibody complexes implies an increase of mass as compared with the antigen or the antibody alone that is detected with piezoelectric devices, such as a quartz crystal balance or a cantilever.

In the following sections, these transducing mechanisms will be reviewed with selected examples from the literature.

4. Electrochemical immunosensors

In electrochemical immunosensors, the event of the formation of antigen-antibody complex is converted into an electrical signal: an electric current (amperometric immunosensors), a voltage difference (potentiometric immunosensors), or a resistivity change (conductimetric immunosensors).

The most common type of amperometric immunosensors can be regarded as ELISA tests with electrochemical detection, where redox species generated by a redox enzyme (enzymatic label) are converted into a measurable current. The aim of the test is to detect the presence of antibodies in serum via the formation of antigen-antibody complexes. An usual strategy is to immobilize the antigen onto the surface of a conductive electrode such as gold through adequate molecular linkers, for instance amino or carboxylic acid thiols. Thiols strongly bond to the gold surface, forming a self-assembled monolayer and providing the amino or carboxylic groups at the end of a small hydrocarbonated chain to which proteins can be covalently bonded. During an incubation time (typically from 30 to 60 minutes) with a positive serum, antigen-antibody complexes are formed. After rinsing, a second incubation is carried out with a solution containing anti-human Ig antibodies labeled with a redox enzyme, such as horseradish peroxidase (HRP). The formation of the antigen-antibody-labeled antibody complex is detected after the addition of the enzyme substrate and a proper redox mediator (cofactor). In the case of HRP, the substrate is hydrogen peroxidase and the redox mediator must be an adequate electron donor (a reduced species such as hydroquinone). HRP enzymatic activity converts the reduced redox mediator (hydroquinone) into an oxidized one (benzoquinone), which is further electrochemically reduced at the electrode surface. Thus, a steady-state current is established in a process schematically shown in Fig. 3. For negative sera, no antigen-antibody-enzyme labeled antibody complexes are formed in the first place so that the measured current values are considerably lower. Thus, high current values are indicative of a positive result.

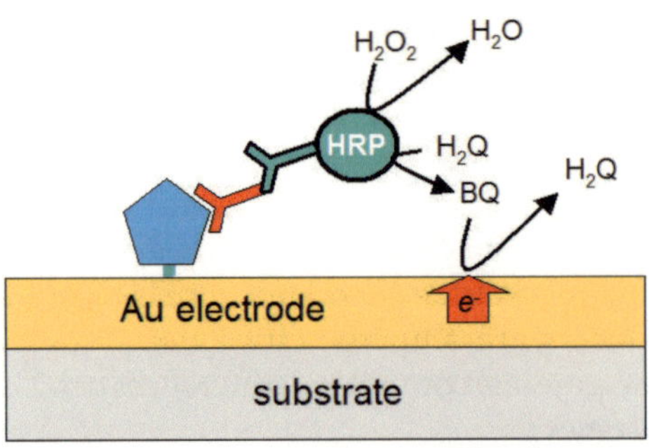

Fig. 3. Schematic representation of the electrochemical detection of enzyme-linked immunoassay with antigens immobilized onto a gold electrode (adapted from Longinotti et al., 2010a).

In order for the immunosensor to work properly, it is necessary that the enzyme employed as a label must be close to the electrode surface. If the antigen is immobilized onto the electrode surface, this requisite is complied. The immobilization of the biological recognition element onto the surface of the transducer is by far the most common configuration employed in biosensors. Nevertheless, it is possible to devise different immobilization carriers, such as magnetic beads, which can be placed onto the electrode surface by applying magnetic fields. Antigens can be immobilized onto the surface of the magnetic beads. The formation of antigen-antibody is more efficient and faster when using nanoparticles with respect to direct electrode immobilization. As a consequence, the incubation time has been reduced to a few minutes (Melli, 2011). After incubation, the magnetic beads can be placed onto the electrode surface by means of a magnet and removed once the test has been completed (Fig. 4). This strategy also allows the electrodes to be re-utilized several times.

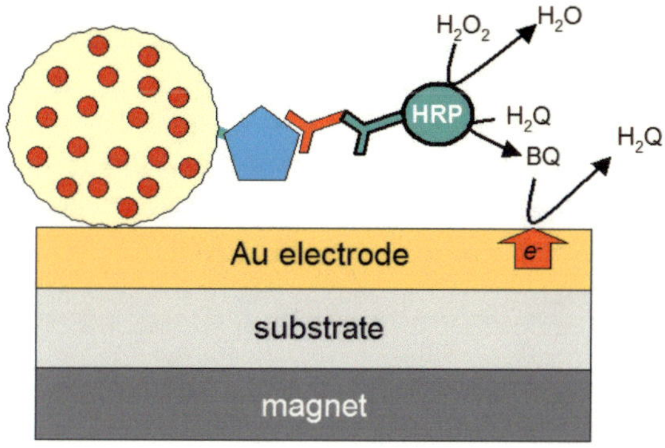

Fig. 4. Schematic representation of the electrochemical detection of enzyme-linked immunoassay with antigens immobilized onto silica-coated iron oxide nanoparticles (adapted from Longinotti et al., 2010b).

A promising type of immunosensors with electrochemical detection employs aptamers as the sensitive biological element. Aptamers are synthetic, single-stranded DNA molecules, which specifically bond to molecular targets, such as proteins and haptens, and can be regarded as synthetic antibodies. An interesting aspect of using aptamers as the recognition element in place of proteic antibodies is that it makes possible label-free biosensors. Plaxco et al. have been pioneering the development of such biosensors, which has been proved effective for the recognition of thrombin by electrochemical methods (aptamers have been previously used for the detection of thrombin in optical biosensors). In this type of biosensors, the single-stranded DNA that forms the aptamer is immobilized onto an electrode surface from one end and linked to a redox label from the other end. The event of formation of aptamer-target molecule complex leads either to an activation or to a deactivation of the redox probe (Fig. 5). In both cases, the change in redox activity can be measured as a current, usually employing a highly sensitive electrochemical technique such as AC voltammetry.

Field-effect transistors (FET), which have found wide application in ion sensing (i.e. ion-selective field-effect transistors, ISFETs), can also be employed in biosensors, and open a very promising field. Briefly, a FET consists of three terminals, called gate, drain, and source. The gate controls the current between the source and the drain and, what is most important in

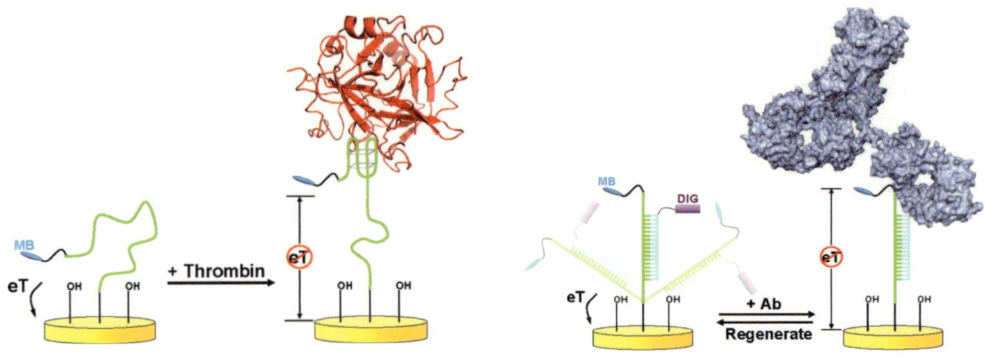

(a) (b)

Fig. 5. (a) An electrochemical, aptamer-based sensor comprises a redox-tagged DNA aptamer directed against the bloodclotting enzyme thrombin. Thrombin binding reduces the current from the redox tag, readily signaling the presence of the target (Xiao et al., 2006). (b) Utilizing double-stranded DNA as a support scaffold for a small molecule receptor, sensors for the detection of protein-small-molecule interactions have been fabricated, for instance, for the detection of low nanomolar concentrations of antibodies against the drug digoxigenin (Cash et al., 2009).

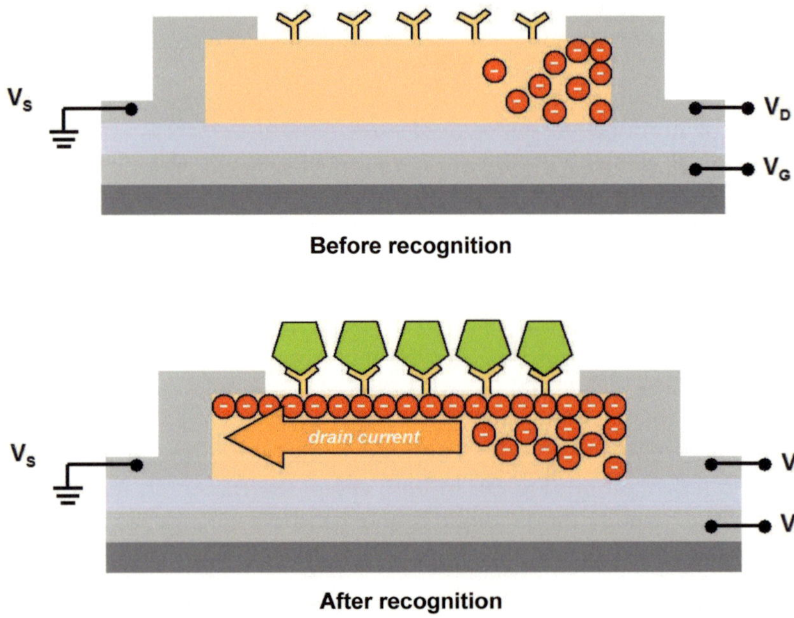

Fig. 6. Schematic of a FET immunosensor. The formation of antigen-antibody complex at the gate terminal modulates the charge carrier flow between source and gate, generating an increase in current (adapted from Ivanoff Reyes et al., 2011).

sensors applications, can be made sensitive to particular substances. For instance, in the scheme shown in Fig. 6, biofunctionalization of gate with antibodies enables the exposed channel direct interaction with the antigens detected. The formation of antibody-antigen complex causes the majority carriers of the n-type channel to accumulate and facilitate a conduction path for the charge carriers' flow from drain to source. It is a compact, label-free immunosensor in which an electrical signal is generated as a consequence of the formation of the antibody-antigen complex. Of course, FET biosensors are compatible with microelectronics technology, which allows a high degree of integration between all components of the biosensors: detection, transducing, and signal processing.

5. Optical immunosensors

In optical biosensors, the biological sensitive element is immobilized onto the surface of the transducer and respond to the interaction with the target analyte either by generating an optical signal, such as fluorescence, or by undergoing changes in optical properties, such as absorption, reflectance, emission, refractive index, and optical path. The optical signals are collected by a photodector and converted into electrical signals that are further electronically processed. There are many reviews on optical biosensors, the one by Borisov & Wolfbeis, 2008, is highly recommended. The main optical phenomena employed in optical immunosensors are summarized in Table 1.

Optical Signal	Transducing technique
Absorbance	Light intensity measurement
Reflectance	Light intensity measurement
Fluorescence	Total internal reflection fluorescence
Refraction index	Interferometry
	Surface plasmon resonance (SPR)
	Total internal reflection
Optical path	Interferometry
Spectroscopies	Surface enhanced Raman scattering (SERS)

Table 1. Main optical phenomena employed in optical immunosensors.

The geometric design of optical platforms is a key point to achieve efficient and integrated optical immunosensors. There are several geometric layouts, the most usual being strips, waveguide fibers (Leung et al., 2007), planar optical waveguide systems, capillary sensors, and arrays. Planar waveguide systems are especially attractive because of the possibility of innovative designs and the integration of multiple functionalities onto a single sensor. Planar geometry is compatible with microfabrication technologies and can be integrated with microfluidic systems (lab-on-a-chip). These attributes have made planar waveguides an ideal platform for development of integrated optical sensors. Several optical transducing techniques can be employed in planar waveguide systems: interferometry, surface plasmon resonance, and light-coupling strategies to transduce refractive index changes. Planar waveguide platforms comprise a planar substrate made of glass, plastic, or silicon that forms the basis of the sensor platform (Yimit et al., 2005). In some cases, this substrate acts as the waveguide, while in others an additional waveguide layer is deposited onto the substrate. All examples given in this section are considered for a planar configuration.

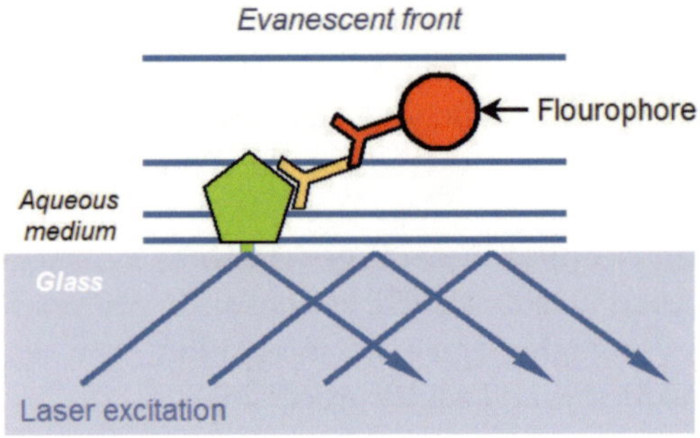

Fig. 7. Principle of the total internal reflection fluorescence. On reflection at dielectric interface, light penetrates into the second phase that has a lower refractive index than that of the core. Intensity decreases exponentially over the penetration (which typically is about as long as the wavelength of the light employed). Any labeled antibodies located close to the glass-aqueous medium interface are excited to produce fluorescence, while those located further into the solution will not.

Fluorescence is one the most widely methods employed in immunosensors, especially in ELISA-like immunosensors where the conjugate antibody is labeled with a fluorescent probe. Using an evanescent wave spectroscopic technique, such as total internal reflection fluorescence, can enhance the sensitivity of the biosensor. When light is transported by total internal reflection in an optical guide, an evanescent field is generated at the interface between the guide and the external medium. The penetration depth of this exponential field is of the order of the incident wavelength. Therefore, if the optical guide is placed in contact with a solution containing fluorophores, only those within the evanescent field are excited by light. In this way, fluorescent labels can be employed in conjunction with total internal reflection in ELISA-like immunosensors as schematically shown in Fig. 7. Unbound labeled species in solution remain unexcited and do not contribute to the background signal. An additional advantage of total internal reflection fluorescence measurements is that it can be performed in absorbing or turbid media.

The measurement of changes in the refractive index that takes place at the interface between the guide and the external medium is the basis for optical transducing techniques employed in refractometric immunosensors (Fig. 8). Surface plasmon resonance is one of the main optical biosensor technologies and has been the subject of numerous reviews (Mullett et al., 2000; Homola, 2003; Scaranoa et al., 2010).

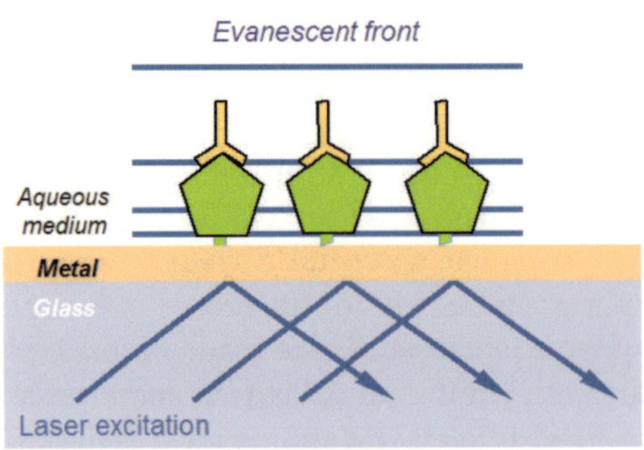

Fig. 8. Schematic representation of the surface plasmon resonance immunosensor.

Many refractometric immunosensors are based on interferometric techniques. The Mach-Zehnder interferometer is one of the most commonly employed interferometers in immunosensors (Fig. 9). In the Mach-Zehnder interferometer, the optical power is transported by a single-input waveguide, which is split equally between two parallel waveguides and recombined by means of two Y-splitters. When used in immunosensors, both branches are coated with the biological sensitive element (antigen or antibody). One of the waveguides is exposed to the sensing environment while the other branch serves as a reference waveguide. Changes in the refractive index of the sensing layer environment influence the effective refractive index in the sensing channel, which induces a phase shift in the optical signal that propagates through this channel. Upon recombination, interference of the two optical signals occurs and the measured output power changes depending on the phase shift between these two signals.

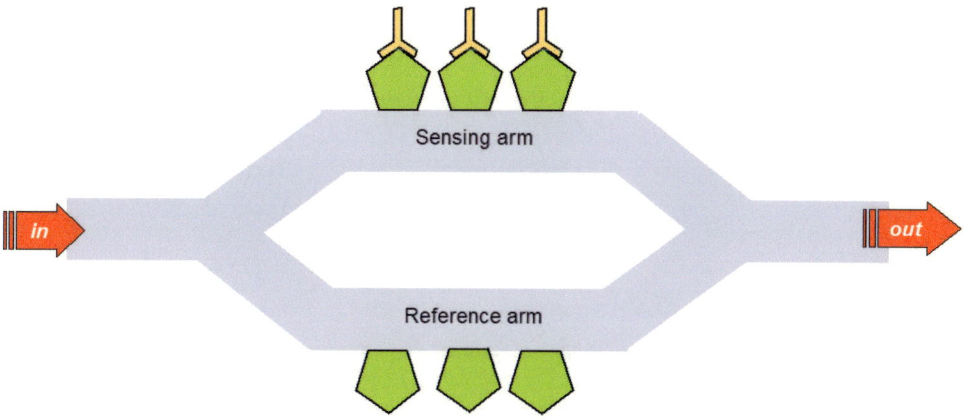

Fig. 9. Schematic of a Mach-Zehnder interferometer used for immunosensing.

Other interferometric immunosensors are based on changes in optical path rather than in the refractive index. Changes in the thickness of the thin film deposited on a substrate due to swelling upon interaction with the analyte of interest can be detected as shifts in the interference pattern.

6. Piezoelectric immunosensors

The mass changes that take place after the formation of antigen-antibody formation can be measured by means of piezoelectric transducers, such as quartz crystal microbalances and microcantilevers, which vibrate at a certain frequency sensitive. Antigens or antibodies can be immobilized onto the surface of piezoelectric devices and the formation of the antigen-antibody complex can be detected as a vibration frequency shift with a high sensitivity (Janshoff et al., 2000; Raiteri et al., 2001).

Microcantilevers are especially attractive for immunosensors because of the possibility of microfabrication at low cost. Microcantilevers can also be employed in a static, non-vibrating mode, detecting the event of formation of antigen-antibody complexes via the deflection of the cantilever as a result of the surface stress it provokes (Fig. 10).

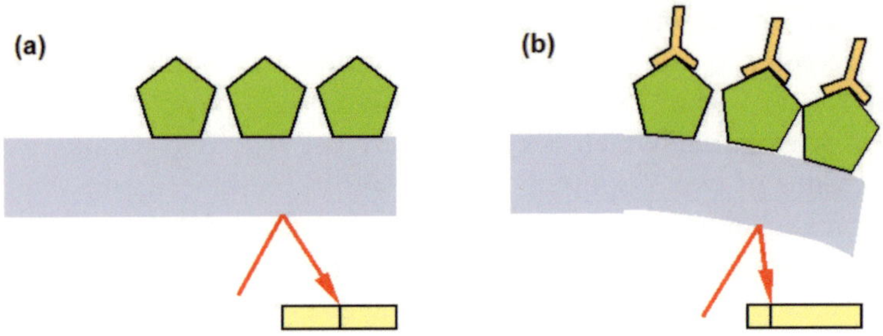

Fig. 10. Microcantilever working in static mode. The formation of the antigen-antibody complexes provokes a surface stress and, consequently, a deflection of microcantilever, which is detected optically.

Analyte	Transducing technique	References
Escherichia coli **O157:H7**		Tokarskyy & Marshall, 2008
	Surface plasmon resonance	Fratamico et al., 1998
	Piezoelectric	Su & Li, Y. 2004
	Electrochemical	Radke & Alocilja, 2005
	Fluorescence	Yu et al., 2002
Antibodies		
Antibody aimed at foot-and-mouth disease	Electrochemical	Longinotti et al., 2010
Various antibodies aimed at Chagas disease	Electrochemical and fluorescence	Melli, 2011
Tumoral markers		Chen et al., 2009
Prostate-specific antigen (PSA)	Amperometric	Meyerhoff et al., 1995
PSA	Amperometric	Rusling et al., 2009
PSA, C-reactive protein	Cantilevers	Wee et al., 2005
PSA, PSA-α1-antichymotrypsin, CEA, mucin-1	Field-effect	Zheng et al., 2005
CA 125, CA 153, CA 199, CEA	Chemiluminescence	Fu et al. 2007
Toxins and pollutants		
Aflatoxins	Electrochemical	Owino et al., 2007
TNT	Fluorescence	Bromage et al., 2007
Clostridium botulinum toxin A	Fluorescence	Ogert et al., 1992

Table 2. Some examples of analytes detected with immunosensors and immunoassays.

7. Prospects and future of immunosensors

Immunosensors have been used for the detection of pathogens, antibodies, toxins, biomarkers, among other analytes (Table 2). The wide spectrum of application of immunosensors ascertains a great future for this type of biosensors. Especially attractive is the possibility of carrying out point of care testing (Skottrup et al., 2008), as discussed previously in the introduction. Although all transducing techniques have advantages and disadvantages, much of the success of immunosensors in point of care testing depends on the intrinsic detection limits, the required sample preparation (e.g. the possibility of direct detection of the analyte), and the degree of integration of the units that conforms a biosensor. All these crucial aspects are conditioned by the type of transducer employed in immunosensors. For instance, the limit of detection of fluorescence is eventually a single molecule (Table 3), but fluorescence transduction in immunosensor usually requires a fluorescent label, and a rather complex optical instrumentation that compromises a high degree of integration among the biological sensitive element, the transducer and the electronic instrumentation. It is in this sense that field-effect transistors seem to be the optimal transducers, because they do not require a label and the biological sensitive element is immobilized onto the surface of the transducer that itself forms part of the electronic instrumentation.

Technique	Limit of detection (molecules per mμ^2)	References
Fluorescence	1	
Hollow cantilevers	10	Burg et al., 2007
Surface plasmon resonance	10^2	Myszka, 2004
Quartz crystal balance	10^3	
Microcantilevers	10^6	Braun et al., 2005

Table 3. Estimated order of magnitude of the limits of detection for different transducing techniques.

A diagram with a comparison of the compromise between the ease of integration and the ease of sample preparation for the different transducing techniques is presented in Fig. 11.

The future of biosensors will be greatly influenced by the inclusion of nanomateriales, which provide new tools to improve the performance of immunosensors (Chen et al., 2009). There is a great interest in including carbon nanotubes in biosensing (Jacobs et al., 2010), taking advantage of their conductive properties. Also nanoparticles can provide new strategies for immunosensors design, and especial interest is in the use of quantum dots in optical transducers, with a higher fluorescence efficiency. Superparamagnetic nanoparticles are also been increasingly used in biosensing (Longinotti et al., 2008; Lloret et al., 2010). A point of care testing device aimed at the diagnosis of foot-and-mouth disease, brucellosis, and Chagas disease has been recently presented (Longinotti et al., 2011, Fig. 12) in which the biological sensitive element is immobilized onto the surface of silica-coated superparamagentic iron oxide nanoparticles. The use of nanoparticles reduces the incubation time to a few minutes, while an analog ELISA usually would require 30-60 minutes incubation.

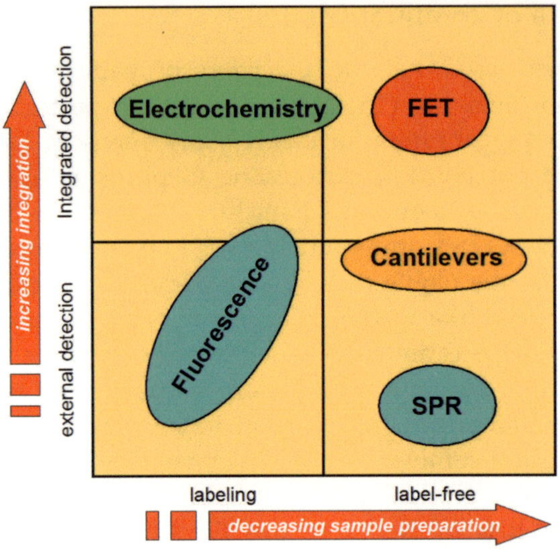

Fig. 11. Comparison of ease of sample preparation and integration for different transducers employed in immunosensors.

Finally, multiple analytes detection (Chen et al., 2009), microfluidics (Bange et al., 2005) and lab-on-a-chip (Hart et al., 2011) concepts are clearly in the future of immunosensors, and many devices have been presented that may also find soon wide application, with great impact in health care assessment, especially in developing countries.

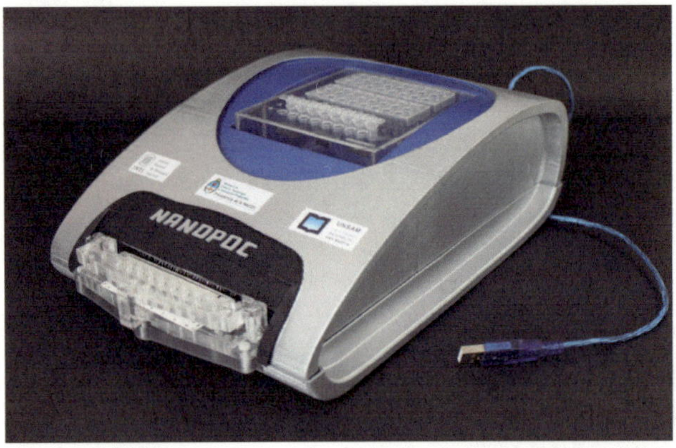

Fig. 12. Point of care electrochemical immunosensing platform Nanopoc®, designed for the diagnosis of foot-and-mouth disease, brucellosis, and Chagas disease (Longinotti et al., 2011). The sample preparation is carried out in the blue sector, which involves magnetic separations. The final amperometric measurement is carried out in the 8-channel electrochemical cells at the front of the device. Data are processed by a PC via a USB connection.

8. Conclusions

The field of immunosensors is an exciting, fast growing one, as can be seen from the evolution of the number of scientific publications from 1990 to 2011 (Fig. 13). Especially, electrochemical immunosensors seem to lead the trend, possibly because of the ease of integration with electronic instrumentation, while optical and piezoelectric transducers are more demanding in this regard. However, due to the high sensitivity of optical and piezoelectric transducers, these kinds of transducers may soon find many practical applications. It is expected that the research in this field will continue to grow in the next years and point of care testing platforms will soon find wide applications that will greatly improve the health caring situation.

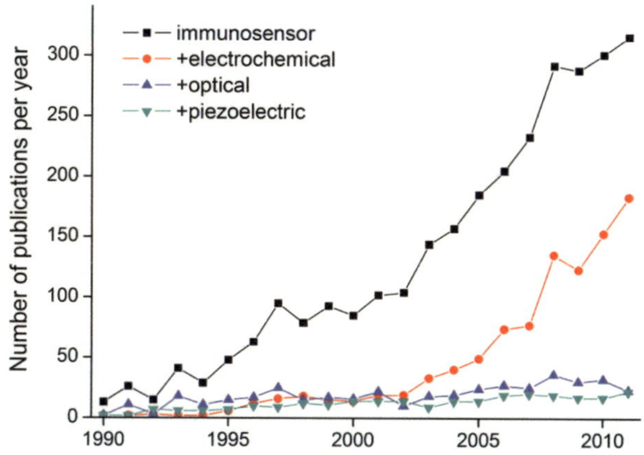

Fig. 13. Evolution of published articles on immunosensors (source: Scopus database).

9. Acknowledgment

This work has been supported by the Instituto Nacional de Tecnología Industrial and by FS Nano 005 granted by the Ministry of Science, Technology and Innovative Production of the Argentine Republic.

10. References

Bange, A.; Halsall, H.B. & Heineman, W.R. 2005. Microfluidic immunosensor systems. *Biosensors and Bioelectronics*. Vol. 20, pp. 2488–2503.

Burg, T.P.; Godin, M.; Knudsen, S.M.; Shen, W.; Carlson, G.; Foster, J.S.; Babcock, K. & Manalis, S.R. 2007. Weighing of biomolecules, single cells and single nanoparticles in fluid. *Nature*. Vol. 446, pp. 1066-1069.

Braun, T.; Barwich, V.; Ghatkesar, M.K.; Bredekamp, A.H.; Gerber, C.; Hegner, M. & Lang, H.P. 2005. Micromechanical mass sensors for biomolecular detection in a physiological environment *Physical Review E (Statistical, Nonlinear, and Soft Matter Physics)*. Vol. 72, pp. 031907.

Borisov, S.M. & Wolfbeis, O.S. 2008. Optical Biosensors. *Chem. Rev.*, Vol. 108, pp. 423-461.

Bromage, E.S.; Vadas, G.G.; Harvey, E.; Unger, M.A. & Kaattari, S.L. 2007. Validation of an antibody-based biosensor for rapid quantification of 2,4,6-trinitrotoluene (TNT) contamination in ground water and river water. *Environ. Sci. Technol.*, Vol. 41, pp. 7067–7072.

Cash, K. J.; Ricci, F.; Plaxco, K.W. 2009. An electrochemical sensor for the detection of protein-small molecule interactions directly in serum and other complex matrices. *J. Am. Chem. Soc.* Vol. 131, pp. 6955–6957.

Chen, H.; Jiang, C.; Yu, C.; Zhang, S.; Liu, B. & Kon, J. 2009. Protein chips and nanomaterials for application in tumor marker immunoassays. *Biosensors and Bioelectronics.* Vol. 24, pp. 3399–3411.

Fratamico, P.M., Strobaugh, T.P., Medina, M.B., Gehring, A.G. 1998. Detection of *Escherichia coli* O157:H7 using a surface plasmon resonance biosensor. *Biotech. Tech.* Vol. 12, pp. 571–576.

Fu, Z.; Yang, Z.; Tang, J.; Liu, H.; Yan, F.& Ju, H. 2007. Channel and substrate zone two-dimensional resolution for chemiluminescent multiplex immunoassay. *Anal. Chem.* Vol. 79, pp. 7376–7382.

Hart, R.W.; Mauk, MG; Liu, C.; Qiu, X; Thompson, J.A.; Chen, D.; Malamud, D.; Abrams, W.R. & Bau, H.H. 2011. Point-of-care oral-based diagnostics. *Oral Diseases.* Vol. 17, pp. 745–75.

Hock, B. 1997. Antibodies for immunosensors. A review. *Analytica Chimica Acta.* Vol. 347 pp. 177-186.

Homola, J. 2003. Present and future of surface plasmon resonance biosensors. *Anal. Bioanal. Chem.* Vol. 377, pp. 528 - 539.

Ivanoff Reyes, P.; Ku, C.-J.; Duan, Z.; Lu, Y.; Solanki, A. & Lee, K.-B. 2011. ZnO thin film transistor immunosensor with high sensitivity and selectivity. *App. Phys. Lett.*, Vol. 98, 173702.

Jacobs, C.B; Peairs, M.J. & Venton, B.J. 2010. Review: Carbon nanotube based electrochemical sensors for biomolecules. *Analytica Chimica Acta.* Vol. 662, pp. 105–127.

Janshoff, A.; Galla, H. & Steinem, C. 2000. Piezoelectric mass-sensing devices as biosensors - An alternative to optical biosensors? *Angewandte Chemie - International Edition.* Vol. 39, pp. 4004-4032.

Lazcka, O.; Del Campo, F.J. & Muñoz, F.X. 2007. Pathogen detection: A perspective of traditional methods and biosensors. *Biosens. Bioelec.*, Vol. 22, pp. 1205-1217.

Lee, J.H.; Kang, D.Y.; Lee, T.; Kim, S.U.; Oh, B.K. & Choil, J.W. 2009. Signal enhancement of surface plasmon resonance based immunosensor using gold nanoparticle-antibody complex for β-amyloid (1-40) detection. *J. Nanosci. Nanotechnol.* Vol. 9, pp. 7155–7160.

Leung, A.; Shankar, P. M. & Mutharasan, R. 2007. A review of fiber-optic biosensors. *Sensors and Actuators B.* Vol. 125, pp. 688–703.

Lloret, P.; Longinotti, G.; Ybarra, G.; Socolovsky, L.; Halac, B. & Moina, C. 2010. Synthesis, characterization, and functionalization of magnetic core-shell flower-like nanoparticles. *Proc. XIX International Materials Research Congress,* Cancún, México, August 15-19, 2010.

Longinotti, G.; Lloret, P.; Peter-Gauna, R.; Ybarra, G.; Ciochinni, A.; Hermida, L.; Malatto, L.; Fraigi, L. & Moina, C. 2010b. Natural polymer coated magnetic nanoparticles for biosensing. *Proceedings of the XIX International Materials Research Congress,* Cancún, México, 15-19/8/2010.

Longinotti, G.; Ybarra, G.; Lloret, P.; Moina, C.; Ciochinni, A.; Hermida, L.; Milano, O.; Roberti, M.; Malatto, L. & Fraigi, L. 2008. Screen-printed electrochemical biosensors based on magnetic core-shell nanoparticles, *Proceedings of the 6th Ibero-American Congress on Sensors*, November 24-26, 2008, São Paulo, Brazil.

Longinotti, G; Ybarra, G.; Lloret, P; Melli, L.; Rey Serantes, D.; Comerci, D.; Ciochinni, A.; Ugalde, J.; Moina, C.; Malatto, L; Mass, M.; Roberti M.; Brengi, D.; Tropea, S; Fraigi, L. & Lloret, M. 2011. Point of care diagnosis of infectious diseases. *INTI Spring Meeting*, Buenos Aires, Argentina, October 2011.

Longinotti, G.; Ybarra, G.; Lloret, P.; Moina, C.; Ciochinni, A.; Rey Serantes, D.; Malatto, L.; Roberti, M.; Tropea, S. & Fraigi, L. 2010a. Diagnosis of foot-and-mouth disease by an electrochemical enzyme-linked immunoassay. *Proceedings of the 32nd Annual International Conference of the IEEE Engineering in Medicine and Biology Society "Merging Medical Humanism and Technology"*, Buenos Aires, Argentina, September 2010.

Melli, L. 2011. Development of optical and electrochemical immunosensors for the diagnosis of Chagas disease. *Thesis*. Universidad Nacional de Gral. San Martín.

Meyerhoff, M.E.; Duan, C. & Meusel, M. 1995. Novel nonseparation sandwich-type electrochemical enzyme immunoassay system for detecting marker proteins in undiluted blood. *Clin. Chem.* Vol. 41, pp. 1378–1384.

Myszka, D.G. 2004. Analysis of small-molecule interactions using Biacore S51 technology. *Anal. Biochem.* Vol. 329, pp. 316.

Mullett, W.M.; Lai, E.P.C; Yeung, J.M. 2000. Surface plasmon resonance-based immunoassays. *Methods.* Vol. 22, pp. 77-91.

Ogert, R.A.; Brown, J.E.; Singh, B.R.; Shriverlake, L.C. & Ligler, F.S. 1992. Detection of *Clostridium botulinum* toxin-A using a fiber optic-based biosensor. *Anal. Biochem.* Vol. 205, pp. 306–312.

Owino, J.H.O.; Ignaszak, A.; Al-Ahmed, A.; Baker, P.G.L.; Alemu, H.; Ngila, J.C. & Iwuoha, E.I. 2007. Modelling of the impedimetric responses of an aflatoxin B1 immunosensor prepared on an electrosynthetic polyaniline platform. *Anal. Bioanal. Chem.* Vol. 388, pp. 1069.

Radke, S.M. & Alocilja, E.C. 2005. A high density microelectrode array biosensor for detection of *E. coli* O157:H7. *Biosens. Bioelectron.* Vol. 20, pp. 1662–1667.

Raiteri, R.; Grattarola, M.; Butt, H.-J. & Skládal, P. 2001. Micromechanical cantilever-based biosensors. *Sens. Actuators B*. Vol. 79, pp. 115-126.

Rusling, J.F., Sotzing, G. & Papadimitrakopoulosa, F. 2009. Designing nanomaterial-enhanced electrochemical immunosensors for cancer biomarker proteins. *Bioelectrochemistry*. Vol. 76, pp. 189–194.

Scaranoa, S.; Mascinia, M; Turnerb, A.P.F. & Minunnia, M. 2010. Surface plasmon resonance imaging for affinity-based biosensors. *Biosensors and Bioelectronics.* Vol. 25, pp. 957–966.

Skottrup, P.D.; Nicolaisen, M. & Justesen A.F. 2008. Towards on-site pathogen detection using antibody-based sensors. *Biosensors and Bioelectronics.* Vol. 24, pp. 339–348.

Su, X.-L. & Li, Y. 2004. A self-assembled monolayer-based piezoelectric immunosensor for rapid detection of *Escherichia coli* O157:H7. *Biosens. Bioelectron.* Vol. 19, pp. 563–574.

Tokarskyy, O. & Marshall, D.L. 2008. Immunosensors for rapid detection of *Escherichia coli* O157:H7 —Perspectives for use in the meat processing industry. *Food Microbiology.* Vol. 25, pp. 1–12.

von Lode, P. 2005. Point-of-care immunotesting: Approaching the analytical performance of central laboratory methods. *Clinical Biochemistry*. Vol. 38, pp. 591 - 606.

Wee, K.W., Kang, G.Y., Park, J., Kang, J.Y., Yoon, D.S., Park, J.H., Kim, T.S. 2005. Novel electrical detection of label-free disease marker proteins using piezoresistive self-sensing micro-cantilevers. *Biosens. Bioelectron.* Vol. 20 , pp. 1932–1938.

Xiao, Y.; Lubin, A. A.; Heeger, A. J.; Plaxco, K. W. 2005. Label-free electronic detection of thrombin in blood serum by using an aptamer-based sensor. *Angew. Chem., Int. Ed.*, Vol. 44, pp. 5456–5459.

Yimit, A.; Rossberg, A.G.; Amemiya, T. & Itoh, K. 2005. Thin film composite optical waveguides for sensor applications: a review. *Talanta.* Vol. 65, pp. 1102–1109.

Yu, L.S.L.; Reed, S.A. & Golden, M.H. 2002. Time-resolved fluorescence immunoassay for the detection of *Escherichia coli* O157:H7 in apple cider. *J. Microbiol. Meth.* Vol. 49, pp. 63–68.

5

Capabilities of Piezoelectric Immunosensors for Detecting Infections and for Early Clinical Diagnostics

Tatyana Ermolaeva and Elena Kalmykova
Lipetsk State Technical University, Department of Chemistry, Laboratory of Chemical and Biochemical Sensors, Russia

1. Introduction

Methods of early laboratory diagnostics which allow the prevention of diseases and their effective treatment, as well as establishing their causes, make a considerable contribution to the prevention and treatment of human diseases. A precise diagnosis is directly connected with the speed and sensitivity of the applied method of clinical diagnostics. Diagnostic tests are also important in pharmacology and pharmacokinetics for estimating the effectiveness of medications used in medical treatment and for controlling their digestion. First of all it concerns the diagnostics of such widespread diseases of civilisation as cardiovascular and coronary heart diseases, diabetes, oncological and infectious diseases. Besides diagnosing diseases, laboratory methods must determine genetic predisposition to serious pathologies, as well as determine - with high reliability - the quantitative indicator of pathologies when they are still in a clinical asymptomatic state.

The speed of measurements with the use of biosensors has been the reason for close attention on the part of experts in clinical laboratory diagnostics. The past decade has seen active development of piezoelectric gravimetric immunosensors that provide for the intensification of work in performing a considerable number of tests and the reduction of the time necessary for medical treatment.

A piezoelectric immunosensor is an analytical device, the sensitive element of which is a piezoelectric resonator with electrodes coated by receptor molecules. An obvious advantage of a piezoelectric immunosensor is the possibility to carry out the direct registration of biochemical interaction without the introduction of additional labels (fluorescent, enzyme, radioactive, luminescent, etc.), which makes it different from other similar devices. Sensors are characterised by their fast response, ease of operation, portability, and possibility to be included in automatic systems of information collecting and processing. A unique feature of piezoelectric immunosensors is the combination of high sensitivity, which is provided by the use of a high-frequency piezoelectric transducer as a physical transducer, and selectivity which is determined by the nature of employed receptor molecules. An electrode's coating is formed on the basis of natural bio-recognizing substances characterized by high selectivity of interaction. In order to increase the selectivity and to widen the range of tested substances, which is especially important in the field of medicine and pharmacology, piezoelectric immunosensors' electrode coatings are formed from natural bio-recognizing compounds which are characterized by high selectivity of interaction.

Currently antibodies - protective proteins formed in the organisms of higher animals in response to the introduction of foreign agents - antigens (nucleic acids DNA and RNA, carbohydrates, etc.) - are most frequently used as key reagents. Both in the living organism and outside it antibodies are capable of forming immune complexes with a complementary antigen (or hapten), despite the presence of a great number of other components in the sample.

A number of reviews (Vaughan et al. 2007, Ermolaeva et al. 2008, Skladal 2003) are devoted to considering the theoretical aspects of piezoelectric immunosensors functioning and the peculiarities of their practical application in determining various analytes.

Gravimetric piezoelectric sensors, named a piezoquartz microbalance (quartz crystal microbalance, QCM), are high-frequency transducers (with the basic frequency of 5-15 MHz) made from an AT-cut quartz crystal. The analytical signal of such a sensor is most commonly the reduction of the oscillation frequency of the resonator with the increase of the receptor layer's mass as a result of its interaction with determined substances. Frequency variation of the oscillating crystal depending on change of the mass fixed on a quartz surface is described by the Sauerbrey equation (Sauerbrey 1959) for rigid, uniform and thin adsorptive layers:

$$\Delta m = C \cdot \Delta f,$$

where m - mass, C - proportionality coefficient, f - crystal oscillation frequency.

There can be a deviation from the Sauerbrey equation and errors in mass measurement for soft or viscous-elastic films which are not fully contacting the oscillatory crystal, therefore it is necessary to standardize (calibrate) a QCM sensor before testing various liquid samples.

The analysis of liquids with the use of piezoelectric sensors can be carried out both in static and flowing modes. In the first case (the procedure being known as «dip and dry») the increase of the receptor layer's mass is measured before and after the contact of the sensor with the analyzed liquid sample and the following air drying up to the constant mass. The use of the sensor as the detector of the flow-injection analysis makes it possible to raise the speed of determination, and also provides the opportunity to observe immunochemical reactions in real time.

The creation of gravimetric biosensors of various designs (test-means, detectors for flow-injection analysis) on the basis of highly specific interactions (antibody-antigen, receptor-ligand, etc.) can expand their range of applications in medicine with the aim of identifying not only toxic micro-organisms, but specific substances that act as a sort of precursors of dangerous diseases.

2. The features of registration of biochemical interactions with the help of piezoelectric immunosensors

The most developed types of immunoassay with the use of piezoelectric transducers are the following: direct, indirect (competitive) and displacing (Ermolaeva et al. 2006, Su et al. 2003).

The sandwich assay and some other ways of amplifying the analytical signal are recommended for increasing the sensitivity of determinations.

Direct detection is used to determine somatic cells, micro-organisms and macromolecules (proteins, antibodies, nucleic acids, glycoproteins, glycolipids, etc.). It is implemented in one step when analyte contacts the sensor's receptor layer. The decrease of resonant frequency due to the formation of the complex on the surface of the electrode is directly proportional to the concentration of the determined component (Fig. 1).

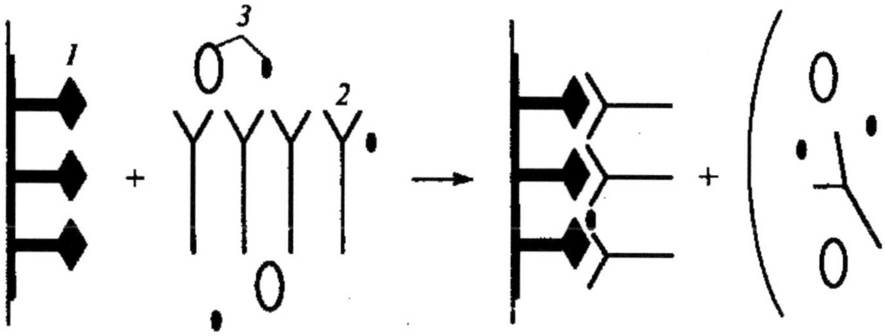

Fig. 1. The scheme of the direct assay of the antibody using piezoelectric immunosensors: 1 - antigen (hapten); 2 - specific antibody; 3 - non-specific components of the mixture

The sensor's electrodes are modified by antigens or antibodies (mono- or polyclonal). Usually the sensor is previously treated with a solution of a non-ionic surfactant or an inactive protein (BSA, gelatine, etc.) in order to increase the selectivity of determination. Such proteins do not cross-interact with the components of the sample but connect with non-specific sites of the sensor's receptor layer. For example, the sensor's receptor layer based on DNA interacts weakly with BSA molecules, causing only a slight frequency signal (not more than 5 Hz), while the serum of patients with symptoms of an autoimmune disease, containing antibodies to DNA, gives an analytical signal on the level of hundreds of Hz (Kalmykova et al. 2002). In order to determine small molecules the indirect/competitive analysis, the sandwiched assay and other types of analysis are used.

The competitive analysis of haptens with the use of piezoelectric sensors (U. S. Patent 4,242,096 1980) was first performed in 1980. While in a routine immunochemical analysis, free and labelled analytes presented in the sample compete for binding with antibodies, in the case of piezoelectric immunosensors the competition takes place between free analyte (hapten) and hapten-protein conjugate immobilized onto the bioreceptor layer. The value of the obtained analytical signal of the sensor is inversely proportional to the concentration of hapten in the sample. The essence of this method is illustrated in Fig. 2.

Such a method has been successfully used for determining different low-molecular-mass haptens: vitamins, drugs, hormones, metabolites, etc. The detection limit of the competitive analysis is lower compared with that of the direct one (Prusak-Sochaczewski et al. 1990), but the range of determined concentrations is narrower by a factor of 10 to 100. In order to apply the competitive analysis, the receptor layer can be formed on the basis of both hapten-protein conjugates and antibodies. In the latter case a fixed quantity of hapten-protein conjugate is added to each sample. This type is known as the **alternative competitive assay** (Fig. 3).

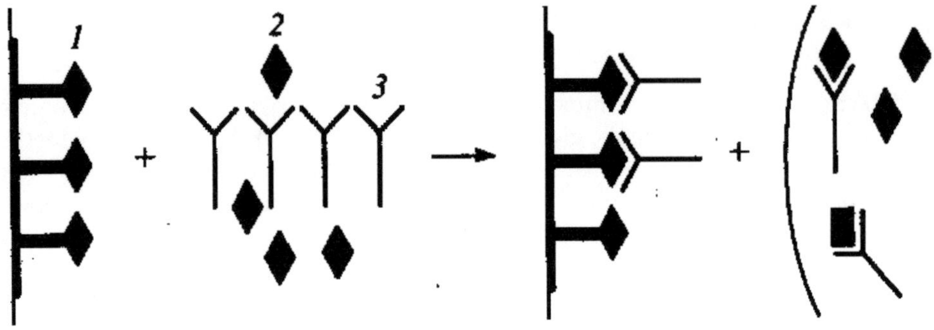

Fig. 2. The scheme of the competitive (indirect) assay using piezoelectric immunosensors: 1 - hapten-protein conjugate; 2 - hapten; 3 - antibody

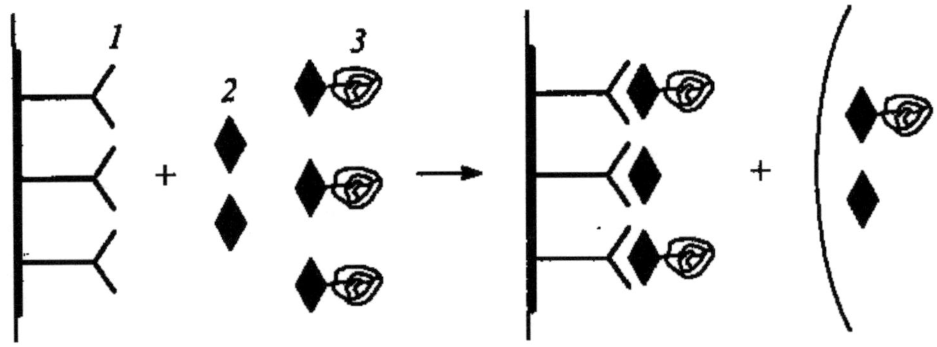

Fig. 3. The scheme of the alternative competitive assay using piezoelectric immunosensors: 1 - antibody; 2 - hapten; 3 - hapten-protein conjugate

Conjugated and free haptens are equally probably bound with the active sites of immobilized antibodies. Therefore, the lower the concentration of free analyte in a sample, the greater the conjugated hapten attached to the sensor's receptor layer. Thus, the sorption of the conjugated analyte provides for a significant amplification of the registered signal. Despite a lower sensitivity, the alternative method is characterized by a wider range of determined concentrations in comparison with the competitive assay.

The displacement assay has been successfully used to characterize the stability of the affine complexes (antibody - antigen, DNA - protein, DNA - RNA, etc.), to study the kinetics of dissociation, and to solve a number of problems dealing with analyte concentration determination. While the competitive assay is preferable for determining low concentrations of small molecules, the **displacement** assay is more convenient for detecting macromolecules. The principle of determination consists of measuring the heterogeneous complex's mass reduction as a result of dissociation under the influence of an excess of one of the components. The analysis is carried out in two stages (Fig. 4).

An example of this type of immunoassay may be the determination of *Listeria monocytogen* (Minunni et al. 1996) micro-organisms in milk (at $2.5{\cdot}10^5$ – $2.5{\cdot}10^7$cells ml^{-1}). The decrease of the frequency of the sensor is caused by binding specific antibodies in a sample of milk with a protein antigen extracted from *L. monocytogenes* cells and pre-immobilized on the electrode surface. In the second stage the *L. monocytogenes* cells additionally introduced into the sample of milk cause the displacement of antibodies in immune complex. The number of displaced antibodies is directly proportional to the concentration of *L. monocytogenes* cells in the sample. A similar method was proposed to determine the *P. aeruginosa* bacteria in samples of milk and drinking water (Bovenizer et al. 1998).

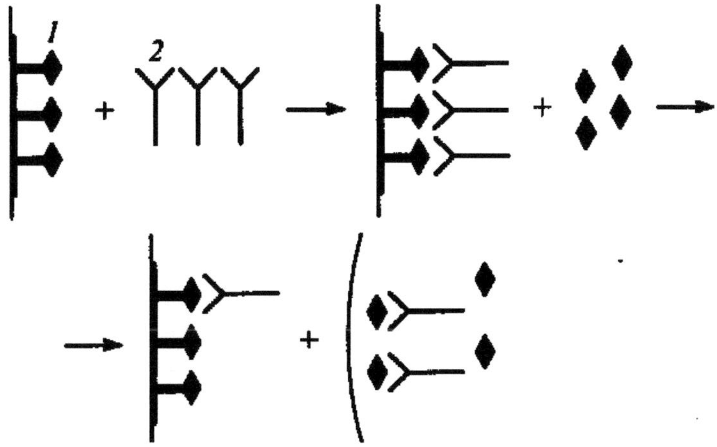

Fig. 4. The scheme of the displacement assay using piezoelectric immunosensors: 1 - antigen, 2 - specific antibody

The sandwich assay is carried out in two stages with the use of two types of antibodies (U.S. Patent, 4,314,821 1982). In the first stage the antibodies immobilized on the electrode surface are bound with the analyte, in the second stage the "sandwich" structure is formed with other types of antibodies being additionally introduced (Fig. 5). A method for determining human serum albumin based on the formation of the complex with two types of antibodies can serve as an illustration of the successful application of the sandwich assay (Saber et al. 2002). In this example the analytical signal of the sensor is 3 times higher than the same value obtained by the direct detection.

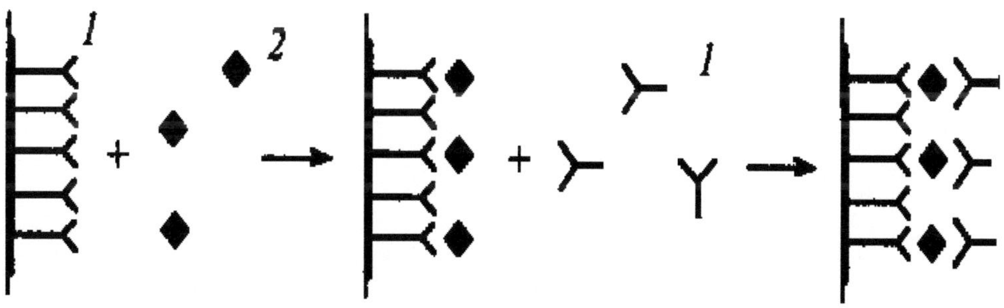

Fig. 5. The scheme of the sandwich assay using piezoelectric immunosensors: 1 - specific antibody; 2 - antigen

In order to reduce the detection limit other methods are used along with the sandwich assay that will increase the value of the analytical signal, e.g. modification of reagents with nanoparticles of different nature (secondary antibodies, metal colloidal particles, polymers nanoparticles and liposomes), which significantly increase the size and mass of the detected complexes formed at the solid phase (Aizawa et al. 2001, Kim et al. 2007, Chu et al. 2006). In (Su et al. 2000), such methods are marked as a separate kind of analysis, namely the analysis with signal amplification (**mass amplified assay**) (Fig. 6.).

The application of secondary (anti-species) antibodies that interact with the antibodies of the immune complex increases the analytical signal and decreases the detection limit only 1.5 - 2 times, since the mass of secondary antibodies does not exceed 150 kDa. For example, the detection limit of steroid hormone was thus reduced from 12 to 7ng ml^{-1} (Kubitschko et al. 1997). The mass-amplified assay is operated in two stages. In the first stage the immobilized antigen is bound with defined antibodies. In the second stage – after the removal of antibodies unbound during the first stage – secondary antibodies are introduced which are bound only to specific antibodies. An example of using this method is the determination of allergen-specific immunoglobulin (IgE) in serum of patients with the symptoms of allergic dermatitis (Su et al. 2000). An allergenic protein is immobilized on the surface of the sensor's electrode. In the first stage antibodies of different classes were bound on the surface of the receptor's layer during the contact of the sensor with the patient's blood serum sample. In the second stage the differentiation of antibodies after adsorption of secondary antibodies to human IgE in the process of contact with the sensor was carried out. The differentiation of allergen-specific antibodies (IgE) from other classes of immunoglobulins (IgG and IgM) contained in blood serum is possible after application of these secondary antibodies.

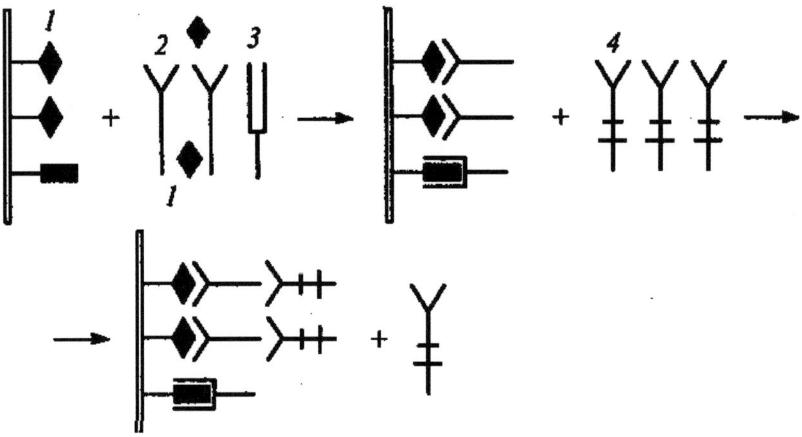

Fig. 6. The scheme of the competitive assay with signal amplification by secondary antibodies using piezoelectric immunosensors: 1 – hapten; 2- anti-hapten antibodies; 3 - non-specific antibody; 4 - secondary antibody

A more significant reduction in the detection limit of analytes (Aizawa et al. 2001, Kim et al. 1996, Liu et al. 2007, Grieshaber et al. 2008, Reyes et al. 2009, Han et al. 2011, Wei et al. 2010, Kim et al. 2010) was observed in the application of colloidal particles of gold, lead, cadmium or zinc sulphides, chromium, titanium and iron oxides, as well as composite particles based on liposomes or latex modified by antibodies.

The colloidal particles modified by antibodies can be applied in all types of analysis reviewed above with the purpose of increasing the signal of the sensor. For example this approach was applied to the determination of the *E. coli* bacteria in the range of 10^6-10^8 cells ml^{-1}(Liu et al. 2007).

Antibodies immobilized on the electrode of the sensor interacted with *E. coli* bacterial cells in the analyzed sample. After that the particles of latex with bound *E. coli*-antibodies were introduced into the reaction mixture to form a sandwich complex with cells that had already been bound with antibodies on the surface of the electrode of the sensor.

Thus, the application of nanoparticles of various masses makes it possible to increase the signal and to change the detection limit of analytes in the sample. However, in choosing the nanoparticles it is necessary to exclude their non-specific interactions with the components of the sample which lead to a distortion of the results of the analysis.

3. Application of piezoelectric immunosensors for medical diagnostics

Various metabolic biomarkers (substances that appear in biological fluids and tissues of the human body during the development of many somatic and infectious pathological processes) can be used in medical and biological research. The determination of these substances allows for diagnosis of diseases at early stages. An urgent problem in the clinical analysis is the need to detect single cells and micro-organisms. In this connection, along with speed, high sensitivity and selectivity, one of the main requirements in performing a large number of routine analyses is the simplicity in preparation of samples for the analysis. Piezoelectric immunosensors are used primarily to identify markers associated with oncological, cardiovascular, autoimmune, allergic and infectious diseases. The nature of molecular markers is quite diverse - they are specific proteins (antibodies, enzymes) and non-specific protein molecules, glycoproteins and glicoconjugates, modified alkaloids, hormones, steroids, drugs and other high- or low-molecular metabolites (Wu et al. 2007, Simon 2010, Martínez-Rivas et al. 2010, Bohunicky et al. 2011, Keusgen 2002, Malhotra et al. 2003, Georganopoulou et al. 2000, Mascini et al. 2008). In addition, sensors can be used to identify microorganisms - bacteria, viruses, and phages. Let us review in more detail the results of research on the sensors for determining the most important groups of biomarkers.

3.1 Tumour markers

Oncological diseases are still the most common threatening ailments, therefore it is not surprising that the search continues for not only new pharmaceutical products but diagnostic methods facilitating the detection of pathology at early stages.

In order to identify certain types of cancer so-called tumour markers are used, conventionally divided into specific and non-specific ones. Tumour markers are complex substances, mainly glyco- or lipoproteins, that are produced by tumour cells much more intensively than normal ones (Wu et al 2007, Guillo et al 2008, Justino et al. 2010). Usually the present marker is determined by a blood test giving a positive result in the presence of malignancy. Different tumour cells produce a variety of markers with different chemical structure.

In creating immunosensors much attention is paid to immobilization of receptor biomolecules in the formation of the detecting layer whose quality determines the basic characteristics of the sensor (Ding et al. 2007, Chang et al. 2010), namely sensitivity, selectivity and stability (reproducibility of measurements and stability for repeated application of the biolayer). The creation of "bioreactors" with high-density and spatial availability of binding sites of receptor biomolecules is a new approach to obtaining detecting electrode coatings of piezoelectric resonators, which allows multiple determinations without the regeneration of the sensor's biolayer.

The largest number of piezoelectric immunosensors presented in the literature is intended for the detection of such specific antigens as the marker of ovarian carcinomas CA 125; pancreatic cancer CA 19-9 and prostate specific antigen (PSA); carcinoembryonic antigen (CEA) that appears with carcinoma of the cervix or with the developing fetus. In order to determine low concentrations of tumour markers, various techniques aimed at increasing detection sensitivity are used. One of the methods of immobilizing bioreceptor molecules is to use nanoparticles of various nature - magnetic (Chen et al 2007, Wei et al. 2010) or gold (Tang et al. 2006, Tang et al. 2008, Uludağ and Tothill 2010), as well as calixarene (Lee et al. 2003).

Magnetic nanoparticles based on $CoFe_2O_4/SiO_2$ are used to obtain a detection layer containing specific antibodies to SEA (Chen et al 2007). It is possible to determine carcinoembryonic antigen using this sensor in the range of 2.5 - 55 ng·ml^{-1} with the detection limit of 0.5 ng·ml^{-1}. Since the normal concentration of tumour marker levels does not exceed 2.5 ng·ml^{-1} for non-smokers and 5 ng·ml^{-1} for smokers, the proposed immunosensor system can detect even a slight increase in the level of antigen in blood, demonstrating stability of work and satisfactory reproducibility of measurements.

In addition to magnetic particles, gold nanoparticles (Tang et al. 2006) and chains on the basis of nanoparticles (Tang et al. 2008) are used to amplify the sensor's signal and increase the number of active sites on the selective surface.

Gold nanoparticles of optimal length with immobilized antibodies are proposed as a biolayer of the sensor (Tang et al. 2008) for the determination of antigen CA 125. These structures are a result of a multi-stage process with the use of 2-aminoethanethiol (AET) bifunctional molecules with amino- and thiol terminal groups and the following reduction of gold by sodium borohydride (Fig. 7).

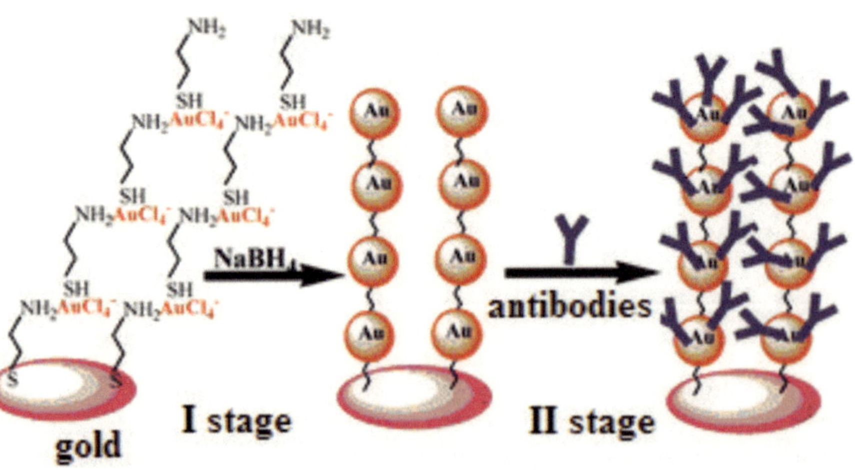

Fig. 7. The formation of the receptor layer on the surface of the gold electrode: Stage I - nano-chains generation of molecules $HAuCl_4$ and AET; Stage II - immobilization of antibodies (Tang et al. 2008).

In the process of the preparation of the biolayer the AET solution (pH 4.5) is put on the clean gold surface of the electrode and exposed for 2 hours at 4°C. Adjustment of AET molecules is achieved by coordinating bindings between sulphur and gold atoms. Chains from gold nanoparticles are formed as a result of multiple successive putting the $HAuCl_4$ solution and AET due to the binding of ions $[AuCl_4]^-$ with NH_2^- and SH-groups of AET and the formation of self-organizing layers $\{AuCl_4^-/AET\}$. This technique of obtaining electrode coating provides the sequence of layers, and after the reduction of anions $[AuCl_4]^-$ by the sodium borohydride ($NaBH_4$) water solution chains from gold nanoparticles are formed. The process is accompanied by a change in the colour of the surface from yellow to deep red. The addition of the antibody solution results in fixation of the molecules of specific immunoglobulins with the space-available active sites on the gold particles.

Therefore the presence of gold nanoparticles and nanochains (nanosequences) on the surface of the sensor's electrode increases the number and density of immobilized antibodies, as well as facilitates the formation of a three-dimensional structure in the biolayer, as confirmed by the methods of atomic force and electron microscopy at stepwise formation on the surface of the receptor layer. The detection layers based on gold nanoparticles and nanochains (nanosequences) exhibit high selectivity which is confirmed by the analysis of solutions containing interfering antigens such as CEA, CA 199, α-fetoprotein and hepatitis B surface antigen. It is shown that even high concentrations of impure antigens do not significantly affect the determination of CA 125, whose concentration in serum does not normally exceed 25 U ml^{-1}. The biolayer obtained with the use of gold nanoparticles has high capacity, satisfactory stability and provides good reproducibility of the analytical signal of the sensor. The linear range of determined concentrations of CEA and CA 17 125 (Tang et al. 2008) is 3.0 - 50 ng ml^{-1} and 1.5 - 180 U ml^{-1} respectively, with the detection limit being 1.5 ng ml^{-1} and 0.5 U ml^{-1}. The results of the analysis of human blood serum obtained with the use of piezoelectric immunosensors correlate with those of enzyme immunoassay. However, an advantage of sensor technologies is higher speed and simplicity of measurement, eliminating the stages of the introduction of an enzyme label, of separation and washing, which is important when conducting a large number of clinical tests.

A new approach to the formation of the detection layer with a higher capacity is realized in the design of the sensor, proposed for determining carbohydrate antigen CA 19-9, which is a marker of pancreatic (Ding et al., 2008, Tanaka et al. 2000), colon (Nakayama et al., 1997), liver (Uenishi et al. 2003) cancer. The possibility of using organo-inorganic hybrid nanomaterials based on hydroxyapatite [HA, $Ca_{10}(PO_4)_6(OH)_2$] and lysine is shown. Hydroxyapatite is the main inorganic component of bones, characterized by exceptional biocompatibility and therefore not causing immune rejection or toxic effects on the body (Ding et al., 2008). However, the use of pure materials on the basis of hydroxyapatite is hampered by instability, fragility and low solubility of the mineral. The addition of an organic component improves physical and chemical properties (such as permeability, solubility, etc.). The biosensor's receptor layer is formed on the basis of specific antibodies attached to a hybrid nanocomposite consisting of poly-L-lysine/hydroxyapatite/carbon nano-tubes (Fig. 8).

In order to obtain the coating, the resonator is initially treated with mercaptopropionic acid, which leads to the functionalization of the gold electrode surface by carboxyl groups as a monolayer. Further addition of 1-(3-dimethylaminopropyl)-N'-ethylcarbodiimide (EDC) and N-hydroxysuccinimide (NHS) provides the activation of carboxyl groups. After washing and drying the resonator a suspension composed of poly-L-lysine, hydroxyappatite, carbon nanotubes is put on the surface of the resonator's electrode and exposed for 2 h at 37°C, then antibodies to CA 19-9 are immobilized after the washing. The biosensor with nanocomposite detecting coating provides the direct registration of the immune complex which is formed in the process of the sorption of the tumour marker (a high molecular glycoprotein with the molecular weight of approximately 20.000) as an increase of the mass of the biolayer in the range from 12.5 to 270 U ml^{-1}. The content of CA 19-9 antigen in healthy people is less than 37 IU ml^{-1}, so a piezoelectric immunosensor can detect even slight deviations from the norm and diagnose the disease at an early stage.

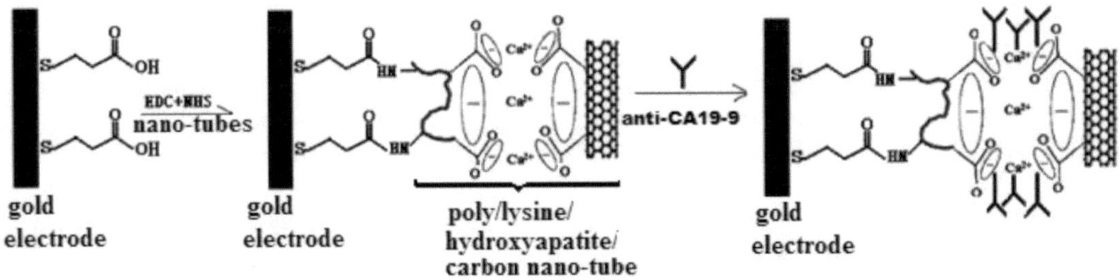

Fig. 8. The formation of the biolayer based on antibodies to CA 19-9, immobilized with poly-L-lysine/hydroxyapatite/carbon nano-tubes (Ding et al. 2008).

The combination of the methods reviewed above (application of new hybrid materials on the basis of gold nanoparticles and hydroxyapatites (*Ding* et al. 2007) and subsequent immobilization of antibodies) increases the sensitivity and widens the range of concentrations of the marker. The authors have shown that the use of selecting surface of the sensor with nanoparticles leads to the increase of the biolayer's binding activity with immobilized antibodies to α-fetoprotein (Ab-AFP). The immunosensor is designed to detect α-fetoprotein (a glycoprotein with a molecular weight of 65 - 70 kDa, which is a marker of trophoblastic tumors (Chou et al. 2002) in the range of 15.3 - 600.0 ng ml^{-1}).

Along with new ways of immobilization, traditional approaches to the formation of the bio-detecting layer of the sensor still remain popular. Methods of immobilizing specific monoclonal Ab-AFP (physical sorption, attachment to substrates based on protein A and concanavalin A, cystamine with the use of a cross-reactant - glutaraldehyde - GA) are studied in detail. The highest stability was shown for the biolayer obtained using the self-organizing monolayers on the basis of cystamine. The sensor provides the detection of even minor deviations of AFP from the norm (20 ng ml^{-1} in human serum), as the linear range of determined concentrations of glycoprotein corresponds to 0.1-100 ng ml^{-1} (Tatsuta et al. 1986). The results of determining AFP in serum samples correlated with the data of the radioimmunoassay.

In order to increase the stability of the biolayer a method of immobilizing protein molecules (antigens or antibodies) is proposed using the bifunctional linkers and calixarenes "Prolinkers" (Lee et al. 2003). It is shown that the activation of a solid surface by Prolinkers (Fig. 9) allows bioreceptor layers to be obtained with high density and vertical position of the molecules and hence a high concentration of spatially available binding sites for immobilized antigens or antibodies.

The active sites of the receptor molecules are not affected, which usually occurs in immunoglobulin covalent fixing. Immobilization is accomplished by including proteins in the calixarene cavity with the formation of the host-guest complex, as well as a result of hydrophobic interactions. The fixation of the linker on the metal surface is achieved by means of sulphur atoms or carbonyl groups comprising Prolinker B or A, respectively. The considered method of forming the biolayer provides high sensitivity of determination of such tumour markers as hCG (chorioiditic gonadotropin), CEA, α-fetoprotein, ferritin, etc. at the fg ml^{-1} level

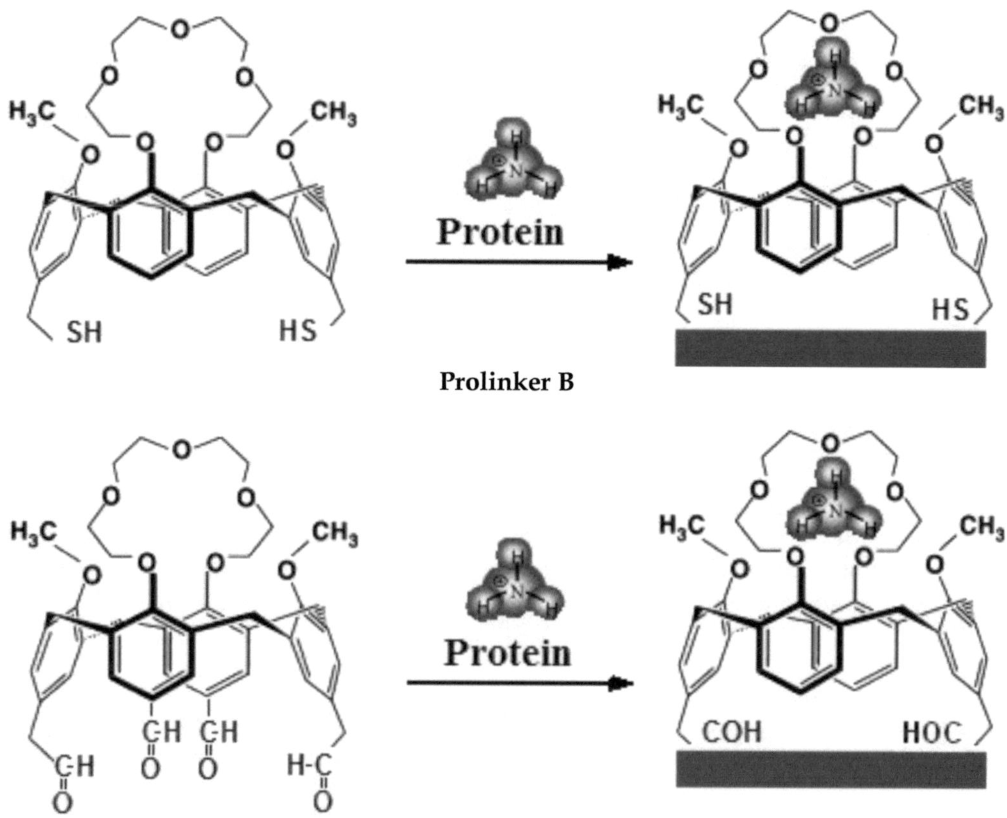

Prolinker A

Fig. 9. The scheme for obtaining the biolayer based on Prolinkers (Lee et al. 2003)

A flow-injection sensor has been designed to determine mezotelin (a glycoprotein with the weight of 40 kDa) which like the C 19-9 antigen is associated with pancreatic cancer processes (Corso et al. 2006) and is present in blood practically in all pancreatic adenocarcinomas. The detecting coating of the sensor is obtained on the basis of mezotelin-specific antibodies immobilized on the self-organized alkanthiol monolayers.

The increase in sensitivity and reliability of tumour marker determination is achieved not only by the formation of the receptor layer with a high concentration of available binding sites but also by improving the methods of determining the equipment, which allow monitoring of immunochemical interactions in real time. The improvement of the "signal-noise" ratio and the reduction of the contribution of nonspecific interactions occur when taking measurements using a system of two sensors: the indicator sensor and the comparison sensor, both placed in individual flow cells (Fig. 10).

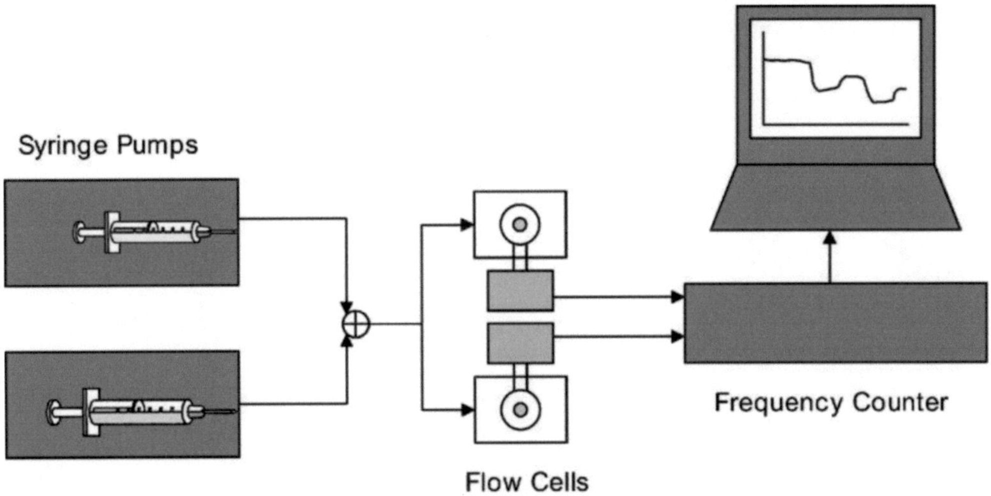

Fig. 10. The diagram of the device for performing the flow analysis (Corso et al. 2006)

The use of two syringe pumps (to feed the carrying solution and the sample solution) reduces pulsations in the system and allows the stabilization of the sensor signal, while determining mezotelin at the nano-level (Corso et al. 2006).

As seen from the above examples, piezoelectric immunosensors are a highly sensitive tool for detecting low concentrations of tumour markers and for identifying the disease at early stages. Most commonly, however, sensors are used for detecting recurrences of cancer previously diagnosed and treated for. This is due to the nature of antigenic tumour markers which can give false positive reactions.

The reliability of diagnosis increases with the use of biochips and multisensor systems consisting of a set of sensors for determining individual tumour markers and metabolites, complicating the diagnosis of cancer. Thus, a multi-sensor system is described designed for highly specific determination of several tumour markers in serum, such as α-fetoprotein, CEA and carcinoma antigen, prostate-specific antigen (Zhang et al. 2007). The possibility of the simultaneous determination of several tumour markers, a perfect combination of high speed and relatively low cost makes the approach attractive compared with traditional diagnostic laboratory methods. The detection limits of PSA, AFP, CEA, and CA125 are 1.5 - 40 ng ml^{-1}, 20 - 640 ng ml^{-1}, 1.5 - 30 mg ml^{-1}, 5 - 150 IU ml^{-1}, respectively. The comparison of the results of the analysis of clinical samples using the multichannel immunosensor and the chemiluminescence method showed no significant differences.

In spite of the fact that specific biomarkers are more informative because they indicate the emergence of specific forms of pathological processes, non-specific tumour markers, however, such as human serum albumin (HSA) and ferritin have also proved useful in assessing the health status of patients.

A number of studies are aimed at creating a piezoelectric immunosensor for the determination of HSA. The focus is on methods of immobilization, as well as increasing the sensitivity of determination from μg ml^{-1} to ppm (for example, signal amplification due to the use of secondary antibodies in the sandwich-analysis (Sakai et al. 1995) or colloidal particles of latex (Xia et al. 1997)). The simplest way to fix biomolecules is the physical adsorption in that it, unlike covalent bonding, preserves the activity of immunoglobulins. This is due to rather mild conditions of protein immobilization, but the stability of the film coating is low, the mass of the bio-layer is already lower after 2 - 4 measuring cycles. Immunosensors (Muratsugu et al. 1993) make it possible to determine HSA with high sensitivity and selectivity in the range of 0.1 - 100 μg ml^{-1} even in the presence of a nonspecific impurity protein – bovine serum albumin (BSA). Further development of immobilization methods was aimed at increasing the strength of the bio-layer due to a substrate on the basis of calixarenes and synthetic polymers (Sakti et al. 2001), which ensures the sensor's long-term operation in analyzing not only sample solutions but real samples of biological fluids (e.g., urine).

At present, the problems of increasing the sensitivity of determining the HSA and the stability of the sensor are fully understood. Considerable attention is paid to both methods of obtaining the biolayer and ways of amplifying the sensor's analytical signal. This can be achieved by increasing the mass of the heterogeneous immune complex. Secondary antibodies whose mass exceeds that of HSA are used in the sandwich assay to amplify the signal, which leads to lowering the HAS detection limit to 20 ppm. With the same purpose the nano-particles of carboxyethyl cellulose polymer (Xia et al. 1997) are used, thus increasing the sensor signal due to latex agglutination.

Along with the HSA determination considerable attention is paid to the creation of sensors for the determination of another non-specific marker – ferritin, a backup protein the level of which increases during the inflammatory processes in the body. Methods of immobilizing poly- and monoclonal antibodies on the electrode surface have been thoroughly researched. They include: physical adsorption, covalent attachment to substrates on the basis of concanavalin A and protein A, and self-organizing monolayers on the basis of cystamine, cystamine/GA (Chou et al. 2002). It has been shown that the biolayer based on cystamine has the highest stability. The sensors remain active for 15 days and can be used up to 10 times in ferritin linear concentration range of 0.1 - 100 ng ml^{-1}. It should be noted that in order to determine tumour markers, monoclonal antibodies are more frequently used. This increases the reliability of determinations and ousts polyclonal antibodies from the laboratory practice.

In diagnosing leukemia whole cells (leukocytes) circulating in blood (*Wang* et al. 2006, *Zeng* et al. 2006*)* are determined. The receptor coating is formed on the basis of Fab'-SH fragments of specific monoclonal antibodies, thus avoiding overloading the sensor. Performing the analysis in the automatic mode involves the measurement and regeneration of the biolayer in one measurement cycle. The application of 8M of urea as a regeneration solution permits keeping the coating stable for up to 17 measurement cycles. Firm fixation of the fragments of immunoglobulins is achieved through the formation of covalent bonds between the biomolecules and thin-film substrates obtained by plasma polarization of n-butyl amine, on the basis of protein A or gold nanoparticles. The sensor is able to quickly and reliably detect normal cells, leukemic blasts and to determine the concentration of leukocytes in the range of 10^4 - 10^6 cells ml^{-1}.

Thus nowadays piezoelectric immunosensors have successfully proved to be promising tools for express determination of blood cells and tumour markers of different chemical structure and biological specificity.

3.2 Cardiac markers

Cardiovascular diseases leading to the growth of cardiac infarctions and strokes remain one of the main causes of death and disablement throughout the world. Myocardial necrosis is accompanied by the appearance of blood-specific biomarkers - proteins released with the destruction of myocytes: myoglobin, cardiac troponin and specific enzymes - creatine kinase, glycogen phosphorylase BB (GPBB), lactate dehydrogenase, etc. (Casey 2004). Despite a wider application of enzymatic methods of analysis in laboratory diagnostics of cardio-pathology, several works of the recent years have described piezoelectric chemical, bio- and immunosensors for determining biomarkers of non-enzymatic nature - myoglobin (Godber et al. 2005), C-reactive protein (CRP) (Kurosawa et al. 2003, Kim et al. 2009), troponin (Wong-ek et al. 2010, Mohammed and Desmulliez 2011), heparin (Cheng et al. 2002), thrombin, etc.

Bi-sensor systems are being developed in order to reduce the impact of non-specific effects. To change the viscous-elastic properties of the receptor films which influence the comprehensiveness of contact of the vibrating crystal with the surface, which in turn causes errors in calculating the adsorbed mass. Bi-sensor systems on the basis of high-frequency resonators (16.5 MHz) have been developed for determining mioglobin, a cytoplasmatic protein with the weight of 17 κDa, a part of muscular cells (Godber et al. 2007), the presence of which in blood serves as a good diagnostic marker of cardiac diseases (Casey 2004). The receptor layer of the indicator sensor includes anti-mouse-Fc-specific antibodies in the rabbit which are immobilized by means of EDC and NHS. Mouse immunoglobulins G are fixed on the surface of the control sensor to control a non-specific interaction of mioglobin with the surface of the protein. The analytical signal caused by the specific interaction is measured relative to the comparison sensor thus providing the opportunity to differentiate between the normal level of mioglobin in blood (100 ng ml^{-1}) and excess at cardio ischemia because mioglobin concentration directly after infarction reaches 1000 ng ml^{-1} and more and decreases to 500 ng ml^{-1} after a time.

The combination of a bi-sensor system and the sandwich assay is directed at increasing the sensitivity in determining C-reactive protein (McBride and Cooper 2008), which is a multifunctional biomarker of an acute phase playing an important role at inflammations, in protection against alien agents, at necroses and autoimmune processes. For a number of years the exceeding concentration of CRP by over 5 mg l^{-1} marked the absence of any systemic inflammatory process in the organism. Now, new data on the diagnostic possibilities of CRP, including participation in the development of various pathologies have been obtained, particularly vascular diseases. The determination of "background" or "base" (hsCRP) concentrations in biological liquids can be used to forecast the degree of risk from acute myocardial infarction, a brain stroke, and sudden death in people not suffering from cardiovascular diseases. Expansion of the diagnostic status of CRP has demanded the development of methods of high-sensitive determination of a biomarker. It is recommended to use the calibration graph obtained with the application of human CRP standard solutions

(0.3 - 116 ng ml^{-1}) on the basis of diluted horse blood to decrease irregularities. Sheep anti-CRP are immobilized on the surface of the indicator sensor, and purified sheep immunoglobulins G are immobilized on the control sensor. Such an approach enhances the reliability of revealing patients predisposed to cardiovascular diseases. The use of secondary antibodies in the second stage of the analysis promotes the increase in specificity and sensitivity of determination in comparison with the results of the traditionally used ELISA.

The works of Japanese researchers are devoted to determining CRP and providing the quantitative characteristic of affinity of monoclonal antibodies and their Fab'-fragments (Kurosawa et al. 2002 and 2004). They studied the influence of the nature of thin plasma-polymerized coatings of gold electrodes (styrene, allylamine and acrylic acid) on the orientation of immobilized antibodies and their fragments. It was shown that the highest analytical signals are observed for biolayers on polyallylamine substrates. Processing the electrode by a polymer based on phosphorylcholine and methylacrylate derivatives increases the affinity of the receptor molecules to the determined substance and decreases the reaction activity in relation to non-specific proteins of human serum. The highest values of affinity constants were seen for Fab'-fragments in comparison with the whole antibodies. The application of fragments of antibodies allows the achievement of the linear range of defined concentrations of C-reactive protein of 0.001 - 100 μg ml^{-1} (Kurosawa et al. 2004) in serum samples.

The suggested approaches increase both the speed of diagnostics and the sensitivity and reliability of determining cardiac markers.

3.3 Detection of infections

The possibility of the spread of epidemic-causing pathogenic germs and the threat of bioterrorism necessitate the development of new express methods for detecting pathogens for early detection of cases and localization of sources of infection. Control over the spread of extremely dangerous, acute intestinal, septic, sexual, viral diseases (influenza, hepatitis, HIV) involves not only the identification of bacteria or viruses in biological fluids of patients but also the determination of markers of infection – specific antibodies and in some cases – toxins (proteins, glycoproteins or glycolipids) produced by pathogenic causative agents.

The application of piezoelectric immunosensors for determining microbial and bacterial antigens, toxins and antibodies (which are large analytes) proved to be more promising not only compared with the traditional methods of analysis (microbiological, immunochemical and molecular-genetic) but also with other biosensors. This is explained by peculiarities of gravimetric detection which does not require the introduction of biochemical markers for the registration of binding. This greatly simplifies and speeds up the analysis procedure. Piezoelectric micro- and nano-weighing makes it possible both to register the mass of a microbe or a biopolymer at μg or ng and to calculate the number of individual cells or viruses according to their mass and size in the concentration range of 10^2 - 10^7 cells ml^{-1} or 10^6 - 10^{10} particles ml^{-1}, respectively (Pathirana et al. 2000, Konig and Gratzel 1992).

In determining microorganisms the direct analysis is used most commonly, while the sandwich and the displacing assays and the analysis with the amplification of the sensor signal are used to increase the sensitivity of determination.

The characteristics of piezoelectric immunosensors for determining microorganisms and protein molecules are given in tables 1-3.

Analyte	Method of immobilizing receptor molecules or assay design (detection format)	Linear range. Detection limit	References
Escherichia coli O157:H7	Immobilization on gold electrode on the basis of N-hydroxysuccinimide and 16-mercaptohexadecanic acid	10^3 - 10^8 CFU ml^{-1} -	Su and Li 2002
Escherichia coli	Covalent immobilization of Ab cross-linked by GA	1.7 ·10^5 - 8.7 ·10CFU ml^{-1} 3 ·10^4 - 3 ·10^7CFU ml^{-1}	Adanyi et al. 2006
Escherichia coli O157:H7	Biotylated Ab immobilized on monolayers on protein A	10^5 - 10^7 CFU ml^{-1} 10^2 CFU ml^{-1}	Liu et al. 2007
	Ab immobilized on monolayers on the basis of 16-mercaptohexadecanic acid (MHDA) with NHS	- 2.0 ·10^2 CFU ml^{-1}	*Wang* et al. *2008*
Francisella tularensis	Ab immobilized *via* protein A	10^4 - 10^9 CFU ml^{-1}; 10^5 CFU ml^{-1}	Pohanka et al. 2007
	Ab immobilized to monolayer cystamine/GA	- -	Pohanka et al. 2007
Mycobacterium tuberculosis	Immobilization of Ab on silver electrode *via* protein A	10^5- 10^8 cells ml^{-1}. 10^5 cells ml^{-1}	He and Zhang 2002
Salmonella sp.	Direct detection, Ab immobilized with cross-linker	ABCD-serogroups 10^5 - 10^8 cells ml^{-1}	Wong et al. 2002
S. typhimurium	Ab immobilized on the films of PEI-GA	- 1.5 ·10^9 CFU ml^{-1}	Babacan et al. 2000
	Ab immobilized on the films of protein A	- 1.5 ·10^9 CFU ml^{-1}	
Staphylococcus aureus	Ab covalently immobilized by GA to self-assembled monolayer of thiolamin	10^5 - 10^9 cells ml^{-1} -	Boujday et al. 2008
Treponema pallidum	Ab immobilized on the latex particle; latex agglutination	- -	Aizawa et al. 2001
Yersinia enterocolitica	Direct detection, Ab immobilized *via* concanavalin A, sulfated polysaccharide	(0.30 - 4.90) ·10^4 cells ml^{-1} 0.04 ·10^4 cells ml^{-}	Kalmykova et al. 2007
Vibrio cholera 0139	Adsorption of Ab	- 10^5 cells ml^{-1}	Carter et al. 1995

Table 1. Piezoelectric immunosensors for the determination of bacteria

Most of the modern sensors are designed to determine the causative agents of a widespread group of intestinal diseases - bacteria *E. coli* (Plomer et al. 1992, Su and Li 2002, Adanyi et al. 2006, Liu et al. 2007, *Wang* et al. 2008, Shen et al. 2011, Jiang et al. 2011, *Li* et al. 2011), *Listeria monocytogenes* (Minunni et al. 1996, Vaughan et al. 2002, *Wang* et al. 2008), *Salmonella* sp. (Su et al. 2001, Su et al. 2005, Yang et al. 2009, Park and Kim 1998, Wong et al. 2002, Fung and Wong 2001, Ying-Sing et al 2000), *Vibrio cholera* (Carter et al. 1995), *Yersinia enterocolitica* (Kalmykova et al. 2007 and 2008), viruses (Konig and Gratzel 1992). (*Adenovirus*, and *Rotavirus*), as well as toxins (e.g. staphylococcus toxin) (Harteveld et al. 1997, Salmain et al. 2011).

Analyte	Method of immobilizing receptor molecules or assay design (detection format)	Linear range. Detection limit	References
Adenovirus	Direct assay, Ab immobilized via protein A, siloxane, polyethylenamine	$1 \cdot 10^6 - 1 \cdot 10^{10}$ particulars ml^{-1} –	Konig et al. 1992
Hepatitis virus A, B	Direct assay, Ab immobilized via protein A	– 10^5 particulars ml^{-1}	Zhou et al. 2002
Hepatitis virus C (HCV)	RNA of HCV immobilized via avidin (streptavidin) to a monolayer of cystamine	– –	Skladal et al. 2004
Human cytomegalovirus	Competitive definition, monolayers of poly-L-lysine and tiosalicylic acid	2.5 - 5 $\mu g\ ml^{-1}$ 1 $\mu g\ ml^{-1}$	Susmel et al. 2000

Table 2. Piezoelectric immunosensors for the determination of viruses and bacteriophages

Salmonellosis diagnostics is successfully carried out with the help of sensors with the biodetecting layer based on both common and thiolated antibodies (Park and Kim 1998, Kim et al. 2003), which are specific for the determined bacteria (*S. typhimurium, S. paratyphi, S. enteritidis*). Along with the traditional ways of antibody immobilization (physical adsorption, specific binding to protein A or covalent attachment using a bifunctional cross-linker to the Langmuir-Blodgett films) in obtaining the biolayer self-organizing monolayers on polyethyleneimine (Wong et al. 2002, Babacan et al. 2000) and electropolymerization techniques are used.

It should be noted that the method of electrode coating does not significantly affect the sensitivity of determining bacterial pathogens (10^5 - 10^9 cells ml^{-1}), but significantly increases the reproducibility and stability of analysis. For example, a sensor has been designed to determine the *Staphylococcus aureus* bacteria causing purulent-septic diseases (Le et al. 1995, Boujday et al. 2008). It is designed on the basis of the chromatographic phase (YWG-$C_{18}H_{37}$) with antibodies immobilized with glutaraldehyde and is meant for repeated use and long-term storage. The sensor (Le et al. 1995) can be used up to 15 times and stored for months without a decrease in biomolecule activity. However, it is characterized by a few cases of cross-binding with bacteria of other genera: *P. aeruginosa, S. epidermidis E. coli*. The formation of the biolayer on the surface of an electropolimerized film increases the resistance of sensors that can be stored for more than 5 weeks. The ability to maintain constant values of the electrode's potential and current provides for obtaining receptor coatings with identical thickness, mass and distribution of functional groups, which is very important for commercial production of sensors.

Despite the fact that most strains of *E. coli* are not harmful to humans, some serotypes (e.g. K12, O157: H7) cause serious food poisoning. Sensors are suggested for the "dip and dry" analysis with a receptor layer on the basis of antibodies to *E. coli* K12, immobilized on a

Analyte	Method of immobilizing receptor molecules or assay design (detection format)	Linear range. Detection limit	References
Ab to bacteria F. tularensis	Direct detection, Antigens are attached by means of GA to the cystamine-monolayer on a gold electrode	Titer 40 - 160 -	Pohanka et al. 2007
Ab to HIV	Direct detection synthetic HIV-peptide or recombinant proteins are immobilized	Tests yes/no	Kosslinger et al. 1995 and 1998
Ab to parasites Shistosoma japonicum	Antigens (SjAg32, mass 32kD) covalently immobilized on 3-mercaptopropionic SAM-to you (MPA) using EDC/NHS	3.6 – 42.0 μg ml^{-1} -	Wu et al. 2003
Ab to bacteria Y.enterocolitica	Direct assay, LPS immobilized on a lipid substrate	3 - 110 μg ml^{-1} 1.3 μg ml^{-1}	Kalmyken et al. 2007
Immuno-globulin E	Direct assay, Physical sorption of protein antigen	0 - 300 ME ml^{-1} 0.1 - 25 μg ml^{-1} 0.15 - 17.5 μg ml^{-1} -	Su et al. 2000
Immuno-globulin E	Direct assay, Affine immobilization to aptomer on the basis of ssDNA	- 0.05 nmol ml^{-1}	Liss et al. 2000
Human IgG	Direct assay, Chemo sorption of protein complex IgG-Ab on polystyrene substrate	- 5 μg ml^{-1}	Liu et al. 2003
Surface antigen of Hepatitis B	Direct assay, Ab linked by method of cross-linkikg to cystimine monolayer	- 4.7 nmol l^{-1}	Chen et al. 2002
Cholera toxin	Sandwich method, amplified by ganglioside-modified liposomes	- 0.0001 nmol l^{-1}	Alfonta and Wilner 2001
Staphylococcus enterotoxin (SEB)	Competitive assay, Ab immobilized on god electrode	- 0.1 μg ml^{-1}	Harteveld et al. 1997

Table 3. Piezoelectric immunosensors for determination of protein molecules

substrate of protein A (Plomer et al. 1992) and monolayers on alkanthiols (Su and Li 2002). The detection limit of bacteria *E. coli* 0157: H7 is 10^3 CFU ml^{-1}. In order to increase the sensitivity of the determination of *E. coli* O157: H7 streptavidin-conjugated nanoparticles gold (145 nm), magnetic, silica and polymer nanoparticles of 30 - 970 nm, immunomagnetic nanoparticles (BIMPs) and affinity-purified antibodies against *E.coli* treated with biotin (Liu et al. 2007, Shen et al. 2011, Jiang et al. 2011) are used. After binding cells with immobilized antibodies nanoparticles of bio-conjugates with streptavidin are injected into the system (Liu et al. 2007), thus amplifying the sensor's signal, with the detection limit of bacteria *E. coli* O157: H7 decreasing to 10^2 CFU ml^{-1}.

Besides the research aimed at determining certain types of bacteria, in microbiological control it is possible to simultaneously determine several of the most dangerous micro-organisms belonging to the same family (Kim and Bhunia 2008). It is perspective to apply antibodies against enterobacterial common antigen (ECA) which represents a phospholipid in the outer membrane and characterized by specificity to the whole *Enterobacteriaceae* family comprising the *Salmonella* and *E. coli* genera. Using monoclonal antibodies to ECA, Plomer et al proposed immunosensors for determining any microorganism of the *Enterobacteriaceae* family in the range of 10^4 - 10^6 cells ml^{-1}.

This displacement analysis is recommended for determining the *Pseudomonas aeruginosa* bacteria which cause postoperative or post-burn complications. In order to determine the bacteria directly in the flow of the solution thiolated antibodies (Kim et al. 2004) were used, which increases its service life by more than 10%.

A method has been suggested for flow-injection determination of pathogenic "fridge bacteria" – the *Yersinia enterocolitica* bacteria, O:3 serotype, in aqueous media. The necessity to determine *Yersinia* is caused by the fact that they are agents of an infectious intestinal disease – yersiniosis which considerably influences human and animal pathology. In order to determine the *Y. enterocolitica* bacteria the biolayer of the sensor is formed on immobilized specific antibodies. The comparative evaluation of methods for obtaining the bio-detecting layer of the sensor (absorption of antibodies on metal surfaces, covalent binding with sulfated polysaccharides substrates, concanavalin A, aminosiloxane using glutaraldehyde) has demonstrated the advantage of polysaccharide substrates, which increase the reproducibility of the analytical signal and reduce the detection limit to $0.02 \cdot 10^4$ cells ml^{-1} (Kalmyken et al. 2007). The widest linear range of determined microorganisms was found for the siloxane biolayer substrate: 0.30 - $4.90 \cdot 10^4$ cells ml^{-1}. The methods of flow-injection determination of the *Y. enterocolitica* bacteria using a piezo-quartz immunosensor with the biolayer based on monoclonal homologous antibodies can reliably detect the presence of microorganisms in aqueous media. The proposed immunosensors can detect bacteria in water solutions with a minimum concentration of $0.10 \cdot 10^4$ cells ml^{-1}.

Despite very rare occurrences of cholera in this day and age, it is an infection which can cause rapid dehydration and death. In order to determine the *Vibrio cholerae* 0139 a highly specific sensor was developed (Carter et al. 1995) showing no cross-interactions with other bacteria, such as *Ogawa, E.coli, L. monocytogenes* and *S. marcescens.*

Piezoelectric biosensors can be applicable not only in determining individual analytes, but also for the study of biochemical processes (agglutination, hybridization) in real time, as well as of the kinetics of reversible reactions. Such sensors can subsequently be used to select antibodies as bioreceptor molecules to create immunosensors. For example, researchers deal with the application of monoclonal antibodies against pathogenic *Francisella tularensis* bacteria causing a zoonotic disease – tularaemia, as well as bacterial endotoxins to determine specific antibodies (Pohanka et al. 2007).

Viruses. Among all infectious diseases the most complicated problems are associated with viral infections. This is mainly due to the prevalence of viruses, their participation in the processes of immunogenesis, difficulty in diagnoses, so it is equally important to create sensors for the determination of pathogenic viruses (hepatitis, herpes, human immunodeficiency - HIV, etc.).

One of the first researchers who reported on the possibility of detecting not only bacterial, but viral pathogens of diarrhea (*Rotavirus* and *Adenovirus*) in liquid were Konig and Gratsel. The sensors designed by these authors allow the determination of both the microbial pathogens in the range of $1 \cdot 10^6$ - $1 \cdot 10^8$ and $1 \cdot 10^6$ - $1 \cdot 10^{10}$ virus ml^{-1}, respectively, as a result of direct increment of the mass of the receptor layer. The direct detection is used to determine the herpes viruses 1 and 2, *Varicella-zoster*, *Epstein-Barr* virus at 10^4 virus ml (Susmel et al. 2001). In the case of hepatitis A and B, the detection limit is 10^5 viral particles ml^{-1} (Konig and Gratsel 1995, Zhou et al. 2002). When testing serum samples for viral presence with the application of specific antibodies absorbed on the surface of the crystal, screening was carried out to determine the content of viral particles; the results were correlated with those of the enzyme-linked immunosorbent assay.

In order to determine human cytomegalovirus the competitive immunoassay (Susmel et al. 2001) is recommended, as direct cooptation of the virus from the solution gives poor results (Konig and Gratsel 1995), while the competitive analysis, performed with a monolayer on poly-L-lysine (covalently bonded to the monolayer of tiosalicylic acid) allows the detection of the antigen in the range of 2.5 to 5 mg ml^{-1}, the detection limit being 1 mg ml^{-1}.

Antibodies and bacteriotoxins. Antibodies of various specificity, and some protein toxins can act as biomarkers of infectious and somatic diseases. The first researches on determining antibodies to human immunodeficiency virus (Kosslinger et al. 1995, Kosslinger et al. 1998) were reported in 1992. Their authors used synthetic peptides of human immunodeficiency virus (HIV) as receptor molecules immobilized on the surface of the electrode of a high-frequency resonator (20 MHz). The influence of the dilution of a serum sample on the reliability of the determination is shown.

The sandwich-analysis with the recombinant protein as receptor molecules and the amplification of the signal by secondary antibodies labelled with an enzyme was used to assess patients' contamination by the *Helicobacter pylori* bacteria, detectable by the presence of specific antibodies in serum (Su and Li 2001). The sensor can be used both in static and flow modes.

Determining specific antibodies in infectious yersiniosis (caused by the *Yersinia enterocolitica* bacteria) allows differentiating an acute intestinal infection from surgical pathology (e.g. acute appendicitis), which provides the correct choice of therapeutic measures and the identification of chronic forms of the disease. A sensor is proposed with the receptor layer on the basis of lipopolysaccharides (LPS) – components of the outer membrane of the cell wall of Gram-negative bacteria, consisting of covalently linked (Kalmykova et al. 2006 and

2007) carbohydrate and lipid parts. In determining specific antibodies it is necessary to provide spatial availability for carbohydrate, and not lipid, LPS (O-specific polysaccharides) macromolecules. Activation of silver electrodes is carried out with lipids of oil, Fig. 11.

The application of a hydrophobic electrode modifier for the immobilization of lipopolysaccharides leads to the interaction of the lipid part of macromolecules with a lipid coating and the orientation of O-specific polysaccharide chains (O-antigenic determinants) in the direction of the hydrophilic eluent (Fig. 11). At the same time the biolayer is characterized by maximum binding activity with corresponding antibodies.

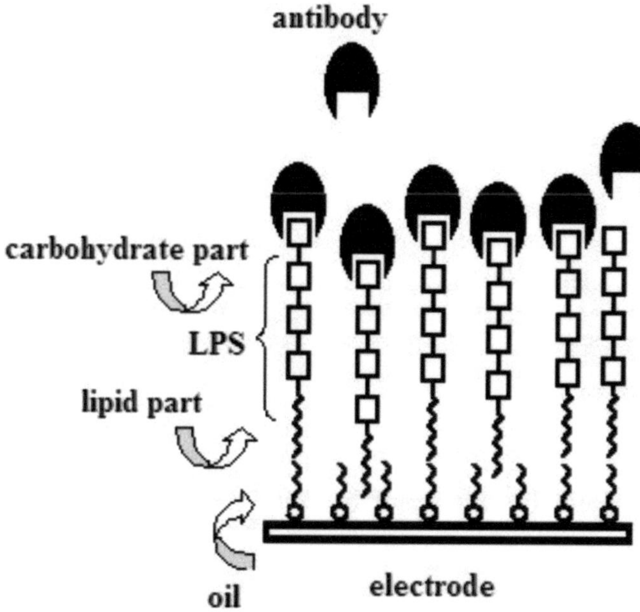

Fig. 11. The interaction of LPS with antibodies immobilized on a hydrophobic substrate (oil) (Kalmykova et al. 2007)

The significance of this research lies in both determining antibodies and establishing a correlation between different ways to express the activity of sera (activity titre and the concentration of specific antibodies). The sensor allows the determination of antibodies in serum with a higher sensitivity compared with the reaction of passive hemagglutination. This is useful for identifying yersiniosis at an earlier stage and monitoring treatment efficiency.

Another area in the application of sensors is the detection of parasites *Shistosoma japonicum* (Wu et al. 2003, Wu et al. 2006, Cheng et al. 2008) when specific antibodies are determined in blood as a result of polymer agglutination.

Of special interest are sensors for the determination of certain classes of antibodies - IgA, IgG, IgM, which can serve as indirect indicators of candidiasis and facilitate the diagnostics of fungal infections.

Determination of antibodies to DNA. One of the clinical forms of yersiniosis is the arthritic one, when patients with rheumatoid arthritis have antibodies to the *Y. enterocolitica* bacteria, serotype O:5. However, more often the arthritic pathology is an indicator of developing autoimmune diseases: systemic lupus erythematosus, rheumatoid arthritis, chronic glomerulonephritis, etc. when antibodies to DNA are formed in the body itself. Immunosensors have been designed based on denatured DNA molecules for determining antibodies to DNA in blood serum (Fakhrullin et al. 2007, Kalmykova et al. 2003) in the range of 0.1 - 25 μg ml^{-1} (0.03 – 8 IU), the detection limit being 0.01 μg ml^{-1} (0.003 IU). Other substances of protein nature in blood plasma does not interfere with the quantitative determination of antibodies to DNA.

4. Conclusion

Possible practical applications of piezoelectric immunosensors are not limited to the examples discussed above. The analysis of papers published over the past 15 years shows that the new research direction, connected with the development and application of piezoelectric immunosensors, causes a growing concern around the world. Sensors are used in clinical diagnostics to identify high and low molecular compounds, to monitor the effectiveness of drugs action and their metabolism, to identify the causes of the intoxication of the body, to detect drug and doping agents in biological fluids.

The relatively low cost combined with high sensitivity and selectivity, plus the possibility to analyze just one drop of blood, saliva, or urine with little or no additional sample preparation, the resumption of the activity of the bioreceptor layer and multiple use make piezoelectric immunosensors a real alternative to the existing methods used in medicine.

Besides, the combination of piezoelectric micro- and nano-weighing with other methods (e.g. optical or electrochemical methods, the surface plasmon resonance method, the method of atomic force microscopy) will contribute to a better understanding of biochemical processes at the cellular level, leading to various diseases.

5. References

Adanyi N., Varadi M., Kim N, Szendro I. (2006). Development of new immunosensors for determination of contaminants in food. Current Appl. Phys. 6. 279-286.

Aizawa H., Kurasawa S., Ogawa K., Yoshimoto M., Miyake J., Tanaka H. (2001). Conventional diagnosis of C-reactive protein in serum using latex piezoelectric immunoassay. Sens. Actuators B. 76. 173-176.

Aizawa H., Kurosawa S., Tanaka M., Wakida S., Talib Z.A., Park J. W., Yoshimoto M., Muratsugu M., Hilborn J.,Miyake J., Tanaka H. (2001). Rapid diagnosis of Treponema pallidum in serum using latex piezoelectric immunoassay. Analytica Chimica Acta. 437(2). 167-169.

Babacan S., Privarnik P., Letcher S., Rand A.G. (2000). Evaluation of antibody immobilization methods for piezoelectric biosensor application. Biosens. Bioelectron. 15. 615 -622.

Bohunicky B., Mousa S. (2011). Biosensors: the new wave in cancer diagnosis. Nanotechnology, Science and Applications. 4. 1–10.

Boujday S., Briandet R., Salmain M., Herry J.M., Marnet P.G., Gautier M., Pradier C.M. (2008). Detection of pathogenic Staphylococcus aureus bacteria by gold based immunosensors. Microchim. Acta. 163 (3-4). 203-209.

Bovenizer J.S., Jacobs M.B., O'Sullivan C.K., Guilbault G.G. (1998), The Detection of Pseudomonas aeruginosa Using the Quartz Crystal Microbalance. Anal. Lett. 31. 1287-1295.

Carter R.M., Mekalanos J.J., Lubrano G.J., Guilbault G.G. (1995). Quartz crystal microbalance detection of Vibrio cholerae O139 serotype. .J. Immunol. Methods. 187. 121- 125.

Casey P. (2004). Markers of myocardial injury and dysfunction. AACN Clin. Issues. 15. 547–557.

Chang C.-C., Shenhsiung L., Yu C.-S., Chii-Wann L. (2011). Using Polyethylene Glycol-Modified Chitosan for Improvement of Carbohydrate Antigen 15-3 Detection on a Quartz Crystal Microbalance Biosensor. Sensor Letters. 9(1). 404-408.

Chen Z.-G., Tang D.-Y. (2007) . Antigen-antibody interaction from quartz crystal microbalance immunosensors based on magnetic CoFe2O4/SiO2 composite nanoparticle-functionalized biomimetic interface. Bioprocess Biosyst Eng. 30. 243-249.

Cheng Ch.-W. , Chen Ch.-.K. , Chen Y.-Sh., Chen L.-Y. (2008). Determination of Schistosoma japonicum circulating antigens in dilution serum by piezoelectric immunosensor and S/N enhancement. Biosens.Bioelectron.24(1).136-140.

Cheng T., Lin T.-M., Chang H.-C. (2002). Physical adsorption of protamine for heparin assay using a quartz crystal microbalance and electrochemical impedance spectroscopy. Anal. Chim. Acta. 462 (2). 261–273.

Chou S.-F., Hsu W.-L,.Wang J.-M., Chen C.-Y. (2002). Determination of [alpha]-fetoprotein in human serum by a quartz crystal microbalance-based immunosensor. Clin. Chemistr. 48. 913 - 918.

Chou S.-F., Hsu W.-L., Hwang J.-M., Chen C.-Y. (2002). Development of an immunosensor for human ferritin, a nonspecific tumor marker, based on a quartz crystal microbalance Anal. Chimi. Acta. 453. 181–189.

Chu X., Zhao Z.L., Shen G.L., Yu R.Q. (2006). Quartz crystal microbalance immunoassay with dendritic amplification using colloidal gold immunocomplex. Sensors and Actuators. B. 114. 696–704.

Corso C.D., Stubbs D.D., Lee S.-H., Goggins M., Hruban R.H., Hunt W.D. (2006). Real-time detection of mesothelin in pancreatic cancer cell line supernatant using an acoustic wave immunosensor. Cancer Detection and Prevention. 30 (2). 180-187.

Ding Y, Liu J.,.Jin X,.Lu H, Shen G., Yu R. (2008). Poly-L-lysine/hydroxyapatite/carbon nanotube hybrid nanocomposite applied for piezoelectric immunoassay of carbohydrate antigen 19-9. Analyst. 133. 184-190.

Ding Y,.Liu .J, Wang H., .Shen G.,Yu R. (2007). A piezoelectric immunosensor for the detection of α-fetoprotein using an interface of gold/hydroxyapatite hybrid nanomaterial. Biomaterials. 28. 2147–2154.

Ding Y., Liu J., Jin X., Shen G., Yu R. (2008). A Novel Piezoelectric Immunosensor for CA125 Using a Hydroxyapatite/Chitosan Nanocomposite-Based Biomolecular Immobilization Method. Australian J. Chem. 61(7). 500-505.

Ermolaeva T. N, Kalmykova E. N, Shashkanova O. Yu. (2008). Piezoquartz Biosensors for the Analysis of Environmental Objects, Foodstuff and for Clinical Diagnostic. Rus. J. General Chem. 78 (12). 2430-2444.

Ermolaeva T.N, Kalmykova E.N. (2006). Piezoelectric immunosensors: analytical potentials and outlooks. Rus. Chem. Rev. 75 (5). 397–409.

Fung Y. S. and Wong Y. Y. (2001). Self-Assembled Monolayers as the Coating in a Quartz Piezoelectric Crystal Immunosensor To Detect Salmonella in Aqueous Solution. Anal. Chem. 73 (21). 5302–5309.

Georganopoulou D.G., Carley R., Jones D.A., Boutelle M.G.. (2000). Development and comparison of biosensors for in-vivo applications. Faraday Discuss. 116. 291-303.

Godber B., Frogley M., Rehak M., Sleptsov A., Thompson K.S.J., Uludag Y., and. Cooper M.A (2007). Profiling of molecular interactions in real time using acoustic detection. Biosens. Bioelectron. 22 (9-10), 2382-2386.

Godber B., Thompson K.S.J., Rehak M,, Uludag Y., Kelling S., Sleptsov A., Frogley M, Wiehler K., Whalen Ch., Cooper M.A. (2005). Direct Quantification of Analyte Concentration by Resonant Acoustic Profiling. Clin. Chem. 10. 1962–1972.

Grieshaber D., de Lange V., Hirt T., Lu Z., Voros J. (2008). Vesicles for Signal Amplification in a Biosensor for the Detection of Low Antigen Concentrations. Sensors. 8. 7894-7903.

Guillo Ch., Roper M.G. (2008). Affinity assays for detection of cellular communication and biomarkers. Analyst. 133. 1481–1485.

Han J., Zhang J., Xia Y., Li S., Long J. (2011). An immunoassay in which magnetic beads act both as collectors and sensitive amplifiers for detecting antigens in a microfluidic chip (MFC)–quartz crystal microbalance (QCM) system Colloids and Surfaces A. 31 (28). 1–9.

Harteveld J.L.N., Nieuwenhuizen M.S., Wils E.R.J. (1997). Detection of staphylococcal enterotoxin B employing a piezoelectric crystal immunosensor. Biosens. Bioelectron. 12 (7). 661-667.

He F.J., Zhang L.D, Zhao J.W, Hu B.L, Lei J.T. (2002). A TSM immunosensor for detection of M-tuberculosis with a new membrane material. Sens. Actuators B. 85 (3). 284–290.

Jiang X, Wang R, Wang Y, Su X, Ying Y, Wang J, Li Y.(2011). Evaluation of different micro/nanobeads used as amplifiers in QCM immunosensor for more sensitive detection of E. coli O157:H7. Biosens Bioelectron.

Justino C., Rocha- Santos T., Armando C., Rocha-Santos T. A. (2010). Review of analytical figures of merit of sensors and biosensors in clinical applications. Trends Anal. Chem. 29(10). 1172-1183.

Kalmykova E. N., Dergunova E. S., Ermolaeva T. N.,Gorshkova R. P., Komandrova N. A. (2007). Piezoquartz immunosensors for assessing the interactions between Yersinia enterocolitica lipopolysaccharides and antibodies to them. Applied Biochemistry and Microbiology. 44 (4).372-377.

Kalmykova E. N., Dergunova E. S., Zubova N. Yu., Gorshkova, R. P., Komandrova N. A., Ermolaeva, T. N. (2007). Determination of antibodies to Yersinia enterocolitica bacteria using a piezoelectric quartz crystal immunosensor. J. Anal. Chem. 62 (10). 970-976.

Kalmykova E.N., Dergunova E.S., Ermolaeva T.N., Gorshkova R.P., Komandrova N.A. (2006). Piezoelectric immunosensors on the basis of immobilized lipopolysaccharides for the determining of antibodies to the Yersenia enterocolitica bacteria. Сорбционные и хроматографические процессы. 6. 415-421.

Kalmykova E.N., Garbusova A.V., Shashkanova O.YU., Zubova N.YU., Ermolaeva T.N. (2007). Flow-injection piezoelectric immunosensors for the phage detection. Вестник ВГУ. Серия Химия. Биология. Фармация. 6. 47-56.

Kalmykova E.N., Garbusova A.V., Shashkanova O.YU., Zubova N.YU., Ermolaeva T.N.(2007). Quartz cristal microbalance immunosensors on the base antibodies immobilized for detection of Yersinia Enterocolitica bacteria in water media. Известия вузов. Химия и химическая технология. 50. 10-15.

Kalmykova, E.N., Ermolaeva, T.N., Eremin, S.A. (2002.) The development of piezoelectric immunosensors for the flow-injection analysis of high- and low-molecular compounds. Вестник МГУ. Серия Химия. 43. 399-403.

Keusgen M. (2002). Biosensors: new approaches in drug discovery. Naturwissenschaften. 89. 433-444.

Kim G.-Ho, A. Garth Rand and Stephen V. Letcher (2003). Impedance characterization of a piezoelectric immunosensor part II: Salmonella typhimurium detection using magnetic enhancement. Biosens. Bioelectron. 18 (1). 91-99.

Kim H., Bhunia A. K. (2008). SEL, a Multipathogen Selective Enrichment Broth for Simultaneous Growth of Salmonella enterica, Escherichia coli O157:H7, and Listeria monocytogenes. Appl. Environ. Microbiol. 74 (15). 4853-4866.

Kim N, Park I.S, Kim D.K. (2004). Characteristics of a label-free piezoelectric immunosensor detecting Pseudomonas aeruginosa. Sens. Actuators B. 100 (3). 432–438.

Kim N. H., Bark T. J., Park H. G., Seong G. H. (2007). Highly Sensitive Biomolecule Detection on a Quartz Crystal Microbalance Using Gold Nanoparticles as Signal Amplification Probes. Anal. Sci. 23. 177-181.

Kim N., Kim D.-K., Cho Y.-J. (2009). Development of indirect-competitive quartz crystal microbalance immunosensor for C-reactive protein. Sens. Actuators B. 143(1). 444-448.

Kim N., Kim D.-K., Cho Y.-J. (2010). Gold nanoparticle-based signal augmentation of quartz crystal microbalance immunosensor measuring C-reactive protein. Current Appl Phys. 10(4). 1227-1230

Konig B. and Gratzel M. (1993). Development of a piezoelectric immunosensor for the detection of human erythrocytes. Anal. Chim. Acta. 276. 329-333.

Kosslinger C., Drost S., Abel F., Wolf H., Koch S., Woias P. (1998). The Quarz Crystal Microbalance (QCM) as an Immunosensor. Methods in Molecular Medicine. 13. II. Part 8. 519-529.

Köβlinger C., Uttenthaler E., Drost S., Aberl F, Wolf H., Brin G., Stanglmaier A, Sackmann E. (1995). Comparison of the QCM and the SPR method for surface studies and immunological applications. Sens. Actuators B. 24(1-3). 107-112.

Kubitschko S., Spinke I., Brucker T., Pol S., Oranth N. (1997). Sensitivity Enhancement of Optical Immunosensors with Nanoparticles. Anal. Biochem. 253. 112-122.

Kurosawa S, Aizawa H, Tozuka M, Nakamura M, Park JW. (2003). Immunosensors using a quartz crystal microbalance. Meas Sci. Technol. 14 (11). 1882–1887.

Kurosawa S., Hirokawa T., Kashima K., Aizawa H., Park J.-W., Tozuka M., Yoshimi Y., Hirano K. (2002). Adsorption of anti-C-Reactive Protein Monoclonal Antibody and Its F(ab')2 fragment on Plasma-Polymerized Styrene, Allylamine and Acrylic Acid Coated with Quartz Crystal Microbalance. J. Photopolym. Sci.Technol. 15. 323 -331.

Kurosawa S., Nakamura M., Park J.W., Aizawa H.,Yamada K., Hirata M. (2004). Evaluation of a high-affinity QCM immunosensor using antibody fragmentation and 2-methacryloyloxyethyl phosphorylcholine (MPC) polymer. Biosens. Bioelectron. 2. 1134–1139.

Le D., He F.-J., Jiang T.J., Nie L., Yao Sh., (1995). A goat-anti-human IgG modified piezoimmunosensor for Staphylococcus aureus detection, J. Microbiol Meth. 23 (2). 229-234.

Lee Y., Lee E.K., Cho Y.W., Matsui T., Kan g I. C., Kim T.S., Han M. H. (2003) . ProteoChip: A highly sensitive protein microarray prepared by a novel method of protein immobilization for application of protein-protein interaction studies. Proteomics. 3. 2289-2304.

Li D, Feng Y, Zhou L, Ye Z, Wang J, Ying Y, Ruan Ch, Wang R, Li Y. (2011). Label-free capacitive immunosensor based on quartz crystal Au electrode for rapid and sensitive detection of Escherichia coli O157:H7. Anal Chim Acta. 68 (1). 89-96.

Liu F., Su X.-L, Li Y. (2007). QCM immunosensor with nanoparticle amplification for detection of Escherichia coli O157:H7. Sensing and Instrumentation for Food Quality and Safety. 1. 161-168.

Malhotra B.D., Chaubey A. (2003) Biosensors for clinical diagnostics industry. Sens. Actuators B. 91. 117–127.

Mao Ch., Liu A. (2009). Virus-Based Chemical and Biological Sensing. Angew. Chem. 48(37). 6790–6810.

Martínez-Rivas A., Chinestra P., Favre G., PinaudS., Séverac Ch., Faye J.-Ch., Vieu Ch. (2010). Detection of label-free cancer biomarkers using nickel nanoislands and quartz crystal microbalance. Int. J Nanomedicine. 5. 661-668.

Mascin M., Tombelli S. (2008). Biosensors for biomarkers in medical diagnostics. *TOC*. 13 (7-8). 637-657.

McBride J.D., Cooper M.A. (2008). A high sensitivity assay for the inflammatory marker C-reactive protein employing acoustic biosensing, J. Nanobiotechnol. 6. 5.

Minunni M., Mascini M., Carter R.M., Jacobs M.B., Lubrano G.J., Guilbault G.G. (1996). A quartz crystal microbalance displacement assay for Listeria monocytogenes. Anal. Chim. Acta. 325. 169-174.

Mohammed M.-I. and Desmulliez M. P. Y. (2011). Lab-on-a-chip based immunosensor principles and technologies for the detection of cardiac biomarkers: a review. Lab Chip. 11. 569-595.

Muratsugu M, Ohta F., Miya Y.,.Hosokawa T, Kurosawa S., Kamo N.,.Ikeda H. (1993). Quartz crystal microbalance for the detection of microgram quantities of human serum albumin: relationship between the frequency change and the mass of protein adsorbed. Anal. Chem. 65 (20). 2933-2937.

Nakayama T., Watanabe M., Teramoto T.,Kitajima M. (1997). Slope analysis of CA19-9 and CEA for predicting recurrence in colorectal cancer patients. Anticancer Res. 17. 1379-1382.

P.Skladal, C.S. Riccardi, H. Yamanaka, P.L. Costa. (2004). Piezoelectric biosensors for real-time monitoring of hybridization and detection of the hepatitis C virus. J. Virol. Meth. 117. 145-151.

Park I.S., Kim N. (1998).Thiolated Salmonella antibody immobilization onto the gold surface of piezoelectric quartz crystal. Biosens. Bioelectron. 13 (10). 1091 - 1097.

Pathirana S.T., Barbaree J.,Chin B.A.,.Hartell M.G,.Neely W.C, Vodyanoy V. (2000). Rapid and sensitive biosensor for Salmonella. Biosens. Bioelectron. 15. 135-141.

Plomer M., Guilbault G.G., Hock B. (1992). Development of piezoelectric immunosensor for the detection of Enterobacteria. Enzyme. Microb. Technol. 14. 230 - 238.

Pohanka M., Pavlis O.,.Skladal P. (2007). Diagnosis of tularemia using piezoelectric biosensor technology. Talanta. 71. 981-985.

Pohanka M., Treml F., Hubál M., Band'ouchová H., Beklová M., Pikula J. (2007). Piezoelectric Biosensor for a Simple Serological Diagnosis of Tularemia in Infected European Brown Hares (Lepus europaeus). Sensors. 7. 2825-2834 .

Prusak-Sochaczewski E., Luong J. (1990). Detection of Human Transferrin by the piezoelectric Crystal. Anal. Lett. 23. 183-194.

Reyes P.I., Zhang Z., Chen H., Duan Z., Zhong J., SarafG., Taratula O., Galoppini E., Boustany N. (2009). A ZnO Nanostructure-Based Quartz Crystal Microbalance Device for Biochemical Sensing. IEEE SENSORS JOURNAL. 9 (10). 1302-1307.

Saber R., Mutlu S., Piskin E. (2002). Glow-discharge treated piezoelectric quartz crystals as immunosensors for HSA detection. Biosens. Bioelectron. 17. 727-734.

Sakai G., Saiki T., Uda T., Miura N., Yamazoe N. (1995). Selective and repeatable detection of human serum albumin by using piezoelectric immunosensor. Sensor Actuator B. 24 (25). 134-137.

Sakti S.P., Hauptmann P.,.Zimmermann B, Buhling F., Ansorge S. (2001). Disposable HSA QCM-immunosensor for practical measurement in liquid. Sens. Actuators B. 78. 257-262.

Salmain M, Ghasemi M, Boujday S, Spadavecchia J, Técher C, Val F, Le Moigne V, Gautier M, Briandet R, Pradier CM. (2011). Piezoelectric immunosensor for direct and rapid detection of staphylococcal enterotoxin A (SEA) at the ng level. Biosens Bioelectron. 26.

Sauerbrey G. (1959). Use of quartz vibrator for weighing thing films on microbalance. Z. Phys. 155. 206-210.

Shen Z., Wang J., Qiu Z., Jin M, Wang X., Chen Z., Li J., Cao F. (2011). QCM immunosensor detection of Escherichia coli O157:H7 based on beacon immunomagnetic nanoparticles and catalytic growth of colloidal gold. Biosens Bioelectron. 29 (7). 3376-3381.

Simon E. (2010). Biological and chemical sensors for cancer diagnosis. Meas. Sci. Technol. 21. 1-15.

Skladal P. (2003). Piezoelectric Quartz Crystal Sensors Applied for Bioanalytical Assays and Characterization of Affinity Interactions. J. Braz. Chem. 14. 491-499.

Su X, Low S, Kwang J, Chew V, Li S. (2001). Piezoelectric quartz crystal based veterinary diagnosis for Salmonella enteritidis infection in chicken and egg. Sens. Actuators B. 75(1–2). 29–35.

Su X., Li S. (2001). Serological determination of Helicobacter pylori infection using sandwiched and enzymatically amplified piezoelectric biosensor Anal. Chim. Acta. 429 (1). 27-36.

Su X., Li Y. (2004). A self-assembled monolayer-based piezoelectric immunosensor for rapid detection of Escherichia coli O157: H7. Biosens. Bioelectron. 19 (6). 563–574.

Su X., Li Y. (2005). A QCM immunosensor for Salmonella detection with simultaneous measurements of resonant frequency and motional resistance. Biosens Bioelectron. 21 (6). 840-848.

Su X.D., Chew F.T., Li S.F.Y. (2000). Design and Aplication of Piezoelectric Quartz Crystal-based Immunoassay. Anal. Sci. 16. 107-114.

Su X.D., Chew F.T., Li S.F.Y. (2000). Piezoelectric quartz crystal based label-free analysis for allergy disease. Biosens. Bioelectron. 15. 629–639.

Susmel S., O'Sullivan C.K., Guilbault G.G. (2000).Human cytomegalovirus detection by a quartz crystal microbalance immunosensor. Enzyme Technol. 27. 639–645.

Tanaka N., Okada S., Ueno H., Okusaka T., Ikeda M. (2000). The usefulness of serial changes in serum CA19-9 levels in the diagnosis of pancreatic cancer. Pancreas. 20. 378-381.

Tang D.-Q., Zhang D.-J., Tang D.-Y., Ai H. (2006). Amplification of the antigen-antibody interaction from quartz crystal microbalance immunosensors via back-filling immobilization of nanogold on biorecognition surface. .J. Immunol. Meth. 316 144 -152.

Tang. D., Yuan R., Chai Y. (2008). Quartz crystal microbalance immunoassay for carcinoma antigen 125 based on gold nanowire-functionalized biomimetic interface. Analys. 133. 933-938.

Tatsuta M., Yamamura H., Iishi H.,.Kasugai H, Okuda S. (1986). Value of Serum Alpha-Fetoprotein and Ferritin in the Diagnosis of Hepatocellular Oncology. 43. 306- 310.

U. S. Patent 4,242,096. Immunoassays for Antigens. Oliveira, R.J. and S.F. Silver, December 30, 1980.

U.S. Patent, 4,314,821. Sandwich Immunoassay Using Piezoelectric Oscillator. T.K. Rice, February 9, 1982.

Uenishi T., Kubo S., Hirohashi K., Tanaka H.,Shuto T,Yamamoto T., Nishiguch S. (2003). Cytokeratin-19 fragments in serum (CYFRA 21-1) as a marker in primary liver cancer. S. Br. J. Cance. 88(12). 1894 -1899.

Uludağ Y, Tothill IE. (2010). Development of a sensitive detection method of cancer biomarkers in human serum (75%) using a quartz crystal microbalance sensor and nanoparticles amplification system. Talanta. 82 (1). 277-282.

Vaughan R.D, Guilbault G.G. (2007). Piezoelectric Immunosensors. In: Steinem C, Janshoff A, eds. Piezoelectric Sensors. Vol. 5. Springer Berlin Heidelberg. 237-280.

Vaughan R.D., O'Sullivan C.K., Guilbault G.G.. (2001). Development of a quartz crystal microbalance (QCM) immunosensor for the detection of Listeria monocytogenes. Enzyme. Microb. Technol. 29. 635-639.

Wang H.,.Zeng H, Liu Z.,.Yang Y, Deng T., Shen G., Yu R. (2004). Immunophenotyping of acute leukemias using quartz crystal microbalance and monoclonal antibodies coated magnetic microspheres. Anal Chem. 76. 2571-2578.

Wang L.J., Wu C.S., Hu Z.Y., Zhang Y.F., Li R, Wang P. *(2008)*. Sensing *Escherichia coli* O157:H7 via frequency shift through a self-assembled monolayer based QCM immunosensor. J. Zhejiang. Univ. Sci. B. 9. 121- 131.

Wang R., Dong W., Ruan Ch., Kanayeva D., Lassiter K., Tian R., Li Y. (2008). TiO2 nanowire Jacobs bundle microelectrode based impedance immunosensor for rapid and sensitive detection of Listeria monocytogenes. Nano Lett. 9 (12). 4570 – 4583

Wei Q., Li T., Wang G., Li H., Qian Z., Yang M. (2010). Fe_3O_4 nanoparticles-loaded PEG–PLA polymeric vesicles as labels for ultrasensitive immunosensors. Biomaterials. 31. 7332-7339.

Wong Y.Y., Ng S.P., Ng M.H., Si S.H., Yao S.Z., Fung Y.S. (2002). Immunosensor for the differentiation and detection of Salmonella species based on a quartz crystal microbalance. Biosens. Bioelectron. 17 (8). 676 -684.

Wong-ek K., Chailapakul O., Nuntawong N., Jaruwongrungsee K., Tuantranont A. (2010). Cardiac troponin T detection using polymers coated quartz crystal microbalance as a cost-effective immunosensor. Biomed Tech (Berl). 55 (5). 279-84.

Wu J., Zhifeng F., Yan F., Ju H. (2007). Biomedical and clinical applications of immunoassays and immunosensors for tumor markers. Trends Anal. Chem. 26 (7). 679-688.

Wu Z.-Y., Jian W., Wang S.-P., Yu R.-Q. (2006). An amplified mass piezoelectric immunosensor for Schistosoma japonicum. Biosens. Bioelectron. 22 (2). 207-212.

Wu Z.-Y., Shen G.-L., Wang S.-P., Yu R.-Q. (2003). Quartz-crystal microbalance immunosensor for Schistsoma japonicum-infected rabbit serum. Anal. Sci. 19. 437-440.

Xia C., Guoli S., Feiye X., Rugin Y. (1997). Polymer Agglutination-Based Piezoelectric Immunoassay for the Determination of Human Serum Albumin. Anal. Lett. 30. 1783-1796.

Yang G.-J., Huang J.-L., Meng W.-J., Ming S., Jiao X.-A. (2009). A reusable capacitive immunosensor for detection of Salmonella spp. based on grafted ethylene diamine and self-assembled gold nanoparticle monolayers. Anal. Chimica Acta. 647 (2). 159-166.

Ying-Sing F., Shi-Hui S., De-Rong Z.(2000). Piezoelectric crystal for sensing bacteria by immobilizing antibodies on divinylsulphone activated poly-m-aminophenol film. Talanta. 51 (1). 151–158.

Zeng H., Wang H., Chen F., Xin H, Wang G., Xiao L.,Song K,.Wu D., He Q., Shen G. (2006). Development of quartz-crystal-microbalance-based immunosensor array for clinical immunophenotyping of acute leukemias. Anal. Biochem. 351. 69-76.

Zhang B., Zhang X., Yan H.H., Xu S.J.,.Tang D.H,.Fu W.L. (2007). A novel multi-array immunoassay device for tumor markers based on insert-plug model of piezoelectric immunosensor. Biosens Bioelectron. 23 (1). 19-25.

Zhou X.D., Liu L.J., Hu M., Wang L.L., Hu J.M.. (2002). Detection of hepatitis B virus by piezoelectric biosensor. J. Pharm. Biomed. Anal. 27. 341–345.

6

Label-Free Detection of Botulinum Neurotoxins Using a Surface Plasmon Resonance Biosensor

Hung Tran and Chun-Qiang Liu
Human Protection and Performance Division,
Defence Science and Technology Organisation,
Australia

1. Introduction

Neurotoxins produced by the *Clostridium* genus are the cause of botulism, a neuroparalytic disease (Dembek et al., 2007). Besides *Clostridium botulinum*, strains of other species such as *Clostridium argentinense, Clostridium baratii* and *Clostridium butyricum* can also produce botulinum neurotoxins (BoNTs) (Aureli et al., 1986; Hall et al., 1985). BoNTs are a complex containing the neurotoxin itself (molecular weight of 150 kDa) and its associated non-toxic proteins (Cai et al., 1999; Inoue et al., 1996). After synthesis, BoNTs are activated by a protease, forming a di-chain molecule consisting of a heavy chain (HC) (100 kDa) and a light chain (LC) (50 kDa) linked by a disulfide bond (Singh, 2000). At its C-terminus, the HC binds to the presynaptic membrane through gangliosides and a protein receptor (Cai et al., 2007). The toxin is then internalised by endocytosis whereby the HC N-terminus aids the translocation of the LC into the cell cytoplasm (Montecucco & Molgo, 2005; Simpson, 2004; Singh, 2006). The internalised LC is then able to block the release of acetylcholine by inhibiting the fusion of synaptic vesicles with the plasma membrane (Montecucco & Molgo, 2005; Simpson, 2004; Singh, 2006; Singh, 2000). This is done by cleaving and thereby inactivating the enzymes that carry out the fusion of synaptic vesicles.

BoNTs are the most potent biological toxin known (Arnon et al., 2001; Gill, 1982). There are seven BoNT serotypes, A through G, which are structurally related but antigenically different proteins (Dembek et al., 2007; Wictome et al., 1999). Botulinum neurotoxin A (BoNT/A) is the most potent of the seven serotypes (Poras et al., 2009). For example, just one gram of BoNT/A crystalline toxin, when evenly dispersed and inhaled, would kill more than one million people (Arnon et al., 2001; Hicks et al., 2005). From extrapolation of animal studies, an estimated human dose (assuming a 70-kg person) of BoNT/A that is lethal to 50% (LD50) of a population exposed is approximately 0.09 to 0.15 μg intravenously or intramuscularly, 0.70 to 0.90 μg by inhalation and 70 μg orally (Gill, 1982; Schantz & Johnson, 1992; Scott & Suzuki, 1988). There are no currently licensed vaccines available to prevent botulism. An investigational vaccine, pentavalent botulinum toxoid (PBT), is accessible only to people who are deemed to be at high-risk, such as laboratory workers and military personnel (Bossi et al., 2004).

The extreme potency and lethality, the ease of distribution, and the need for prolonged intensive care among affected individuals make BoNTs ideal bioterror agents and bioweapon threats. A deliberate release of BoNTs in a civilian population may originate from a point-source aerosol release or contamination of a food supply. If successful, such bioterrorist attack would very likely overwhelm the existing public health system (Dembek et al., 2007), leading to public fear and social unrest (Cai et al., 2007). As a result, the US Centers for Disease Control and Prevention (CDC) has classified BoNTs as one of the six highest risk threat agents (Category A agent) for bioterrorism (Arnon et al., 2001). Like many other biological threats, rapid detection of BoNTs, in particular in the environment, food and/or clinical samples, is crucial not only to aid in early supportive care for those affected, but also as the key in minimising and managing the impact of a bioterrorism attack involving such potent toxins.

Currently, the mouse bioassay is the widely accepted standard and approved test for laboratory confirmation of botulism (Barr et al., 2005; Ferreira et al., 2003; Kautter & Solomon, 1977; Sharma et al., 2006; Sugiyama, 1980). In this assay, mice after being given suspected BoNT samples were observed for symptoms of botulism for a period up to four days (Barr et al., 2005; Kulagina et al., 2007). Although sensitive, the mouse bioassay is cumbersome, time–consuming and expensive, and it also presents an ethical dilemma due to the use of large numbers of laboratory animals (Lindstrom & Korkeala, 2006; Varnum et al., 2006). As a result, there has been a concerted effort over the last few decades to develop alternative detection methods, some of which have surpassed the detection limit of the mouse bioassay (Lindstrom & Korkeala, 2006). The majority of these alternative assays are immunoassays, and the specificity and sensitivity of the assays are greatly dependent on the quality of the antibodies used.

In this chapter, we describe the development of a new immunoassay based on a surface plasmon resonance (SPR) biosensor for the detection of botulinum toxin serotypes A and B, using formalin-inactivated toxoids (BoTds). We demonstrate that the SPR assay does not cross-react with other closely-related BoTds, and is able to detect BoTds in environmental aerosol samples.

2. Surface Plasmon Resonance technology

Surface plasmon resonance (SPR) is a biophysical method that monitors real-time biomolecular interaction of two interacting molecules (often named ligand and analyte). Besides real time detection, SPR technology is also able to offer kinetic parameters of the measured biomolecular interaction. It allows the direct determination of separate association (k_a) and dissociation (k_d) rate constants; only a few techniques to date are able to offer this kind of information (Hahnefeld et al., 2004). The knowledge of separate k_a and k_d rate constants is valuable in characterising and selecting the most effective binding partners whether they are for applications of drug discovery or detection. Another major advantage of the SPR over other traditional methods is its label-free detection. Fluorescence and luminescence detections in enzyme-linked immunosorbent assays (ELISA) or radioactive labelling in radioimmunoassays (RIA), in some cases, may not seem favourable, as the labelled tag may occupy important binding sites or cause steric hindrance which could interfere with the biomolecular recognition and interaction events (Gopinath, 2010). Another drawback in labelling of materials for biomolecular interaction is the additional steps required; some can be difficult.

SPR enables real time monitoring of a binding event between an immobilised ligand and a free flowing analyte in solution. It is the measurement of this interaction that underpins the basis of how a SPR biosensor works. To understand the optical phenomenon of SPR, one must understand the physics of light and its behaviours under certain conditions. When a beam of light at a particular angle (termed as the angle of incidence, θ) strikes at the interface of two materials with different refractive indices; one material (glass) having a refractive index higher than the other material (biological buffer solution), the light is completely reflected. This is known as total internal reflection. This total internal reflection continues until the angle of incidence reaches a critical angle, θ_C; at this angle some of the light is refracted across the interface (Figure 1a). If a semi-transparent noble metal (in this example, gold) film is thinly coated on one side of the glass surface (the side that is exposed to buffer solution) then under conditions described above for total internal reflection, surface plasmon resonance can occur. The reason is that at a particular light incident angle, known as the surface plasmon resonance angle, θ_{spr}, total internal reflection will not occur (Figure 1b), because some of the light energy is 'transferred' to the metallic gold film. If the intensity of the reflected light is plotted against the angle of incidence, we will observe that at θ_{spr} angle the intensity of reflected light is at its minimum (Figure 1c).

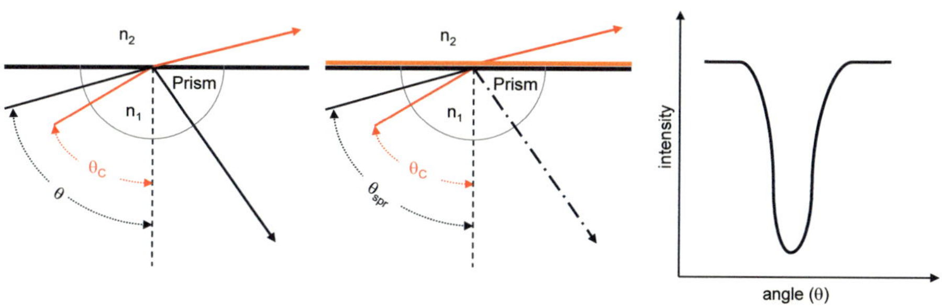

a. b. c.

Fig. 1. Schematic diagram of surface plasmon resonance phenomenon. The refractive indices of glass and buffer solution are n_1 and n_2, respectively; where $n_1 > n_2$. Refracted beam at the critical angle, θ_c, is shown in red. At angles greater than θ_c, light is completely reflected (**a**). When a thin metallic gold film is coated onto one side of the glass surface, at the surface plasmon resonance angle, θ_{spr}, light will not be completely reflected (**b**). Instead, some of the light energy is transferred to the gold film causing a drop in the intensity of the reflected light at θ_{spr} angle (**c**).

The θ_{spr} angle is sensitive to a number of factors such as the incident light wavelength, the nature and thickness of the conducting film and the temperature (Hahnefeld et al., 2004). If all these factors are kept constant, then any shift in the θ_{spr} angle will purely be dependent on the refractive index of the buffer solution medium at close proximity to the interface. Changes in the refractive index of this medium during binding events of immobilised ligands and free flowing analytes can then be closely monitored via any shifts in the θ_{spr} angle by a photo-detector array equipped as a biosensor instrument. The measurement of the photo-detector array can be visually plotted (Figure 2a). The biosensor instrument processor would convert and quantify these small changes in the θ_{spr} angle to absolute resonance units or response units (RU), and plot them against time as sensorgrams (Figure

2b), where 1 RU is equivalent to a small change in the θ_{spr} angle of about 10^{-4} degrees (Hahnefeld et al., 2004).

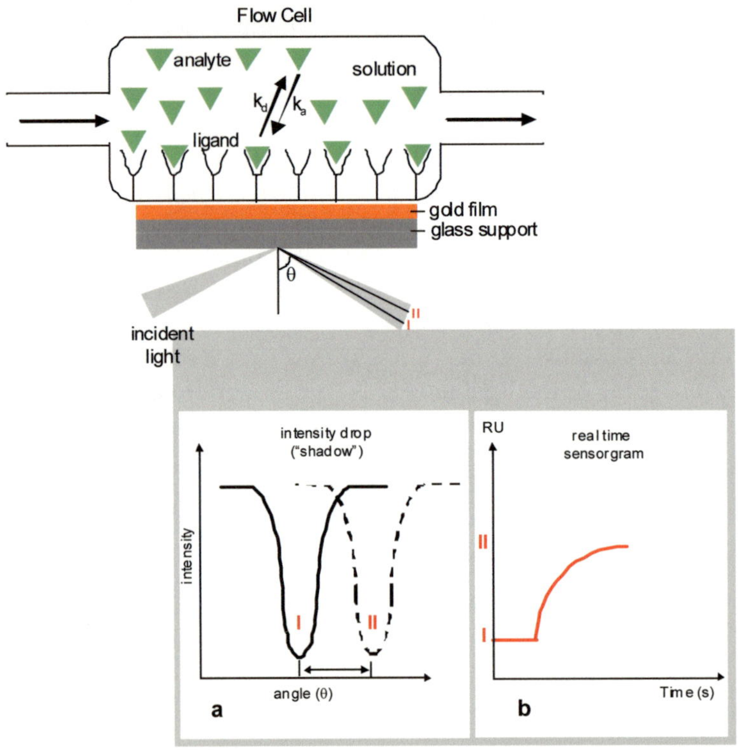

Fig. 2. Schematic illustration of a surface plasmon resonance biosensor. The direction flow of analyte solution is as indicated. As analytes come into contact with immobilised ligands, associations (k_a) and dissociations (k_d) between the molecules occur. These binding interactions, monitored in real time, will shift the θ_{spr} angle from I to II – visually plotted as reflected light intensity against angle of incidence (**a**). The biosensor will process this change in θ_{spr} angle to absolute resonance or response units (RU) and plots the result as a sensorgram (**b**).

SPR-based biosensors have been used increasingly in the past decade, especially in the post-genomic era where the need to understand the function of biologically important molecules are ever increasing (Gopinath, 2010). The technology is widely used to generate bio-recognition information from protein-protein, lipid-protein, nucleic acids and molecular interactions. This information will aid in the screening, discovery and development of therapeutic antibodies and new drugs, the detection and analysis of human pathogens and toxins; and also as a research tool in aptamer selection, epitope mapping, antibody development, ligand fishing and mutant analysis to name a few.

In any application of SPR technology, a single or multiple ligands of interest will need to be firstly immobilised onto the surface of a sensorchip. Ligands can be chemically immobilised onto the sensorchip surface by covalent coupling via primary amines, aldehydes or reactive thiols. Alternatively, high-affinity and specific capture of ligands can also be performed via streptavidin interactions, fusion tags, interactions between antibodies or ligand-specific interactions. This step aims to change the surface chemistry in preparation for subsequent interaction with injected free-flowing analytes. When analyte solution is flown over ligands; immobilised or captured, the interactions between the molecules are monitored in real time. A sensorgram is shown in Figure 3, three phases are involved in a typical biomolecular interaction study on a SPR biosensor.

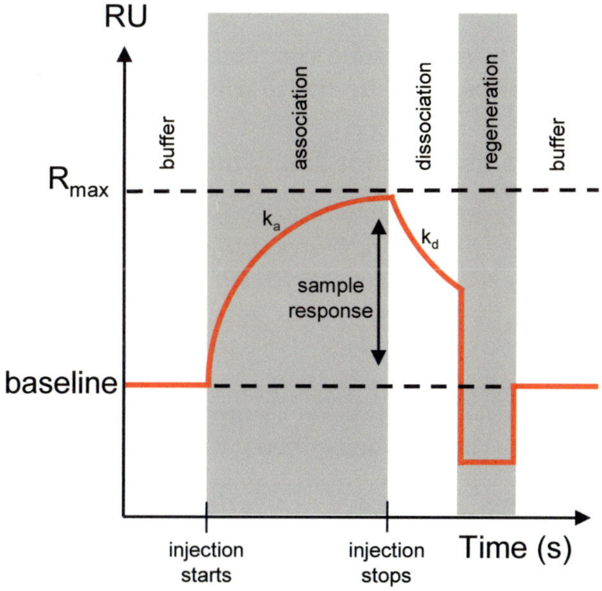

Fig. 3. A typical SPR sensorgram showing the three phases involve in a biomolecular interaction study. The three phases are: association, dissociation and regeneration.

These phases are association, dissociation and regeneration. Understanding the events and significance of each phase is important, as they are required in obtaining kinetic data about the interaction; such as the association (k_a) and dissociation (k_d) rate constants as well as the apparent equilibrium binding constant (k_D or k_A). In an SPR experiment, biomolecular interaction analysis can only be performed after a stable sensorgram baseline is achieved with continuous running buffer flown over immobilised or captured ligands. In the association phase, an analyte solution is injected and flown over the ligand surface where biomolecular interaction between the two, if exists, will occur. This interaction is amplified by an increase in the response unit (RU) on the sensorgram as shown in Figure 3. As more interactions take place between analytes and ligands this will also translate to a corresponding increase in the RU on the sensorgram, which will continue until it reaches its highest binding RU value, usually at the end of an analyte injection. This highest RU sometime can also be the maximum binding capacity (R_{max}). This occurs when analytes are fast and strong binders to the ligand causing these analytes to fully occupy all available ligand binding sites.

Dissociation phase starts when the injection of the analyte solution stops and the system switches to continuous flow of running buffer. Under this condition, dissociation between analytes and ligands is greatly favoured over association. As analytes dissociate from ligands, this event is reflected by a decrease in RU on the sensorgram as shown in Figure 3. In many cases, analyte dissociation is never complete or it takes far too long to observe complete dissociation. Hence, an additional step to aid this process may be incorporated into the regeneration phase, which involves the injection of an appropriate regeneration solution to remove excess bound analytes that have not yet dissociated. The ultimate goal is to elute non-covalently bound analytes but at the same time not adversely disrupt the biological activity of the ligand in the process. At the end of the regeneration phase, a baseline RU is reached and ready for subsequent use, hence saving time and resources. However, it is often that ideal regeneration conditions are hard and time consuming to establish, in which cases it may be more effective to settle for non-ideal regeneration.

3. Reagents and instruments used for assay development

Several anti-BoNT rabbit polyclonal antibodies (PAb), purchased from Metabiologics Inc (Wisconsin, USA), were used as the ligands in this study; they were Anti-BoNT/A PAb (Lot. No. A011708-01) and Anti-BoNT/B PAb (Lot No. B082203-01), each supplied in 100 mM Tris/glycine buffer (pH 7.9). Purified botulinum toxins (BoNTs) and formalin-inactivated toxoids (BoTds) (also from Metabiologics Inc) were used as the analytes, including BoNT/A (Lot No. A031009-01), BoNT/B (Lot No. B031009-01), BoTd/A (Lot No. A090805-01) and BoTd/B (Lot No. B090705-01). The toxins were supplied in 0.22 μm filtered phosphate-buffered saline (PBS) (pH 7.0). All toxins and antibodies were kept refrigerated before use.

For enzyme linked immunosorbent assay (ELISA), the following buffers were prepared: coating buffer [0.05 M carbonate-bicarbonate buffer, pH 9.6]; wash buffer [PBS containing 0.05% Tween 20 (PBST)]; blocking solution and reagent diluent [3% skim milk in PBST (M-PBST)]. Substrate para-nitrophenyl phosphate (pNPP) tablets were purchased from Sigma-Aldrich (Sydney, Australia). A working volume of 100 μl per well was used in the ELISA, except for the blocking step, which was 350 μl per well. BoNTs or BoTds, diluted in coating buffer, were coated onto the wells of a Nunc-Immuno MaxiSorp microtitre plate (Invitro Technologies, Melbourne, Australia, cat. no. 43954) and incubated overnight at 4°C (~ 16 hours). Antibodies were subsequently added, all of which were diluted in M-PBST. Incubations of primary (anti-BoNT PAb at 0.5 μg/ml) and secondary (anti-rabbit IgG-AP diluted 1:10,000) antibodies were carried out for 1 hour at room temperature with shaking. After each incubation step, the plate was washed with PBST (3 X 350 μl per well). The final washing step (after anti-rabbit IgG-AP incubation) involved PBST washes (3 times) and a distilled water wash. This was followed by the addition of substrate solution. Substrate incubation was 1 hour at room temperature with shaking before the plate was read at wavelength 405 nm.

The instruments used included the SPR BIAcore® X (GE Healthcare, NSW, Australia), Labsystems Wellwash Mk2 plate washer (Pathtech, Melbourne, Australia), Ratek plate shaker (Ratek Instruments, Melbourne, Australia) and Labsystems Multiskan Ascent Photometric plate reader (Pathtech, Melbourne, Australia). The BIAcore® X system comprises the BIAcore® X instrument, BIAcore® X Control Software (Version 2.2) and BIAevaluation software (Version 4.1). The following reagents were also purchased from GE Healthcare: CM5 sensor chip (research grade), HBS-EP running buffer (0.01 M HEPES pH 7.4, 0.15 M NaCl, 3 mM EDTA and 0.005% v/v Surfactant P20), and amine coupling kit containing 115 mg/ml N-hydroxysuccinimide (NHS), 750 mg/ml 1-ethyl-3-(3-dimethylamino-propyl) carbodiimide hydrochloride (EDC) and 1.0 M ethanolamine-HCl, pH 8.5. All other chemicals used for buffer preparations were purchased from Sigma-Aldrich (Sydney, Australia).

4. Surface functionalisation

In the SPR assay system, specific antibodies need to be immobilised onto the surface of a SPR sensor chip in order to create favourable surface chemistry that is necessary for interaction between BoTd and its antibody. In this study, commercial PAbs produced in rabbits immunised with BoNT/A and BoNT/B were immobilised onto a CM5 sensor chip. Firstly, carboxymethylated dextrans covalently attached to the gold surface of the sensor chip were activated by chemical treatment to form N-hydroxysuccinimide esters. This was performed with an injection (35 μl) of a mixture of equal volumes of EDC and NHS at a flow rate of 5 μl/min. This activation permitted the reactive succinimide ester surface to covalently bind injected anti-BoNT PAbs (50 μl at concentration of 50 μg/ml diluted in immobilisation buffer, 10 mM sodium acetate, pH 4.5) via its free amino groups. A final 35 μl injection of 1 M ethanolamine, pH 8.5 was passed over the sensor chip surface to deactivate and block residual active esters from any further reaction.

The assay procedure involved injecting a continuous flow of sample solution (50 μl at a flow rate of 5 μl/min), over a sensor chip surface immobilised with a specific antibody. This sample solution first passed over a blank control channel (Flow Cell 1) before flowing over an anti-BoNT PAb immobilised surface channel (Flow Cell 2). Interactions between the injected BoTd and the immobilised anti-BoNT PAb were monitored by plotting the output signal as a sensorgram. During the injection period, BoTd detection could be observed in real-time from rising sensorgram signal. At the completion of sample injection, the final observed sensorgram signal in resonance units (RU) corresponded to the maximum binding that had occurred for a particular sample. At the chosen flow rate of 5 μl/min, an assay took approximately 10 minutes to complete. At the completion of an assay, the sensor chip was regenerated for further assays. This was performed by injecting short pulses of a regeneration buffer over the sensor chip surface to remove non-covalently bound BoTd. The regeneration buffer chosen for this assay was 10 mM glycine-HCl, pH 1.75 with 0.01% (v/v) Tween 20. The generated sensorgram data was analysed by the BIAevaluation software (Version 4.1).

5. Assay development and optimisation

Our preliminary ELISA results revealed that the two anti-toxin PAbs could recognise both the native toxins and the formalin-inactivated toxoids for serotypes A and B (data not shown). For safety reasons, only the toxoids were used for the BIAcore® X system. Each CM5 sensor chip contained two flow cells, but only one of which (i.e. Flow Cell 2) had anti-BoNT PAbs immobilised. The difference in Resonance Units (ΔRU) obtained between pre-ligand (anti-BoNT PAb) injection and post sensor chip deactivation indicates the amount of anti-BoNT PAb immobilised. As a general rule, 1 ng of immobilised antibodies per mm^2 equates to approximately 1,000 RU. For our anti-BoNT PAbs used, ΔRU values in the range of 2,500 to 3,500 RU were obtained consistently using the immobilisation conditions described above. This corresponds to approximately 2.5 to 3.5 ng of anti-BoNT PAbs immobilised per mm^2 for either serotype. On the same sensor chip, Flow Cell 1 was used as a negative control, for which the same immobilisation procedure was carried out without ligand injection. This means the surface on Flow Cell 1 was activated, exposed to ligand-free immobilisation solution and deactivated. Flow Cell 1 was required for non-specific and background signal corrections as sample solution was injected onto the sensor chip flowing through Flow Cell 1 first and then onto Flow Cell 2.

A flow rate of 5 μl/min was selected in order to enhance binding conditions of the assay. This slow flow rate allowed sufficient time for the injected BoTds and the immobilised anti-BoNT PAbs to interact. Samples containing BoTd/A or BoTd/B at various concentrations were each assayed in triplicate to determine the assay's standard deviation and co-efficient of variation. After each sample injection, sensorgram signals (RU) at intervals of 50 μl and 100 μl were recorded and plotted (Figure 4). Similar detection signals were obtained with each serotype SPR assay even though each sensor chip had different anti-BoNT PAbs immobilised on it. As predicted, at the same BoTd concentration, SPR detection signals observed at 100 μl of the loaded sample were greater than that of 50 μl. The increase in detection signals obtained from injections of 100 μl of sample compared to 50 μl was less than two-fold. This increase was not deemed significant to justify doubling of the assay time (at flow rate of 5 μl/min, an assay of 100 μl injection would take 20 minutes to complete). On the other hand, a 50 μl sample injection would only require 10 minutes to complete an assay and still produced considerable and observable RU signals. Therefore, it was concluded that a sample injection volume of 50 μl, corresponding to an assay time of just 10 minutes, would be appropriate, sufficient and beneficial for rapid detection methods such as this SPR assay.

The co-efficient of variations amongst the triplicate results varied from 5% to 13% (data not shown). Compared to other similar SPR assays, these values were considered to be relatively high although they were still acceptable. Ineffective regeneration conditions could be a reason for this higher than expected variation. Ideally, conditions for sensor chip regeneration should be such that they are harsh enough to dissociate all bound analytes while at the same time having minimal to neutral effects on immobilised antibodies of the assay. Despite repeated efforts, the final procedure developed for the assay regeneration in this study does not appear to be optimal and effective (data not shown). This could result in (i) ineffective dissociation of the bound BoTds and/or (ii) partial inactivation of the anti-BoNT PAbs immobilised on the sensor surface. Either or both of these could reduce the number of accessible binding sites after each regeneration cycle, hence leading to higher than expected variations in replicate results.

Based on experimental results, the assay's limit of detection (LOD) was estimated to be less than 50 ng of loaded BoTd amounts, for either serotype (Figure 4). For BoTd amounts below the LOD, RU signals were found to be in the range of 1 to 4 RU. This RU signal range was similar to or below that of the assay LOD signal. This indicates that the assay signal had reached its lower limit, hence stabilising around this RU range even at sub LOD levels. Compared to a blank control injection, negative RU values were often observed.

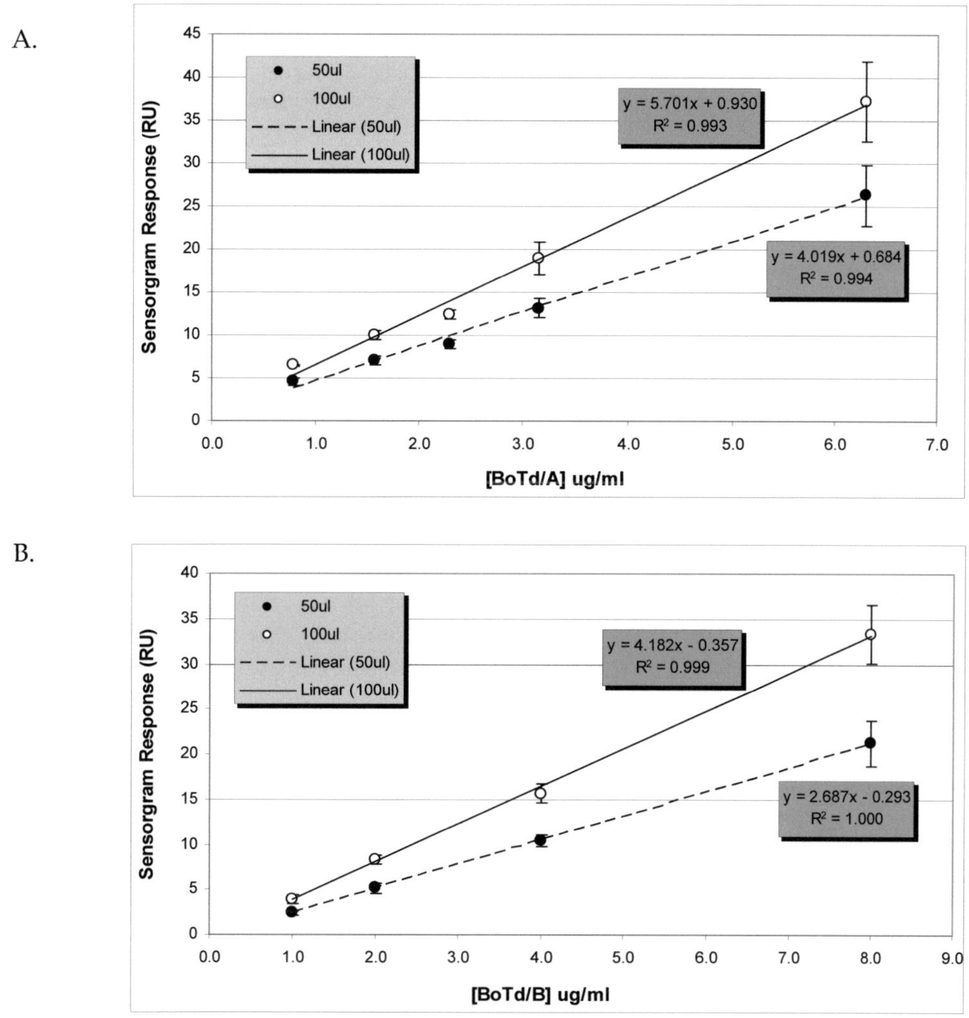

Fig. 4. SPR assay derived standard curves for BoTds; serotypes A (A) and B (B). Error bars are mean ± standard deviation where n = 3.

6. Detection of environmental samples and cross-reactivity

Environmental aerosol samples were collected at different Melbourne sites using a horizontal wet wall cyclone (HWWC). The cyclone is a large volume air sampler that collects ambient aerosol particles at the rate of ~800 litres of air per minute and concentrates these particles into a 10 ml solution. This solution, termed cyclone buffer, was made up of water and Tween 80 (0.01% v/v). These liquid samples were centrifuged and the supernatants were collected as environmental samples (ES). Five ES were assayed, each sample was spiked with BoTds (50 ng loading amounts). Table 1 shows that the assay could be used to detect BoTds, albeit with reduced sensitivity, in environmental aerosol samples. The reduced signals obtained from these spiked ES, compared to spiked cyclone buffer, may suggest inhibitory effects on assay sensitivity from ES testing.

Sample	Recovery (%)	
	BoTd/A	BoTd/B
cyclone buffer	100.0 (13.3)	100.0 (7.7)
ES00338	59.3 (15.2)	72.6 (6.5)
ES00352	45.3 (11.5)	26.3 (5.0)
ES00285	58.7 (8.9)	51.6 (8.4)
ES00316	59.3 (7.2)	51.6 (5.1)
ES00304	87.3 (9.8)	90.7 (5.2)

Table 1.BoTd-spiked environmental samples. An amount of 50 ng of toxoid was loaded onto the sensor chip for each sample. Percentage recovery was calculated based on spiked cyclone buffer signal. Each sample was assayed in duplicate. Values next to recovery percentage, in brackets, are the calculated percentage CV.

A simple examination of the assay for cross-reactivity was performed by observing the detection signal generated by another closely related serotype toxoid, in this case, an injection of BoTd/A onto anti-BoNT/B PAb immobilised sensor chip, and vice-versa. Neither SPR assay showed any cross-reactivity with its related serotype BoTd. The RU signals generated are shown in Table 2. Visually, there was little or no cross-reactivity in either SPR assay, as illustrated by the respective sensorgrams, shown in Figure 5.

Immobilised Sensor Chip	RU signal	
	BoTd/A	BoTd/B
Anti-BoNT/A PAb	22.0	2.3
Anti-BoNT/B PAb	3.6	44.0

Table 2. SPR assay cross-reactivity testing using toxoids BoTd/A and BoTd/B, each loaded at 250 ng onto the sensor chip.

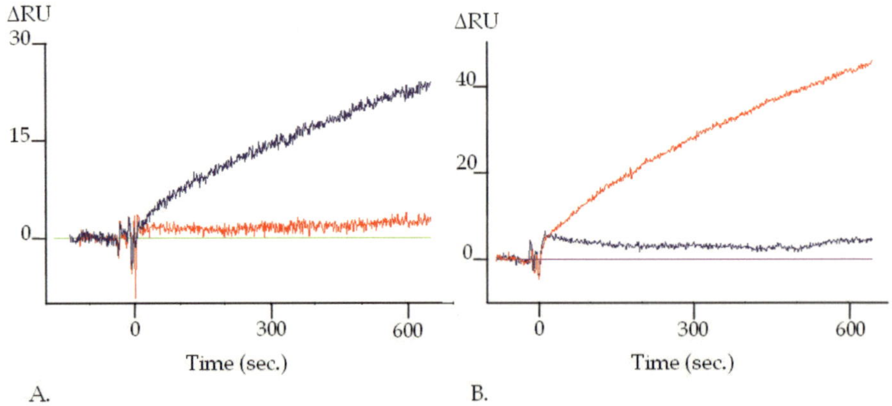

Fig. 5. SPR assay sensorgrams showing minimal cross-reactivity for (A) toxoid BoTd/A and (B) BoTd/B.

7. Estimation of assay sensitivity for active toxins

To estimate the sensitivity of the SPR assay to detect active toxins, ELISA was used to evaluate the two anti-BoNT PAbs used in the SPR assay for their relative binding affinities to the toxins and their toxoids. Toxins BoNT/A and BoNT/B and their corresponding toxoids were coated separately onto the wells of microtitre plates. These analytes were then assayed using their respective anti-BoNT PAbs. ELISA detection signals, measured as optical density (OD) at 405 nm, at various BoNT and BoTd concentrations were plotted for comparisons. Typical ELISA signal curves of BoNTs and BoTds are shown in Figure 6. The anti-BoNT PAbs were found to have a higher binding affinity for the toxins than for the toxoids for both serotypes. Based on the data obtained, both BoNTs were calculated to be at least 40-fold more reactive than their counter-part BoTds with the anti-BoNT PAbs. This was to be expected because the anti-BoNT PAbs were raised specifically against the BoNTs, hence they recognised the BoNTs more favourably and effectively than the BoTds. From the correlation curves, the detection limit of our SPR assay of 50 ng for toxoids can be estimated to an approximate amount of 1.3 ng for BoNTs.

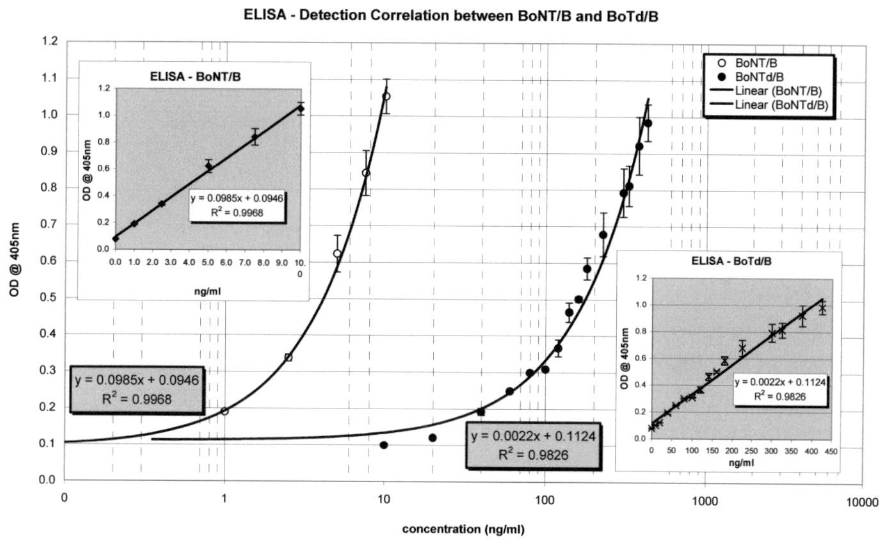

Fig. 6. Correlations in detection sensitivity between toxin BoNT/B and toxoid BoTd/B. ELISA signal, OD at 405 nm, plotted against coated toxin or toxoid concentrations.

The stability of the toxins stored at 4 °C was also investigated. It was found that ELISA signals obtained for 5 ng/ml of coated toxins were gradually reduced over a period of a year, despite refrigeration storage of the toxins. The signals reduced significantly, more than 50 percent, within 6 months of toxin production and it appeared that the rate of degradation was greater for BoNT/A than for BoNT/B (data not shown). This is in agreement with other publications that BoNT itself is less stable than BoNT complex (Brandau et al., 2007). The complex consists of BoNT and its non-toxic associated proteins, which is believed to protect the neurotoxin against damage from exposure to extreme conditions. The increased thermal stability of the BoNT complex may have risen from the internal structure of the complex generated by interactions between BoNT itself and the associated non-toxic proteins (Brandau et al., 2007).

8. Discussion and concluding remarks

Here, we report the development of a real-time optical SPR assay using formalin inactivated toxins, BoTds. The data were then correlated back to their active toxin BoNT values by assessing the same anti-BoNT PAbs for their binding affinities to both BoNTs and BoTds in an ELISA setting. This indirect evaluation of an SPR assay for BoNT detection is less than ideal, but it is a requirement for the SPR instrument due to safety concerns. Unlike other models, the BIAcore® X does not have an enclosed sample injection compartment or an automatic injector. Therefore, samples need to be manually injected into the BIAcore® X in an open area environment where toxin aerolisation and inhalation would pose a possible risk.

The SPR assay developed has several advantages over other assays in that it is rapid, provides real-time detection following sample injection, and requires no reagents to be labelled. The assay has an estimated LOD of 1.3 ng of loaded BoNTs for both serotypes, a value obtained based on BoTd experimental data. A similar SPR assay has been previously reported by Ladd et al (Ladd et al., 2008), which, however, requires at least 60 minutes to complete an assay plus a further 2 hours for preparation prior to the actual assay. In comparison, our SPR assay takes only 10 minutes to complete, and in fact, the entire procedure from antibody immobilisation to completing an SPR assay takes less than 40 minutes. Furthermore, our assay does not require the preparation for antibody biotinylation, purification and immobilisation and the addition of another antibody to achieve the LOD.

Examples of other technologies being used for BoNT detection include ELISA (Ferreira et al., 2003; Poli et al., 2002; Sharma et al., 2006; Wictome et al., 1999; Wictome et al., 1999), mass spectrometry (Barr et al., 2005; Boyer et al., 2005; Kalb et al., 2005; Kalb et al., 2006), enzyme-amplified protein micro-array immunoassay (Varnum et al., 2006), fluorometric biosensor (Dong et al., 2004), and a modified immunoassay (Bagramyan et al., 2008), which measures the intrinsic metalloprotease activity with a fluorogenic substrate. Although some of these assays are more sensitive than the SPR assay, they do not offer real-time detection, often require antibodies to be labelled, which can create problems in antibody-antigen recognition, and most importantly these assays are laborious. Assays based on polymerase chain reaction (PCR) have also been reported; however, these assays can only detect the presence of residual bacterial DNA if present in BoNT samples (Fach et al., 2009; Lindstrom & Korkeala, 2006). Therefore, they are not applicable to toxin samples of high purity (i.e. toxin samples where they do not contain any residual bacterial DNA).

The option of incorporating another antibody into our SPR assay was not investigated. This additional step would theoretically provide a larger SPR response, effectively amplifying the output signal and increasing the assay sensitivity. The significance of enhanced sensitivity should be investigated to determine whether the benefit warrants a longer assay time.

Successful regeneration of sensor chip surface is critical for any SPR assay as it allows multiple assays to be performed. An ideal regeneration condition should be such that it dissociates and removes all bound molecules but does not damage the biological activity of immobilised antibodies on the chip. The present assay has a coefficient of variation ranging from 5% to 13 %, which was a rather high value compared to other SPR assays. This could be caused by an ineffective regeneration of the chip surface. It was also possible that the immobilised antibody surface might have been damaged or that the bound BoTds might have not been effectively removed. Either, or both, of these would contribute to a reduction in the number of accessible binding sites after each regeneration cycle.

The cross reactivity of the assay was evaluated against two closely related serotypes BoTd/A and BoTd/B. Although the experiment was simple and limited, our results showed that the assay did not cross-react with its closely related BoTd serotype, suggesting minimal cross-reactivity issues with other non-related toxins. Both assays also detected BoTd-spiked environmental samples, although all signals were reduced when compared to spiked cyclone buffers. The signal reduction suggests possible inhibitory effects of the sample on the immobilised anti-BoNT PAbs, and consequently on their assay sensitivity. Further studies with a larger number of environmental samples should be performed to provide more information concerning the detection of native toxins in different sample matrices and cross-reactivity with other toxins or contaminants. In addition, more stable anti-BoNT antibodies should be sought because like other immunoassays, the SPR assay also relies heavily on the use of high quality antibodies that are not only highly specific for their targets but are also able to withstand the harsh regeneration process.

9. Acknowledgement

We thank Dr Ray Dawson for critical reading of the manuscript.

10. References

Arnon, S. S., Schechter, R., Inglesby, T. V., Henderson, D. A., Bartlett, J. G., Ascher, M. S., Eitzen, E., Fine, A. D., Hauer, J., Layton, M., Lillibridge, S., Osterholm, M. T., O'Toole, T., Parker, G., Perl, T. M., Russell, P. K., Swerdlow, D. L. & Tonat, K. (2001). Botulinum toxin as a biological weapon: medical and public health management. *Jama*, 285(8), 1059-70.

Aureli, P., Fenicia, L., Pasolini, B., Gianfranceschi, M., McCroskey, L. M. & Hatheway, C. L. (1986). Two cases of type E infant botulism caused by neurotoxigenic Clostridium butyricum in Italy. *J Infect Dis*, 154(2), 207-11.

Bagramyan, K., Barash, J. R., Arnon, S. S. & Kalkum, M. (2008). Attomolar detection of botulinum toxin type A in complex biological matrices. *PLoS One*, 3(4), e2041.

Barr, J. R., Moura, H., Boyer, A. E., Woolfitt, A. R., Kalb, S. R., Pavlopoulos, A., McWilliams, L. G., Schmidt, J. G., Martinez, R. A. & Ashley, D. L. (2005). Botulinum neurotoxin detection and differentiation by mass spectrometry. *Emerg Infect Dis*, 11(10), 1578-83.

Bossi, P., Tegnell, A., Baka, A., van Loock, F., Hendriks, J., Werner, A., Maidhof, H. & Gouvras, G. (2004). Bichat guidelines for the clinical management of botulism and bioterrorism-related botulism. *Euro Surveill*, 9(12), E13-4.

Boyer, A. E., Moura, H., Woolfitt, A. R., Kalb, S. R., McWilliams, L. G., Pavlopoulos, A., Schmidt, J. G., Ashley, D. L. & Barr, J. R. (2005). From the mouse to the mass spectrometer: detection and differentiation of the endoproteinase activities of botulinum neurotoxins A-G by mass spectrometry. *Anal Chem*, 77(13), 3916-24.

Brandau, D. T., Joshi, S. B., Smalter, A. M., Kim, S., Steadman, B. & Middaugh, C. R. (2007). Stability of the Clostridium botulinum type A neurotoxin complex: an empirical phase diagram based approach. *Mol Pharm*, 4(4), 571-82.

Cai, S., Sarkar, H. K. & Singh, B. R. (1999). Enhancement of the endopeptidase activity of botulinum neurotoxin by its associated proteins and dithiothreitol. *Biochemistry*, 38(21), 6903-10.

Cai, S., Singh, B. R. & Sharma, S. (2007). Botulism diagnostics: from clinical symptoms to in vitro assays. *Crit Rev Microbiol*, 33(2), 109-25.

Dembek, Z. F., Smith, L. A. & Rusnak, J. M. (2007). Botulism: cause, effects, diagnosis, clinical and laboratory identification, and treatment modalities. *Disaster Med Public Health Prep*, 1(2), 122-34.

Dong, M., Tepp, W. H., Johnson, E. A. & Chapman, E. R. (2004). Using fluorescent sensors to detect botulinum neurotoxin activity in vitro and in living cells. *Proc Natl Acad Sci U S A*, 101(41), 14701-6.

Fach, P., Micheau, P., Mazuet, C., Perelle, S. & Popoff, M. (2009). Development of real-time PCR tests for detecting botulinum neurotoxins A, B, E, F producing Clostridium botulinum, Clostridium baratii and Clostridium butyricum. *J Appl Microbiol*, 107(2), 465-73.

Ferreira, J. L., Maslanka, S., Johnson, E. & Goodnough, M. (2003). Detection of botulinal neurotoxins A, B, E, and F by amplified enzyme-linked immunosorbent assay: collaborative study. *J AOAC Int*, 86(2), 314-31.

Gill, D. M. (1982). Bacterial toxins: a table of lethal amounts. *Microbiol Rev*, 46(1), 86-94.

Gopinath, S. C. B. (2010). Biosensing applications of surface plasmon resonance-based Biacore technology. *Sensors and Actuators B*, 150, 722-723.

Hahnefeld, C., Drewianka, S. & Herberg, F. W. (2004). Determination of kinetic data using surface plasmon resonance biosensors. *Methods Mol Med*, 94, 299-320.

Hall, J. D., McCroskey, L. M., Pincomb, B. J. & Hatheway, C. L. (1985). Isolation of an organism resembling Clostridium barati which produces type F botulinal toxin from an infant with botulism. *J Clin Microbiol*, 21(4), 654-5.

Hicks, R. P., Hartell, M. G., Nichols, D. A., Bhattacharjee, A. K., van Hamont, J. E. & Skillman, D. R. (2005). The medicinal chemistry of botulinum, ricin and anthrax toxins. *Curr Med Chem*, 12(6), 667-90.

Inoue, K., Fujinaga, Y., Watanabe, T., Ohyama, T., Takeshi, K., Moriishi, K., Nakajima, H., Inoue, K. & Oguma, K. (1996). Molecular composition of Clostridium botulinum type A progenitor toxins. *Infect Immun*, 64(5), 1589-94.

Kalb, S. R., Goodnough, M. C., Malizio, C. J., Pirkle, J. L. & Barr, J. R. (2005). Detection of botulinum neurotoxin A in a spiked milk sample with subtype identification through toxin proteomics. *Anal Chem*, 77(19), 6140-6.

Kalb, S. R., Moura, H., Boyer, A. E., McWilliams, L. G., Pirkle, J. L. & Barr, J. R. (2006). The use of Endopep-MS for the detection of botulinum toxins A, B, E, and F in serum and stool samples. *Anal Biochem*, 351(1), 84-92.

Kautter, D. A. & Solomon, H. M. (1977). Collaborative study of a method for the detection of Clostridium botulinum and its toxins in foods. *J Assoc Off Anal Chem*, 60(3), 541-5.

Kulagina, N. V., Anderson, G. P., S., L. F., M., S. K. & Taitt, C. R. (2007). Antimicrobial Peptides: New Recognition Molecules for Detecting Botulinum Toxins. *Sensors*, 7, 2808-2824.

Ladd, J., Taylor, A. D., Homola, J. & Jiang, S. (2008). Detection of botulinum neurotoxins in buffer and honey using surface plasmon resonance (SPR) sensor. *Sensors and Actuators B*, 130, 129-134.

Lindstrom, M. & Korkeala, H. (2006). Laboratory diagnostics of botulism. *Clin Microbiol Rev*, 19(2), 298-314.

Montecucco, C. & Molgo, J. (2005). Botulinal neurotoxins: revival of an old killer. *Curr Opin Pharmacol*, 5(3), 274-9.

Poli, M. A., Rivera, V. R. & Neal, D. (2002). Development of sensitive colorimetric capture ELISAs for Clostridium botulinum neurotoxin serotypes E and F. *Toxicon*, 40(6), 797-802.

Poras, H., Ouimet, T., Orng, S. V., Fournie-Zaluski, M. C., Popoff, M. R. & Roques, B. P. (2009). Detection and quantification of botulinum neurotoxin type a by a novel rapid in vitro fluorimetric assay. *Appl Environ Microbiol*, 75(13), 4382-90.

Schantz, E. J. & Johnson, E. A. (1992). Properties and use of botulinum toxin and other microbial neurotoxins in medicine. *Microbiol Rev*, 56(1), 80-99.

Scott, A. B. & Suzuki, D. (1988). Systemic toxicity of botulinum toxin by intramuscular injection in the monkey. *Mov Disord*, 3(4), 333-5.

Sharma, S. K., Ferreira, J. L., Eblen, B. S. & Whiting, R. C. (2006). Detection of type A, B, E, and F Clostridium botulinum neurotoxins in foods by using an amplified enzyme-linked immunosorbent assay with digoxigenin-labeled antibodies. *Appl Environ Microbiol*, 72(2), 1231-8.

Simpson, L. L. (2004). Identification of the major steps in botulinum toxin action. *Annu Rev Pharmacol Toxicol*, 44, 167-93.

Singh, B. R. (2006). Botulinum neurotoxin structure, engineering, and novel cellular trafficking and targeting. *Neurotox Res*, 9(2-3), 73-92.

Singh, B. R. (2000). Intimate details of the most poisonous poison. *Nat Struct Biol*, 7(8), 617-9.

Sugiyama, H. (1980). Clostridium botulinum neurotoxin. *Microbiol Rev*, 44(3), 419-48.

Varnum, S. M., Warner, M. G., Dockendorff, B., Anheier, N. C., Jr., Lou, J., Marks, J. D., Smith, L. A., Feldhaus, M. J., Grate, J. W. & Bruckner-Lea, C. J. (2006). Enzyme-amplified protein microarray and a fluidic renewable surface fluorescence immunoassay for botulinum neurotoxin detection using high-affinity recombinant antibodies. *Anal Chim Acta*, 570(2), 137-43.

Wictome, M., Newton, K., Jameson, K., Hallis, B., Dunnigan, P., Mackay, E., Clarke, S., Taylor, R., Gaze, J., Foster, K. & Shone, C. (1999). Development of an in vitro bioassay for Clostridium botulinum type B neurotoxin in foods that is more sensitive than the mouse bioassay. *Appl Environ Microbiol*, 65(9), 3787-92.

Wictome, M., Newton, K. A., Jameson, K., Dunnigan, P., Clarke, S., Gaze, J., Tauk, A., Foster, K. A. & Shone, C. C. (1999). Development of in vitro assays for the detection of botulinum toxins in foods. *FEMS Immunol Med Microbiol*, 24(3), 319-23.

7

Immunoassays Using Artificial Nanopores

Paolo Actis, Boaz Vilozny and Nader Pourmand
Department of Biomolecular Engineering, Baskin School of Engineering, University of California Santa Cruz, USA

1. Introduction

1.1 Scope

Artificial nanopores can be loosely defined as materials possessing one or more nanometer-size pores (1-100 nm in diameter). This recent class of nanostructures is generating great interest in the scientific community as a platform for biomolecular analysis. The first fabrication of an artificial nanopore with true nanometer control dates to 2001 (Li et al., 2001) but the application of nanopores for biological studies started 10 years earlier. Following a rapid review of the highlights of 20 years of nanopore science, we explore the advancement of nanofabrication techniques that allowed the creation of individual nanopores, nanopore arrays, and nanoporous materials. Although most of the methods currently used to fabricate nanopores require expensive equipment and highly-skilled technicians, we focus here upon those technologies that allow the fabrication of nanopores at the bench and discuss signal transduction mechanisms that allow nanopores to be used as biosensors. In particular, we review the creative application of nanopipettes, artificial nanopores that can be easily fabricated from inexpensive glass capillaries, as a biosensing platform and discuss their potential for immunosensing.

1.2 History of nanopores

The concept of employing a nanopore for biological studies was initiated in the early 1990's by David Deamer (UC Santa Cruz) in collaboration with Daniel Branton (Harvard University), and independently by George Church and Richard Baldarelli (Harvard Medical School). Their hypothesis was that a DNA molecule threaded through a nanopore would perturb the ionic current in a sequence-specific fashion. This concept, however, required a very small pore of molecular dimensions to thread a long strand of DNA.

The first experimental evidence of whether a nanopore could detect nucleic acids was reported by Kasianowicz and coworkers in 1996 (Kasianowicz et al., 1996). The authors threaded single stranded DNA and RNA molecules through an α-haemolysin pore by means of an external applied voltage. Isolated from *Staphylococcus aureus*, α-haemolysin is a 33 kDa membrane pore protein whose channel remains open at neutral pH and high ionic strength and whose pore diameter is ~2 nm (Song et al., 1996). The passage of each molecule was detected as a transient decrease of ionic current whose duration was proportional to the polymer length. From the very first paper published using nanopore technology, the authors envisioned that such a device would allow direct, ultra-fast DNA sequencing. The initial optimism was boosted by the discovery that one can distinguish adenine from cytosine within an RNA molecule with a heterosequence $A_{30}C_{70}$ (Akeson et al., 1999).

The initial excitement diminished when scientists realized that the signal-to-noise ratio was insufficient to ever reach single-base resolution in translocation experiments under typical conditions. The main obstacle is that translocation through α-haemolysin occurs at such a high rate that statistical fluctuations mask subtle differences among the four different bases. The fact that well-defined chemical and structural changes can be introduced to α-haemolysin by genetic engineering still offers the promise that a sequencing device can be built out of a biological nanopore. However, biological nanopores hold some inherent limitations. In particular, they need to be embedded in a supporting lipid bilayer whose stability is closely dependent on pH, temperature, electrolyte concentration, and mechanical stress. Even as research on these protein-based pores was progressing, improved nanofabrication techniques have made it possible to artificially sculpt nanopores into inorganic surfaces with nanometer precision. The possibility of precisely tuning nanopore size and geometry has made possible an expansion of nanopore-sensing technologies (Fig. 1). Applications include the detection of small molecules, peptides, enzymes, proteins and protein complexes (Siwy&Howorka, 2010).

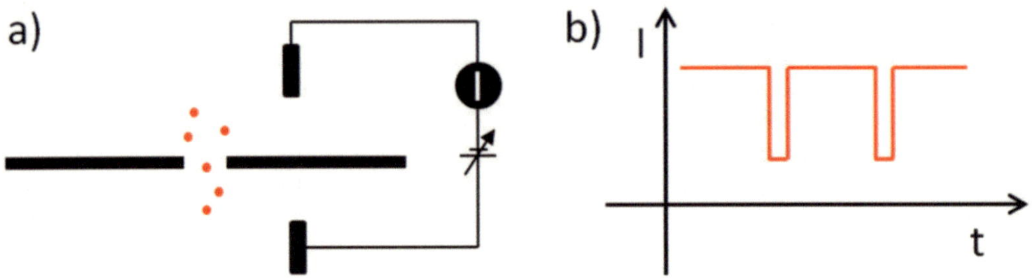

Fig. 1. Scheme illustrating the principle of nanopore measurements. a) A transmembrane potential causes a constant ion flow which is b) temporary perturbed by analytes passing through the nanopore.

Until now, DNA sequencing has been the application of choice for nanopores. The potential of a sequencing device that doesn't require (labelled) nucleotides, polymerases or ligases, requires a minimal sample preparation and allows long reads (>10,000 nt) still inspires several research groups (Branton et al., 2008). Nanopore research is, however, by no means limited to DNA sequencing, and the goal of this chapter is to highlight the recent advances in immunosensing using artificial nanopores, a platform that has the potential for myriad applications.

2. Fabrication of artificial nanopores

Naturally occurring and synthetic zeolites are perhaps the archetypical nanoporous materials, but their sub-nm pores make them more suitable for gas storage rather than for biosensing (Morris&Wheatley, 2008). In this section, we review the fabrication of nanopores and nanoporous materials with cavities of ~2 nm and above. We will first discuss the fabrication of individual nanopores and nanopore arrays using nanolithography, while we dedicate separate sub-sections to bench-top fabrication methods and fabrication of nanoporous materials.

2.1 Ion and electron-beam sculpting

In 2001, Li and coworkers (Li, et al., 2001) reported the first fabrication of a nanopore with true nanometer control using a method called ion beam sculpting. The authors developed a focused ion beam (FIB) machine that uses ions to mill a tiny hole in a silicon nitride membrane. Their system was equipped with ion detectors as a milling feedback-control. Interestingly, they observed that ion rate and temperature affected pore dimensions, causing shrinkage and enlargement, fine-tunable with nanometer precision. Cees Dekker's group (Storm et al., 2003) developed a different approach based on electron beam lithography followed by etching. As with Li's method, pore size could be modified, in this case by exposure of the nanopore to a high-intensity wide field illumination (Fig. 2D). Holes with a diameter greater than the membrane thickness grew in size, whereas smaller holes shrank. Several other groups reported the use of a transmission electron microscope (TEM) to drill nanopores in thin membranes thus making the laborious preparation for electron-beam lithography unnecessary (Zandbergen et al., 2005) (Kim et al., 2006) (Krapf et al., 2005). Traditionally, insulating oxides were used as the material of choice for nanopore fabrication due to their robustness, chemical stability, and wide availability. More recently, scientists started fabricating nanopores into conductive or semi-conductive materials.

Graphene is a two-dimensional layer of carbon atoms packed into a honeycomb lattice with a thickness of only one atomic layer (~0.3 nm). Despite its minimal thickness, graphene is robust as a free-standing membrane. In addition, graphene is an excellent electrical conductor (Geim&Novoselov, 2007). Independently, three groups showed the fabrication of nanopores in graphene (Garaj et al., 2010, Merchant et al., 2010, Schneider et al., 2010) by electron beam milling (Fig. 2E). Preliminary results showed that current blockades due to DNA translocation through graphene nanopores are larger than what has been observed for silicon nanopores of the same diameter. On the other hand, the authors showed that bare graphene devices exhibited large ion current noise and suffered from low yields.

Another very popular technique to fabricate artificial nanopores is the track-etching method (Fig. 2B,C). This technique is based on the irradiation of a polymer foil with energetic heavy ions followed by preferential chemical etching of the particle tracks (Siwy et al., 2003). Cylindrical or conical pores with diameters from a few nanometers to the micrometer range can be obtained. Individual nanopores can be fabricated by masking the polymer foil with a metal during the ion irradiation. Track-etched nanopores can be coated with gold to create individual conical gold nanotubes or nanotube arrays (Martin et al., 2001).

2.2 Bench top fabrication

All nanopore fabrication methods described above require expensive equipment, such as TEM or FIB, or access to heavy ion accelerators. Nanopipettes are a class of artificial nanopores that can be easily fabricated at the bench starting from inexpensive glass capillaries (Fig. 2A). Quartz is the material of choice to fabricate nanopipettes. It possesses many advantages compared to other glasses in term of optical transparency, electrical noise, and mechanical properties. The most widely adopted fabrication method for nanopipettes is

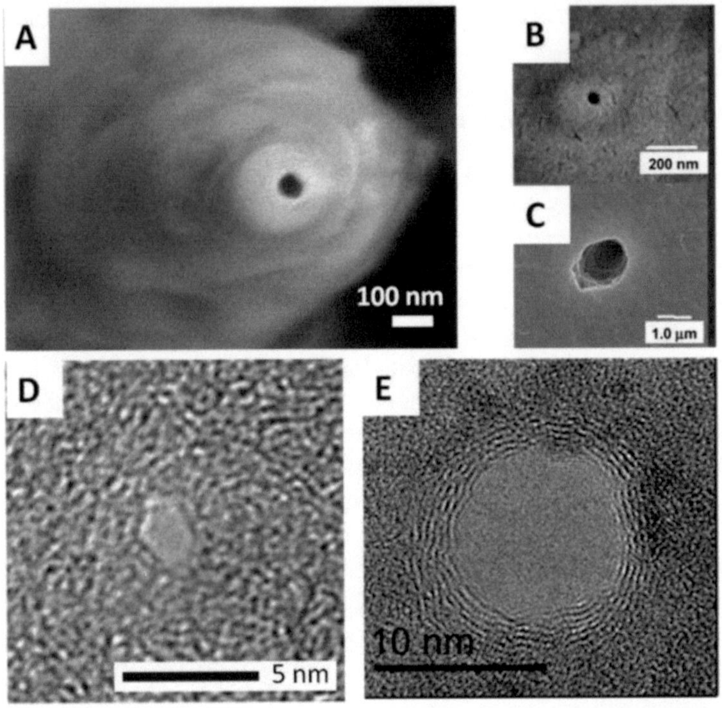

Fig. 2. Electron microscopy of nanopores A) laser-pulled nanopipette, adapted with permission from (Umehara et al., 2006). Copyright 2006 American Chemical Society. Track-etched nanopore in polycarbonate showing respectively B) surface of the membrane exposed to the etch solution and C) surface exposed to the stop solution showing tip opening, adapted with permission from (Harrell et al., 2006). Copyright 2006 American Chemical Society. D) Nanopore in a SiO_2 membrane. Adapted with permission from (Storm, et al., 2003) and E) graphene nanopore. Adapted with permission from (Merchant, et al., 2010). Copyright 2010 American Chemical Society.

laser pulling of a glass capillary. A laser beam is focused on the glass tubing until it reaches its softening point. A hard pull is then applied with a preset delay to generate two identical nanopipettes. The major advantage of the laser pulling method is the simplicity of the approach; there is no need for expensive equipment, clean rooms, or specialized technicians.

Fabrication of nanopipettes with nanometer precision remains technically challenging and alternative methods have been proposed to increase the reproducibility of pore dimensions. Ding and colleagues (Ding et al., 2009) reported an etching protocol to enhance the reproducibility of the nanopore size. First the capillary was pulled into a micropipette and then the very tip was sealed by a heat treatment. A nanopore was opened by external etching and monitored through electrochemical measurements, in order to attain the desired pore size.

Significant effort has been invested in fabricating nanopipettes from materials other than glass. Kim and colleagues (Kim et al., 2005) fabricated carbon nanopipettes with large aspect ratios (length/diameter) based on the glass pulling technique. First, they created an aluminosilicate nanopipette with a conventional laser puller, after which they catalytically deposited carbon layers onto the exterior and interior of the nanopipette. The exterior carbon layer and the glass layer are subsequently removed by chemical etching, exposing the interior carbon nanopipette tip structure. Freedman and coworkers (Freedman et al., 2007) employed magnetic techniques to affix a magnetized carbon nanotube (mCNT) to the tip of a conventional glass nanopipette. The resulting mCNT-tipped nanopipettes were sufficiently robust that they could be used to penetrate cell membranes and to allow fluidic transport.

Zhang and coworkers (Zhang et al., 2004) developed the "nanopore electrode" which consists of atomically sharp platinum wire sealed into a glass capillary. By fine polishing, they exposed a platinum disk of nanometer dimension, and a subsequent etching step produced a truncated cone shaped nanopore embedded in glass, where the bottom of the pore is defined by the platinum disk.

2.3 Nanoporous materials

Numerous methods have been developed to fabricate nanoporous films and materials. We will limit the description to materials already employed for immunosensing whose applications will be described in the Section 3: "Nanoporous structures as loading materials for immunoassays".

Anodized aluminum oxide (AAO) has been one of the substrates of choice for the fabrication of nanoporous materials. AAO membranes are fabricated by anodic oxidation of an aluminum substrate in acidic solutions. The resulting membrane consists of densely packed hexagonal pores of 10–200 nm in diameter, whose size depends on the oxidation conditions (Stroeve&Ileri, 2011). Architectures consisting of long-range ordered nanochannel arrays can be fabricated out of AAO on the millimeter scale (Masuda et al., 1997).

Nanoporous films can be prepared by template-assisted synthesis as well. The self-assembly of polystyrene nanospheres and 5 nm SiO_2 nanoparticles on a glass slide followed by a calcination process produces an ordered array of nanopores embedded in a SiO_2 matrix (Yang et al., 2008). The application of more volatile template materials was used to create both carbon (Lee et al., 2001) and silica (Schmidt-Winkel et al., 1998) mesocellular foams. Moreover, nanoporous structures can be fabricated out of metallic materials. Ding and coworkers (Ding et al., 2004) demonstrated the synthesis of nanoporous gold film by selective dissolution (dealloying) of silver from a silver/gold alloy. Upon silver dissolution, gold atoms re-organize into an interconnected network of nanopores whose size can be tuned in the nanometer range via simple room-temperature post-processing.

Lin and coworkers (Lin et al., 2010) developed a very original method based on biogenic silica to create a nanoporous film on top of electrode materials. Diatoms are eukaryotic, unicellular photosynthetic algae that are ubiquitous in nearly every aquatic habitat. Diatoms produce diverse three-dimensional, regular silica structures (a.k.a. "frustules") with pores from nanometer to micrometer dimensions.

3. Nanoporous structures as loading materials for immunoassays

As discussed in the previous section, nanoporous materials are fundamentally different than solid state, "single-track" nanopores due to fabrication methods, size and geometry of the nanopores. A distinguishing feature is that nanoporous materials have a very large surface area, a property used in many immunoassay applications. Herein, we will review the application of nanoporous materials for immunosensing.

Piao and co-workers constructed a highly stable immunoassay using signal-generating enzyme (as ELISA label) immobilized in mesocellular carbon foam (Piao et al., 2009). Mesoporous carbon possesses large pores (D ~ 31 nm), interconnected by smaller windows (D ~ 21 nm) that are surrounded by small pores (D ~ 5.6 nm). Acid treatment can easily introduce carboxylic moieties at the surface of mesoporous carbon, thus enabling immobilization of horseradish peroxidase (HRP) by cross-linking with glutaraldehyde. HRP can readily enter the large pores while small pores can act as a substrate transporting channel, facilitating the enzymatic reaction. Furthermore, the immobilization of enzyme into nanoporous materials leads to high enzymatic activity and stability, and protection from proteolysis while enhancing mass transport (Wang&Caruso, 2004). The same group demonstrated that this approach give similar results when mesoporous silica was used (Piao et al., 2009).

Li et al (Li et al., 2011) used ultra-thin nanoporous gold leaf to enhance the electrochemiluminescent detection of carcinoembryonic antigen (CEA). Nanoporous gold leaves are large-area, highly conductive and ultra-thin nanoporous gold membranes with uniform pore size distribution centered around 20–30 nm. The authors showed that the nanoporous film reduces electron injection barrier to quantum dots thus enhancing electrochemiluminescence. Shulga and coworkers synthesized a nanoporous gold (NPG) film by selective dissolution (dealloying) of silver from silver/gold alloy. Upon silver dissolution, gold atoms re-organize into an interconnected network of nanopores. Antibodies were immobilized within the nanoporous gold allowing the spectrophotometric detection of prostate specific antigen (PSA) (Shulga et al., 2008). Wei and coworkers employed the same material for the detection of PSA but used a label-free electrochemical transduction (Wei et al., 2011). Li and coworkers constructed a composite material from a nanoporous gold film and graphene sheets. The synergy between these two materials yielded to a highly conductive composite that could detect human serum chorionic gonadotropin (hCG) within the range 0.5–40.00 ng/ml with a detection limit of 0.034 ng/mL (Li et al., 2011). Ding et al. developed an electrochemical immunoassay using nanoporous gold (NPG) electrodes and enhanced the sensitivity of the method by using gold nanoparticles conjugated with horseradish peroxidase (HRP) labeled secondary antibody. They demonstrated the detection of hepatitis B surface antigen (HBsAg) with a dose response in the range of 0.01–1.0 ng/mL with a detection limit of 2.3 pg/mL (Ding et al., 2010).

Yang and coworkers constructed a highly efficient chemiluminescent immunoassay based on a biofunctionalized three-dimensional ordered nanoporous SiO_2 film (Yang, et al., 2008). Lin and coworkers employed biogenic nanoporous silica (diatoms) to create a high density of nanowells where capture antibodies were immobilized. The performance of the biogenic silica membrane biosensor was tested in comparison with nanoporous alumina and plain metallic thin film biosensor. The authors showed an impressive linear range spanning 6 orders of magnitude, from 1 pg/mL up to 1 μg/mL. Significant enhancement in the sensitivity and response time was attributed to enhanced diffusion of fluids within the diatoms nanochannels (Lin, et al., 2010).

4. Methods of detection using nanopores

Because nanopores comprise a wide variety of materials, there are many possible mechanisms to measure a signal for a nanopore-based assay. The most common techniques involve measuring electrolyte flux, or ionic current, through a pore that bridges two chambers. These methods are discussed in detail below (Section 4.1), as they often involve properties that only arise with nanopores. Other methods, employing functionalized nanopore sensors, are discussed in Section 4.2.

4.1 Resistive-pulse sensing

The technique known as resistive-pulse sensing derives from the well-known Coulter counter, in which particles such as individual cells pass through an aperture. If the aperture bridges two electrolyte-filled chambers containing polarized electrodes, then a particle causes a "pulse" of electrical resistance as it passes through the opening. By definition, then, this is a single-channel technique. Performing this technique with nanopores provides the exciting potential for the particles to include many types of biomolecules, including proteins and nucleic acids (Siwy&Howorka, 2010).

For the purposes of immunoassays, the resistive-pulse technique offers a way to analyze biomolecules without labelling. The shape and duration of pulses can discriminate biomolecules, reveal conformational states of proteins, and show antibodies that are bound to antigens. As described by Charles Martin's group (Sexton et al., 2010), the size of proteins as well as their affinity with the pore walls contribute to their electrical translocation signature (Fig. 3). Techniques for analyzing proteins with artificial and biological pores have been recently reviewed (Movileanu, 2009). The wide range of sizes covered by proteins, antibodies, and even viruses makes artificial pores an important tool for analyzing biomolecules.

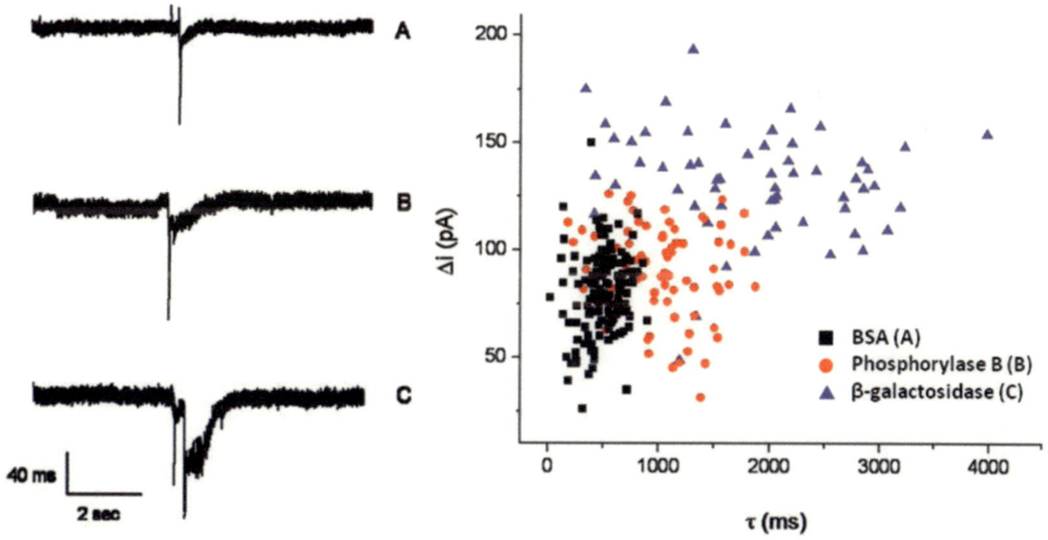

Fig. 3. Left: Ion current pulses arising from translocation of three proteins from tip to base of a conical nanopore with tip diameter of 17 nm. The proteins are bovine serum albumin (A), phosphorylase B (B), and beta-galactosidase (C). Right: scatter plot of the pulse amplitude (ΔI) and pulse duration (τ) for the three proteins. Reprinted with permission from (Sexton, et al., 2010). Copyright 2010 American Chemical Society.

Several recent examples in the literature demonstrate the potential of resistive-pulse sensing to develop powerful immunoassays. In the context of translocation through a nanopore, "immunoprecipitation" can simply mean a change in pore blockade properties compared to individual antigens or individual antibodies. Also, because particles such as viruses can be on the order of 500 nm, we will include micron-scale pores in our consideration of resistive-pulse assays. Using 600 nm pores in glass, Uram, et al. were able to determine antibody binding to a virus based on translocation (Uram et al., 2006). The virions, with diameter of 200 nm, increased in size roughly 60% on antibody binding. A few years earlier, pores of comparable size (1 micron diameter in PDMS) were used to detect binding of antibodies to biotin-derivatized colloids (Saleh&Sohn, 2003).

Moving to pores less than 100 nm in diameter brings the technique of resistive pulse sensing into the realm of detecting native proteins and antibodies. These applications require no labelling of the protein, which can sometimes change binding properties. For example, the Martin group has shown that the electrical signature of a protein can be distinguished from that of the protein bound to an antibody fragment (Sexton et al., 2007). In that report, track-etched nanopores were coated with gold to make a conical nanotube of tip opening 9 to 27 nm in diameter. Electrophoretic translocation of biomolecules from tip-to-base of the nanopores gave characteristic pulse durations that were significantly longer for the immunocomplex than for protein or antibody fragment alone. Silicon nitride pores have been used in several studies of protein translocation. Using 28 nm pores in a membrane 20 nm thick, protein-protein interactions were observed in real-time (Han et al., 2008). More recently, 20 nm pores prepared using the focused ion beam (FIB) technique in silicon nitride membranes were used to discriminate native from unfolded proteins (Oukhaled et al., 2011). Another dimension was recently added to the resistive pulse nanopore techniques, in which artificial nanopores were coated with a "fluid wall" within which biotin was attached (Yusko et al., 2011). The translocation of streptavidin was markedly influenced by the interaction with the antigen. The promise of these new techniques is that they may one day replace immunoassays that require labelling, such as ELISA, and offer greater sensitivity and discriminatory power.

4.2 Ion current modulation methods

The resistive pulse technique measures brief translocation events recorded as "pulses" of resistance (or current). However, ion current can be modulated in other ways in order to give an analytical signal. For example, if a receptor is immobilized to the nanopore surface, then the presence of the target will cause a change in ion current as long as the target is bound. There is a growing arsenal of techniques for chemically modifying the surface of nanopores (Nguyen et al., 2011, Sexton, et al., 2007, Wanunu&Meller, 2007). There is nothing about this particular sensing mechanism that requires nanoscale pores. But as with resistive pulse sensing, bringing the opening down to the scale of biomolecules provides increased sensitivity. Furthermore, there are some properties of ion current in nanopores that are not present in larger structures, and these can be exploited as a signalling mechanism.

The sensitivity of receptor-appended nanopores as analytical instruments depends not only on the binding affinity of the receptor for the analyte, but also on the ability for the binding to result in a modulation of ion current. Predictably, binding many large particles such as antibodies will increase resistance to ion flux through a pore. This was demonstrated with biotin-modified conical nanopores which showed a dramatic decrease in ion current in the presence of streptavidin at concentrations as low as 1 pM (Ali et al., 2008). Quartz nanopipettes functionalized with biotin likewise responded to streptavidin, and were also responsive to the 18 kD protein VEGF after immobilization of antibodies to the pore surface (Umehara et al., 2009) .

Another important consideration is the property of ion current rectification in conical and other types of asymmetric nanopores. This is a true nanoscale effect, and results from the interaction of ions with the electrical double layer formed at the surface of charged nanopores (Wei et al., 1997). The result is a "nanofluidic diode" (Vlassiouk et al., 2009) in which the ion current shows nonlinear dependence on applied voltage. This property is highly sensitive to surface charge, and thus such conical nanopores lend themselves to detection of charged analytes such as polyelectrolytes (Actis et al., 2011, Fu et al., 2009, Umehara, et al., 2006). To date, polyelectrolytes have been the primary targets for assays using this mechanism. Furthermore, it should be possible to target any analyte in which the binding results in a modulation of surface charge.

The use of receptor-appended nanopores for ion current modulation, rather than Coulter counting methods, broadens the technique to include all manner of nanoporous materials and is not limited to single-channel technique (Gyurcsányi, 2008). Despite the availability of many types of functionalized nanoporous materials, there are few examples of these used as ion current-based biosensors (Wang&Smirnov, 2009). Two recent reports illustrate how nanoporous materials can be used for label-free immunosensing. Using a suspension of nanoparticles functionalized with streptavidin, biotin could be detected at a concentration as low as 1 nM (Lei et al., 2010). This method is particularly versatile because there are many established techniques to functionalize nanoparticles. It is also noteworthy that in this case the analyte is very small compared to the receptor. In another example of modulating ion current with a small molecule analyte, glucose was detected using a receptor protein obtained from E. *coli* (Tripathi et al., 2006) where the histidine-tagged receptor was immobilized to a hybrid material consisting of nanoporous polycarbonate onto which gold was deposited using electroless plating. While the measurement of ion current through such membranes is relatively straightforward, reports in the literature of such sensors are scarce. This could be due to the difficulty in functionalizing nanomaterials, or perhaps to insufficient sensitivity in modulations of ion current.

A more common electrochemical technique for biosensing with nanoporous materials is to perform voltammetry using a redox indicator which can be detected as it diffuses through the nanoporous material. The nanoporous membrane can be affixed directly to the working electrode. A recent example is the measurement of biomarkers in whole blood using a nanoporous membrane derivatized with antibodies (de la Escosura-Muñiz&Merkoçi, 2011). To amplify the signal, a secondary antibody was tagged with gold nanoparticles, which then catalyzed the deposition of silver to further block the pores. While this added some complexity to the assay, the device was able to perform using whole, unfiltered blood. Simpler schemes measuring diffusion of a redox active species have also been successful with a variety of nanoporous materials (Lin et al., 2009, Nguyen et al., 2009, Wei, et al., 2011). Singh and co-workers also showed the application of electrochemical impedance spectroscopy to detect peanut protein Ara h1 with an antibody-functionalized nanopore (Singh et al., 2010).

5.1 Label-free immunoassays with functionalized nanopipettes

Our group pioneered the application of nanopipettes as a platform for label-free biosensing (Umehara, et al., 2009). The principles that govern transport properties through nanopipette are similar to conical nanopores in general. The ion current is rectified due to the surface charge and the conical shape of the pore (Wei, et al., 1997). When receptors are attached, the nanopipette can become an electrical biosensor.

We named this technology STING, as Signal Transduction by Ion Nano-Gating. The tip of a nanopipette was functionalized with protein A/G, a commercially available chimeric protein that captures the Fc region of an IgG molecule. This strategy allows the control over the orientation of antigen-binding sites which are always exposed to the analyte. As a proof of concept, two proteins associated with human colorectal cancer were detected, interleukin-10 (IL-10) and vascular endothelial growth factor (VEGF). Exogenously added antigens instantly reduced the ionic flow through the nanopipette, an effect that was not detected in the control nanopipette functionalized with nonspecific antiferritin IgG. Unfortunately, a lack of reproducibility of pore dimensions and lot-to-lot variations in the surface functionalization did not allow for a more quantitative analysis of the observed current reduction. Theoretically, the limit of detection of the nanopipette platform is determined by the number of molecules that generate a detectable signal at the 50-nm tip. In practice, however, consumption of target molecules on surfaces of no sensitivity, such as the outer nanopipette sidewalls, could prevent devices from achieving the theoretical detection limit. Once the protocols were improved to limit the nanopipette functionalization to its inner walls, we were able to demonstrate the analytical applications of nanopipettes for the detection of mycotoxins (Actis et al., 2010)(Fig. 4).

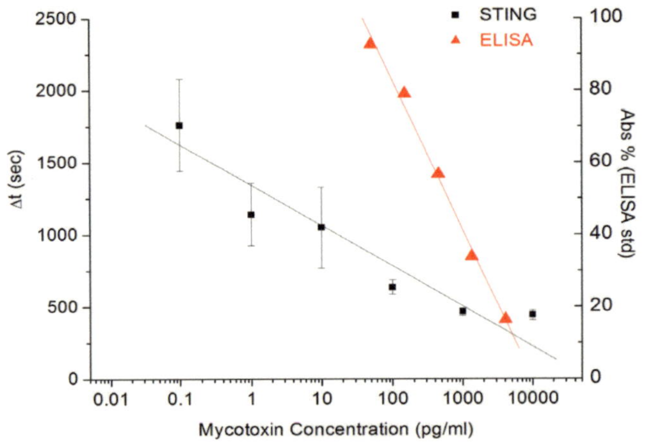

Fig. 4. Comparison between standard curves from ELISA kit (red triangles) and the STING sensor (black squares) for mycotoxin detection. Results show a dynamic range for the STING platform of at least 2 orders of magnitude with a detection limit 3 orders of magnitude lower than ELISA. Adapted with permission from (Actis, et al., 2010).

Mycotoxins are small, non polar molecules produced by fungi and are extremely toxic to mammals even in low concentrations. Using a nanopipette functionalized with antibodies specific to a mycotoxin, we showed a concentration dependent response. Indeed, the nanopipette platform achieved a dynamic range of 5 orders of magnitude with a detection limit 3 orders of magnitude lower than that of a commercially available ELISA kit for mycotoxin.

Despite these successes, antibody-based detection schemes suffer from several drawbacks including: production, cost, limited target analytes, and limited shelf life. To address these imitations, the use of aptamers instead of antibodies as specific receptors was explored. Aptamers are single-stranded oligonucleotides, designed through an in vitro selection process called SELEX (Systematic Evolution of Ligands by Exponential Enrichment) (Ellington&Szostak, 1990, Tuerk&Gold, 1990). Aptamers have similar affinity and selectivity for targets as antibodies, but they can be chemically synthesized, stored in ambient conditions, and easily regenerated. In addition, they can be engineered to undergo a large-scale conformational response to specific molecules, largely affecting the ion transport through the nanopipette.

As a proof-of-concept, a thrombin-binding aptamer was immobilized on the surface of a nanopipette using standard carbodiimide coupling. The interaction of thrombin with its specific aptamer tethered on the nanopipette caused a partial occlusion of the nanopipette pore thus decreasing the ion flow. The decreased ion current can be directly correlated with thrombin concentration in both pure buffer solution and diluted serum. A major advantage of aptamers over antibodies is their ability to reverse the analyte binding. We showed that nanopipette sensors can be reused up to 5 times with minimal degradation of the sensor performance (Actis et al., 2011). In the long term, nanopipette technology promises to open new avenues for biomedical research, and promises breakthroughs in understanding of diseases at the single cell level.

5.2 Potential of nanopipettes for single-cell immunoassay

Nanotechnology-based tools having high sensitivity and low invasiveness hold great promises as new biomedical devices for single cell manipulation and intracellular analysis. We are currently developing a single-cell manipulation platform based on nanopipettes. As a nanopipette approaches the surface of a cell the ionic current through the pore will decrease due to "current squeezing", a well known effect, exploited to great benefit in scanning ion conductance microscopy (Hansma et al., 1989). By monitoring the ionic current the precise position of the nanopipette can be determined and controlled within ~200 nm of the cell membrane. After initial positioning above the cell membrane the nanopipette can either be scanned over the cell membrane to render a topographical image (Klenerman & Korchev, 2006) or inserted into the cell. The comparatively small size of the nanopipette combined with controlled penetration conditions maximizes cell viability.

By employing functionalized nanopipettes, detection of the interaction of intracellular, soluble antigens with antibodies immobilized on the nanopipette pore should be possible.

6. Other detection methods

To round out the discussion of nanopores and nanoporous materials in immunoassays, we will mention some non-electrochemical techniques. As with redox indicators, the diffusion of an optical indicator can be measured through a nanoporous membrane (Jágerszki et al., 2007). Such sensing schemes can potentially take advantage of distinctive recognition/transport phenomena that occur in nanostructures. Many of the other properties of nanoporous materials, such as high surface area, can also be exploited for sensing schemes. A recent example is the use of porous alumina functionalized with a capture protein (Alvarez et al., 2009). The binding of an antibody can be detected by optical interferometry. In theory, this method can be used with many types of nanomaterials and is not restricted to nanoporous structures.

7. Conclusions

Artificial nanopores represent a fundamental technological breakthrough. As with many new technologies, nanopores required interdisciplinary collaboration. Fittingly, then, the potential applications of this new technology are equally broad, ranging from sequencing to diagnostics, cell biology to biophysics. Going forward, the integration of nanopores with microfluidic or optofluidic platforms may generate self-contained biodetectors with single molecule sensitivity (Holmes et al., 2010). The fabrication of nanopores into materials of atomic thickness, such as graphene can dramatically improve signal-to-noise ratio in biosensing experiments. Graphene nanopores may lead to sensing devices where the electric potential is controlled locally at the nanopore and transverse current can be measured across the pore aperture. Although artificial nanopore technology is at its infancy, we believe that it holds a tremendous potential for single-molecule sensing as well as single-cell analysis and manipulation.

8. Acknowledgements

Xiang Li, and Michelle Maalouf are gratefully acknowledged for critical reading of the manuscript. This work was supported in part by grants from the National Aeronautics and Space Administration Cooperative Agreements NCC9-165 and NNX08BA47A, and the National Institutes of Health [P01-HG000205].

9. References

Actis, P.; Jejelowo, O. & Pourmand, N. (2010). Ultrasensitive mycotoxin detection by STING sensors. *Biosensors and Bioelectronics*, Vol.26, No.2, pp. 333-337, 0956-5663

Actis, P.; Vilozny, B.; Seger, R. A.; Li, X.; Jejelowo, O.; Rinaudo, M. & Pourmand, N. (2011). Voltage-Controlled Metal Binding on Polyelectrolyte-Functionalized Nanopores. *Langmuir*, Vol.27, No.10, pp. 6528-6533, 0743-7463

Akeson, M.; Branton, D.; Kasianowicz, J. J.; Brandin, E. & Deamer, D. W. (1999). Microsecond Time-Scale Discrimination Among Polycytidylic Acid, Polyadenylic Acid, and Polyuridylic Acid as Homopolymers or as Segments Within Single RNA Molecules. *Biophysical Journal*, Vol.77, No.6, pp. 3227-3233, 0006-3495

Actis, P.; Rogers, A.; Nivala, J.; Vilozny, B.; Seger, R. A.; Jejelowo, O. & Pourmand, N. (2011) Reversible Thrombin Detection by Aptamer functionalized STING sensors. *Biosensors and Bioelectronics*, Vol.26, No.11, pp. 4503-4507, 0956-5663.

Ali, M.; Yameen, B.; Neumann, R.; Ensinger, W.; Knoll, W. & Azzaroni, O. (2008). Biosensing and Supramolecular Bioconjugation in Single Conical Polymer Nanochannels. Facile Incorporation of Biorecognition Elements into Nanoconfined Geometries.

Journal of the American Chemical Society, Vol.130, No.48, (2008/12/03), pp. 16351-16357, 0002-7863

Alvarez, S. D.; Li, C.-P.; Chiang, C. E.; Schuller, I. K. & Sailor, M. J. (2009). A Label-Free Porous Alumina Interferometric Immunosensor. *ACS Nano*, Vol.3, No.10, pp. 3301-3307, 1936-0851

Branton, D.; Deamer, D. W.; Marziali, A.; Bayley, H.; Benner, S. A.; Butler, T.; Di Ventra, M.; Garaj, S.; Hibbs, A.; Huang, X.; Jovanovich, S. B.; Krstic, P. S.; Lindsay, S.; Ling, X. S.; Mastrangelo, C. H.; Meller, A.; Oliver, J. S.; Pershin, Y. V.; Ramsey, J. M.; Riehn, R.; Soni, G. V.; Tabard-Cossa, V.; Wanunu, M.; Wiggin, M. & Schloss, J. A. (2008). The potential and challenges of nanopore sequencing. *Nat Biotech*, Vol.26, No.10, pp. 1146-1153, 1087-0156

de la Escosura-Muñiz, A. & Merkoçi, A. (2011). A Nanochannel/Nanoparticle-Based Filtering and Sensing Platform for Direct Detection of a Cancer Biomarker in Blood. *Small*, Vol.7, No.5, pp. 675-682, 1613-6829

Ding, C.; Li, H.; Hu, K. & Lin, J.-M. (2010). Electrochemical immunoassay of hepatitis B surface antigen by the amplification of gold nanoparticles based on the nanoporous gold electrode. *Talanta*, Vol.80, No.3, pp. 1385-1391, 0039-9140

Ding, S.; Gao, C. & Gu, L.-Q. (2009). Capturing Single Molecules of Immunoglobulin and Ricin with an Aptamer-Encoded Glass Nanopore. *Analytical Chemistry*, Vol.81, No.16, pp. 6649-6655, 0003-2700

Ding, Y.; Kim, Y. J. & Erlebacher, J. (2004). Nanoporous Gold Leaf: "Ancient Technology"/Advanced Material. *Advanced Materials*, Vol.16, No.21, pp. 1897-1900, 1521-4095

Ellington, A. D. & Szostak, J. W. (1990). In vitro selection of RNA molecules that bind specific ligands. *Nature*, Vol.346, No.6287, pp. 818-822,

Freedman, J. R.; Mattia, D.; Korneva, G.; Gogotsi, Y.; Friedman, G. & Fontecchio, A. K. (2007). Magnetically assembled carbon nanotube tipped pipettes. *Applied Physics Letters*, Vol.90, No.10, pp. 103108,

Fu, Y.; Tokuhisa, H. & Baker, L. A. (2009). Nanopore DNA sensors based on dendrimer-modified nanopipettes. *Chem Commun (Camb)*, No.32, (Aug 28), pp. 4877-4879, 1364-548X (Electronic) 1359-7345 (Linking)

Garaj, S.; Hubbard, W.; Reina, A.; Kong, J.; Branton, D. & Golovchenko, J. A. (2010). Graphene as a subnanometre trans-electrode membrane. *Nature*, Vol.467, No.7312, pp. 190-193, 0028-0836

Geim, A. K. & Novoselov, K. S. (2007). The rise of graphene. *Nat Mater*, Vol.6, No.3, pp. 183-191, 1476-1122

Gyurcsányi, R. E. (2008). Chemically-modified nanopores for sensing. *TrAC Trends in Analytical Chemistry*, Vol.27, No.7, pp. 627-639, 0165-9936

Han, A.; Creus, M.; Schürmann, G.; Linder, V.; Ward, T. R.; de Rooij, N. F. & Staufer, U. (2008). Label-Free Detection of Single Protein Molecules and Protein–Protein Interactions Using Synthetic Nanopores. *Analytical Chemistry*, Vol.80, No.12, (2008/06/01), pp. 4651-4658, 0003-2700

Hansma, P.; Drake, B.; Marti, O.; Gould, S. & Prater, C. (1989). The scanning ion-conductance microscope. *Science*, Vol.243, No.4891, (February 3, 1989), pp. 641-643,

Harrell, C. C.; Choi, Y.; Horne, L. P.; Baker, L. A.; Siwy, Z. S. & Martin, C. R. (2006). Resistive-Pulse DNA Detection with a Conical Nanopore Sensor†. *Langmuir*, Vol.22, No.25, pp. 10837-10843, 0743-7463

Jágerszki, G.; Gyurcsányi, R. E.; Höfler, L. & Pretsch, E. (2007). Hybridization-Modulated Ion Fluxes through Peptide-Nucleic-Acid- Functionalized Gold Nanotubes. A New Approach to Quantitative Label-Free DNA Analysis. *Nano Letters*, Vol.7, No.6, (2007/06/01), pp. 1609-1612, 1530-6984

Kasianowicz, J. J.; Brandin, E.; Branton, D. & Deamer, D. W. (1996). Characterization of individual polynucleotide molecules using a membrane channel. *Proceedings of the National Academy of Sciences*, Vol.93, No.24, (November 26, 1996), pp. 13770-13773,

Kim, B. M.; Murray, T. & Bau, H. H. (2005). The fabrication of integrated carbon pipes with sub-micron diameters. *Nanotechnology*, No.8, pp. 1317, 0957-4484

Kim, M. J.; Wanunu, M.; Bell, D. C. & Meller, A. (2006). Rapid Fabrication of Uniformly Sized Nanopores and Nanopore Arrays for Parallel DNA Analysis. *Advanced Materials*, Vol.18, No.23, pp. 3149-3153, 1521-4095

Klenerman, D. & Korchev, Y. (2006). Potential biomedical applications of the scanned nanopipette. *Nanomedicine (Lond)*, Vol.1, No.1, (Jun), pp. 107-114, 1748-6963 (Electronic) 1743-5889 (Linking)

Krapf, D.; Wu, M.-Y.; Smeets, R. M. M.; Zandbergen, H. W.; Dekker, C. & Lemay, S. G. (2005). Fabrication and Characterization of Nanopore-Based Electrodes with Radii down to 2 nm. *Nano Letters*, Vol.6, No.1, pp. 105-109, 1530-6984

Lee, J.; Sohn, K. & Hyeon, T. (2001). Fabrication of Novel Mesocellular Carbon Foams with Uniform Ultralarge Mesopores. *Journal of the American Chemical Society*, Vol.123, No.21, pp. 5146-5147, 0002-7863

Lei, Y.; Xie, F.; Wang, W.; Wu, W. & Li, Z. (2010). Suspended nanoparticle crystal (S-NPC): A nanofluidics-based, electrical read-out biosensor. *Lab on a Chip*, Vol.10, No.18, pp. 2338-2340, 1473-0197

Li, J.; Stein, D.; McMullan, C.; Branton, D.; Aziz, M. J. & Golovchenko, J. A. (2001). Ion-beam sculpting at nanometre length scales. *Nature*, Vol.412, No.6843, pp. 166-169, 0028-0836

Li, R.; Wu, D.; Li, H.; Xu, C.; Wang, H.; Zhao, Y.; Cai, Y.; Wei, Q. & Du, B. (2011). Label-free amperometric immunosensor for the detection of human serum chorionic gonadotropin based on nanoporous gold and graphene. *Analytical Biochemistry*, Vol.414, No.2, pp. 196-201, 0003-2697

Li, X.; Wang, R. & Zhang, X. (2011). Electrochemiluminescence immunoassay at a nanoporous gold leaf electrode and using CdTe quantun dots as labels. *Microchimica Acta*, Vol.172, No.3, pp. 285-290, 0026-3672

Lin, J.; He, C. & Zhang, S. (2009). Immunoassay channels for α-fetoprotein based on encapsulation of biorecognition molecules into SBA-15 mesopores. *Analytica Chimica Acta*, Vol.643, No.1-2, pp. 90-94, 0003-2670

Lin, K.-C.; Kunduru, V.; Bothara, M.; Rege, K.; Prasad, S. & Ramakrishna, B. L. (2010). Biogenic nanoporous silica-based sensor for enhanced electrochemical detection of cardiovascular biomarkers proteins. *Biosensors and Bioelectronics*, Vol.25, No.10, pp. 2336-2342, 0956-5663

Martin, C. R.; Nishizawa, M.; Jirage, K. & Kang, M. (2001). Investigations of the Transport Properties of Gold Nanotubule Membranes. *The Journal of Physical Chemistry B*, Vol.105, No.10, pp. 1925-1934, 1520-6106

Merchant, C. A.; Healy, K.; Wanunu, M.; Ray, V.; Peterman, N.; Bartel, J.; Fischbein, M. D.; Venta, K.; Luo, Z.; Johnson, A. T. C. & Drndić, M. (2010). DNA Translocation through Graphene Nanopores. *Nano Letters*, Vol.10, No.8, pp. 2915-2921, 1530-6984

Morris, R. E. & Wheatley, P. S. (2008). Gas Storage in Nanoporous Materials. *Angewandte Chemie International Edition*, Vol.47, No.27, pp. 4966-4981, 1521-3773

Movileanu, L. (2009). Interrogating single proteins through nanopores: challenges and opportunities. *Trends in Biotechnology*, Vol.27, No.6, pp. 333-341, 0167-7799

Nguyen, B. T. T.; Koh, G.; Lim, H. S.; Chua, A. J. S.; Ng, M. M. L. & Toh, C.-S. (2009). Membrane-Based Electrochemical Nanobiosensor for the Detection of Virus. *Analytical Chemistry*, Vol.81, No.17, pp. 7226-7234, 0003-2700

Nguyen, G.; Howorka, S. & Siwy, Z. (2011). DNA Strands Attached Inside Single Conical Nanopores: Ionic Pore Characteristics and Insight into DNA Biophysics. *Journal of Membrane Biology*, Vol.239, No.1, pp. 105-113, 0022-2631

Oukhaled, A.; Cressiot, B.; Bacri, L.; Pastoriza-Gallego, M.; Betton, J.-M.; Bourhis, E.; Jede, R.; Gierak, J.; Auvray, L. c. & Pelta, J. (2011). Dynamics of Completely Unfolded and Native Proteins through Solid-State Nanopores as a Function of Electric Driving Force. *ACS Nano*, Vol.5, No.5, (2011/05/24), pp. 3628-3638, 1936-0851

Piao, Y.; Lee, D.; Kim, J.; Kim, J.; Hyeon, T. & Kim, H.-S. (2009). High performance immunoassay using immobilized enzyme in nanoporous carbon. *Analyst*, Vol.134, No.5, pp. 926-932, 0003-2654

Piao, Y.; Lee, D.; Lee, J.; Hyeon, T.; Kim, J. & Kim, H.-S. (2009). Multiplexed immunoassay using the stabilized enzymes in mesoporous silica. *Biosensors and Bioelectronics*, Vol.25, No.4, pp. 906-912, 0956-5663

Saleh, O. A. & Sohn, L. L. (2003). Direct detection of antibody–antigen binding using an on-chip artificial pore. *Proceedings of the National Academy of Sciences*, Vol.100, No.3, (February 4, 2003), pp. 820-824,

Schmidt-Winkel, P.; Lukens, W. W.; Zhao, D.; Yang, P.; Chmelka, B. F. & Stucky, G. D. (1998). Mesocellular Siliceous Foams with Uniformly Sized Cells and Windows. *Journal of the American Chemical Society*, Vol.121, No.1, pp. 254-255, 0002-7863

Schneider, G. g. F.; Kowalczyk, S. W.; Calado, V. E.; Pandraud, G. g.; Zandbergen, H. W.; Vandersypen, L. M. K. & Dekker, C. (2010). DNA Translocation through Graphene Nanopores. *Nano Letters*, Vol.10, No.8, pp. 3163-3167, 1530-6984

Sexton, L. T.; Horne, L. P.; Sherrill, S. A.; Bishop, G. W.; Baker, L. A. & Martin, C. R. (2007). Resistive-Pulse Studies of Proteins and Protein/Antibody Complexes Using a Conical Nanotube Sensor. *Journal of the American Chemical Society*, Vol.129, No.43, pp. 13144-13152, 0002-7863

Sexton, L. T.; Mukaibo, H.; Katira, P.; Hess, H.; Sherrill, S. A.; Horne, L. P. & Martin, C. R. (2010). An Adsorption-Based Model for Pulse Duration in Resistive-Pulse Protein Sensing. *Journal of the American Chemical Society*, Vol.132, No.19, (2010/05/19), pp. 6755-6763, 0002-7863

Shulga, O. V.; Zhou, D.; Demchenko, A. V. & Stine, K. J. (2008). Detection of free prostate specific antigen (fPSA) on a nanoporous gold platform. *Analyst*, Vol.133, No.3, pp. 319-322, 0003-2654

Singh, R.; Sharma, P. P.; Baltus, R. E. & Suni, I. I. (2010). Nanopore immunosensor for peanut protein Ara h1. *Sensors and Actuators B: Chemical*, Vol.145, No.1, pp. 98-103, 0925-4005

Siwy, Z.; Apel, P.; Dobrev, D.; Neumann, R.; Spohr, R.; Trautmann, C. & Voss, K. (2003). Ion transport through asymmetric nanopores prepared by ion track etching. *Nuclear Instruments and Methods in Physics Research Section B: Beam Interactions with Materials and Atoms*, Vol.208, pp. 143-148, 0168-583X

Siwy, Z. S. & Howorka, S. (2010). Engineered voltage-responsive nanopores. *Chemical Society Reviews*, Vol.39, No.3, pp. 1115-1132, 0306-0012

Song, L.; Hobaugh, M. R.; Shustak, C.; Cheley, S.; Bayley, H. & Gouaux, J. E. (1996). Structure of Staphylococcal α-Hemolysin, a Heptameric Transmembrane Pore. *Science*, Vol.274, No.5294, (December 13, 1996), pp. 1859-1865,

Storm, A. J.; Chen, J. H.; Ling, X. S.; Zandbergen, H. W. & Dekker, C. (2003). Fabrication of solid-state nanopores with single-nanometre precision. *Nat Mater*, Vol.2, No.8, pp. 537-540, 1476-1122

Stroeve, P. & Ileri, N. (2011). Biotechnical and other applications of nanoporous membranes. *Trends in Biotechnology*, Vol.29, No.6, pp. 259-266, 0167-7799

Tripathi, A.; Wang, J.; Luck, L. A. & Suni, I. I. (2006). Nanobiosensor Design Utilizing a Periplasmic E. coli Receptor Protein Immobilized within Au/Polycarbonate Nanopores. *Analytical Chemistry*, Vol.79, No.3, (2007/02/01), pp. 1266-1270, 0003-2700

Tuerk, C. & Gold, L. (1990). Systematic evolution of ligands by exponential enrichment: RNA ligands to bacteriophage T4 DNA polymerase. *Science*, Vol.249, No.4968, (August 3, 1990), pp. 505-510,

Umehara, S.; Pourmand, N.; Webb, C. D.; Davis, R. W.; Yasuda, K. & Karhanek, M. (2006). Current Rectification with Poly-l-Lysine-Coated Quartz Nanopipettes. *Nano Letters*, Vol.6, No.11, pp. 2486-2492, 1530-6984

Umehara, S.; Karhanek, M.; Davis, R. W. & Pourmand, N. (2009). Label-free biosensing with functionalized nanopipette probes. *Proceedings of the National Academy of Sciences*, Vol.106, No.12, (March 24, 2009), pp. 4611-4616,

Uram, J. D.; Ke, K.; Hunt, A. J. & Mayer, M. (2006). Submicrometer Pore-Based Characterization and Quantification of Antibody–Virus Interactions. *Small*, Vol.2, No.8-9, pp. 967-972, 1613-6829

Vlassiouk, I.; Kozel, T. R. & Siwy, Z. S. (2009). Biosensing with Nanofluidic Diodes. *Journal of the American Chemical Society*, Vol.131, No.23, (2009/06/17), pp. 8211-8220, 0002-7863

Wang, X. & Smirnov, S. (2009). Label-Free DNA Sensor Based on Surface Charge Modulated Ionic Conductance. *ACS Nano*, Vol.3, No.4, (2009/04/28), pp. 1004-1010, 1936-0851

Wang, Y. & Caruso, F. (2004). Enzyme encapsulation in nanoporous silica spheres. *Chemical Communications*, No.13, pp. 1528-1529, 1359-7345

Wanunu, M. & Meller, A. (2007). Chemically Modified Solid-State Nanopores. *Nano Letters*, Vol.7, No.6, pp. 1580-1585, 1530-6984

Wei, C.; Bard, A. J. & Feldberg, S. W. (1997). Current Rectification at Quartz Nanopipet Electrodes. *Analytical Chemistry*, Vol.69, No.22, pp. 4627-4633, 0003-2700

Wei, Q.; Zhao, Y.; Xu, C.; Wu, D.; Cai, Y.; He, J.; Li, H.; Du, B. & Yang, M. (2011). Nanoporous gold film based immunosensor for label-free detection of cancer biomarker. *Biosensors and Bioelectronics*, Vol.26, No.8, pp. 3714-3718, 0956-5663

Yang, Z.; Xie, Z.; Liu, H.; Yan, F. & Ju, H. (2008). Streptavidin-Functionalized Three-Dimensional Ordered Nanoporous Silica Film for Highly Efficient Chemiluminescent Immunosensing. *Advanced Functional Materials*, Vol.18, No.24, pp. 3991-3998, 1616-3028

Yusko, E. C.; Johnson, J. M.; Majd, S.; Prangkio, P.; Rollings, R. C.; Li, J.; Yang, J. & Mayer, M. (2011). Controlling protein translocation through nanopores with bio-inspired fluid walls. *Nat Nano*, Vol.6, No.4, pp. 253-260, 1748-3387

Zandbergen, H. W.; van Duuren, R. J. H. A.; Alkemade, P. F. A.; Lientschnig, G.; Vasquez, O.; Dekker, C. & Tichelaar, F. D. (2005). Sculpting Nanoelectrodes with a Transmission Electron Beam for Electrical and Geometrical Characterization of Nanoparticles. *Nano Letters*, Vol.5, No.3, pp. 549-553, 1530-6984

Zhang, B.; Zhang, Y. & White, H. S. (2004). The Nanopore Electrode. *Analytical Chemistry*, Vol.76, No.21, pp. 6229-6238, 0003-2700

Part 3

Multiplexing Technologies

Multiplexed Immunoassays

Weiming Zheng[1,*] and Lin He[2]
[1]*BioPlex Division, Clinical Diagnostics Group, Bio-Rad Laboratories, Hercules, CA*
[2]*Department of Chemistry, North Carolina State University, Raleigh, NC*
USA

1. Introduction

Immunoassay has been widely used for quantification of proteins and small molecules in medical diagnostics, proteomics, drug discovery, and various biological research.[1] ELISA (Enzyme-Linked ImmunoSorbant Assay) is the most commonly used immunoassay format.[2] Traditional ELISA assays used in clinical settings are laborious and expensive and often consume large quantities of reagents and patient specimen. Meanwhile, armed with the knowledge from genomic and proteomic study, there is an increasing demand for technologies that are capable of extracting high density of bio-information from limited sample volume for better disease diagnosis, prognosis and treatment.[3] This demand has driven the development of low-cost, flexible and high throughput methods for simultaneous detection of multiple proteins in parallel in a single assay (multiplexed immunoassay). Although the first concept towards multiplexed immunoassay was already described in 1961 by Feinberg for "microspot' test of antibody-antigen reaction in the thin agar films[4], it was not demonstrated until 1989 when Ekins described microarray technology principles in the 'ambient analyte theory' and envisioned the immense potential application in biomedical research and clinical diagnostics[5]. Since then, a great number of multiplexing platforms have been developed. Particularly, recent advances in technology (*e.g.* fluidics, optics, automated sample handling device) and informatics have enabled a real high-throughput multiplexed immunoassay.[6-8] Today, multiplexed immunoassays are becoming popular and have been widely used in basic biomedical research due to their advantages in performing a large number of different assays all in a single reaction vessel from a relatively smaller sample volume with high efficiency. Multiplexed immunoassays are also becoming important for clinical diagnostic purpose by identifying multiple biomarkers for a wide range of diseases. Patterns of several biomarkers have better predictive value compared to detection of single analyte using ELISAs. Although there are still some challenges (*e.g.* complexity, expensive, validation requirement) for these tests, multiplexed protein test panels are now slowly penetrating into clinical diagnostics market and the time of their significant implementation is probably about to come. Several commercial multiplexed immunoassay platforms are available on this emerging market, including Luminex bead based platform, Meso Scale Discovery's Multi Array Technology, and protein array platforms from Whatman, ArryIt and others.

This article will provide an overview of multiplexed immunoassays, and will evaluate existing platforms with multiplexing capabilities and their applications in biomedical research and clinical diagnostics, and will also discuss technical challenges and future prospective.

2. Principle of multiplexed immunoassays

Current multiplexed immunoassays are based on multi-marker strategies, in which high-affinity capture ligands (antibodies or proteins/peptides) are immobilized in parallel assays. When incubated with biological samples, target analytes are bound to corresponding capture ligands, respectively. After washing to remove unbound proteins, captured targets are usually detected by using various labeled reporter ligands. Then target analytes are quantified by measuring the signal intensity of the detection label, which is either converted to mass units of target analyte using calibration curves (i.e. quantitative assay) or evaluated using cutoff calibrator (i.e. qualitative assay). Generally, there are two major approaches to realize multiplexed immunoassay: the use of planar microarrays or encoded-microparticle arrays.

2.1 Planar microarrays

Planar microarrays, such as protein microarrays,[9, 10] are characterized by surface-immobilized capture ligands in microspots onto a two dimensional grid. The identity of capture ligand at each microspot in the array is distinguished by its physical coordinates (x, y) in the grid (**Figure 1A**). Planar microarrays are highly miniaturized and parallelized assays, which consist of high density of microspots (usually ~300 μm in diameter; ~2000 spots/cm^2). Recent development of nanotechnology has enabled the fabrication of highly dense protein nanoarray (~10^6 spots/mm^2).[11] Fluorescence and chemiluminescence reporters are common used in planar arrays due to their high sensitivity and wide dynamic range. Planar microarray systems are perfect tools for ultra high-throughput screening of proteins due to their simplicity in preparing an array of high density of elements and in subsequent signal readouts. Many companies have produced protein microarrays for research purpose (www.biochipnet.com), and these protein based microarrays have been applied in the detection of many protein biomarkers, such as viral infection, cancers, and auto-immune diseases.[12-16]

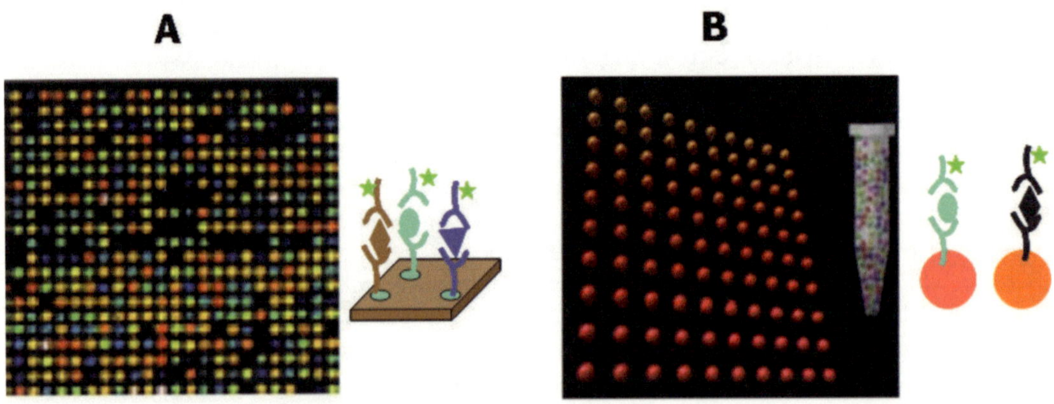

Fig. 1. **(A)** A scheme of planar microarray, which consists of two-dimensional grid of probe molecules (antibodies, peptides, or oligonucleotides). The identity of the probes at each spot in the array is known from its location in the grid. **(B)** An encoded particle array is composed of probe molecules attached to encoded particles. The identity of the probes is revealed by reading the particle code (Reprinted with permission of ref. **17**)

However, planar microarrays are limited by some disadvantages, including slow reaction kinetics (due to surface diffusion), problems with localization of capture ligands bound to the 2D chip (due to the use of physical coordinates to indentify), and inflexibility of probe combinations used in an array (due to pre-fabricated flat surface).

2.2 Encoded-microparticle arrays

Encoded-microparticle array based systems (so called suspension arrays) have emerged as a very interesting alternative.[17, 18] They are composed of encoded mciroparticles suspended in solution and pre-attached with capture ligands (**Figure 1B**). The nature of the capture ligands attached to each particle is revealed by deciphering the particle code. Encoded-microparticle arrays have several advantages over planar microarrays. First, an encoded mciroparticle array exhibits greater sensing flexibility where different capture ligands can be mix-and-matched at different combinations at will. Second, suspended particles with curved surfaces benefit from faster diffusion and smaller steric hindrance whereas the reaction kinetics on a planar array is limited by a flat surface. Third, encoded microparticle arrays have greater reproducibility due to the use of hundreds to thousands of replicates for each target molecule in the same assay, which allows for high precision measurements. Accordingly, in this review, we will focus more on encoded microparticle array based multiplexed immunoassay.

Encoded microparticle based multiplexed immunoassays use microparticles as solid phase and therefore require the encoding of microparticle arrays used for the efficient simultaneous measurement of large numbers of biological binding events in a single sample. An ideal microparticle encoding technique must satisfy a number of requirements, it must be: 1) machine-readable (decoding); 2) unaffected by the biochemical reactions; 3) robust, with low error rate; 4) able to encode large numbers of particles, each with a unique code; 5) are compatible with biomolecule attachment; and 6) able to mass production with low-cost. To this end, since the 1990s, different technologies for multiplexing have emerged (optical[19-28], graphical[29-33], electronic[34, 35], or physical[36, 37] encoding) for different platforms (flow cytometry or fluorescence microscopy). The features of each encoding strategy are listed in **Table 1**.

Of the many encoded technologies developed for multiplexing, optical encoding is the most well established encoding technique, in which the identity of the probe molecules attached to particles is uniquely correlated to the absorbance, fluorescence, Raman, or reflection spectrum of particles. The most common optical encoding method is using polymer microspheres internally doped with one or more fluorescent dyes.[19, 20] By using fluorescent dyes with different emission spectra and doping at different intensity levels, microspheres of different codes can be obtained **(Figure 2).** The maximum number of codes that can be achieved in this way is determined by the formula: $C = N^m\text{-}1$, where C is the number of codes, N is the number of intensity levels and m is the number of dyes. For a typical multiplexed immunoassay, each set of microspheres with unique combinations of fluorescent spectral is used to attach specific capture ligand and constitutes the platform for specific molecular reaction (like each ELISA microwell). After coupling with the appropriate capture ligands, different sets of encoded microspheres can be pooled and multiplexed immunoassay is then carried out in a single reaction vial. The presence of bound targets to their respective capture ligands on the different microsphere sets can be detected with an

Encoding Strategies	Encoding Materials	Decoding & Detection Methods	Limitations	Ref.
Optical	Fluorescent dye	Fluorescence	• Limited codes • Relied on sophisticated instruments for readouts, • Potential interference of encoding and detection spectra	16,17
	Quantum dots	Fluorescence		18
	Chromophores	Absorption		19
	Multiple wavelength/spatial fluorescence	Fluorescence		20
	Raman tags	Raman		21-24
	Silicon photonic crystals	Fluorescence and reflectivity		25
Graphical	Metal strips	Reflectance and fluorescence	• Sequential particle synthesis • Decoding are time-consuming • High throughput limited	26
	Selective Photobleaching code	Fluorescence; confocal microscope		27
	Structural pattern particles	Physical pattern		28-30
Electronic	Radio frequency memory tags	Radio frequency	• Size limited • Instrument limited • Synthesis of the particle are expensive and slow	31,32
Physical	Particle size	Physical pattern	• Limited codes	33
	Particle shape	Physical pattern	• Special instrument	34

Table 1. Summary of different microparticles encoding methods

antibody conjugate coupled to a reported fluorescent dye. The signal intensities of reported dye are measured, which is used to quantify the amount of captured targets on each individual microsphere. Each microsphere type and thus each binding target are identified using the color code measured by a second fluorescence signal. Flow cytometric principle is the basic technology used in the analysis of optically encoded microsphere based multiplexed immunoassay, which generates robust, rapid, high-throughput, sensitive, and reproducible results for a wide range of biomedical application.

To date, several multiplexed immunoassay platforms that based on optically encoded microspheres have been developed and commercialized. Three major companies market the instruments and materials that required for optically encoded microsphere based multiplexed immunoassay: the xMAP technology by Luminex, the CBA technology by Becton Dickinson BioSciences, and the VeraCode™ technology by Illumina, as summarized in **Table 2**.

The Luminex xMAP (Multi-Analyte Profiling) technology uses 5.5-μm microspheres that are internally doped with two fluorescent dyes (red and infrared) at ten different concentrations to produce up to 100 different sets of microspheres.[38, 39] Each set of microspheres can then be derivatized by a specific type of capture ligand. As shown in **Figure 3** for a typical sandwiched

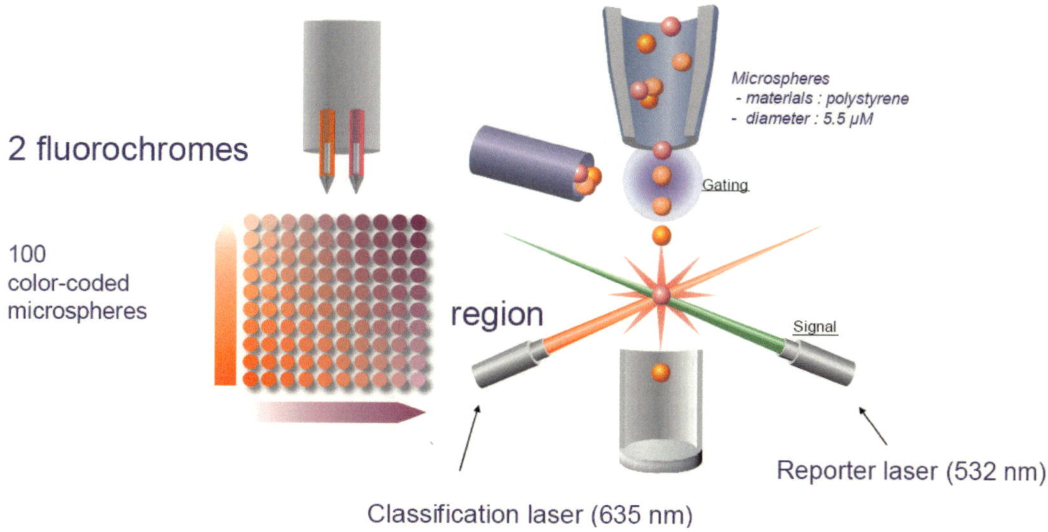

Fig. 2. Optically encoded microspheres: unique microsphere sets are optical coded using a blend of different fluorescent intensities of two dyes and decoded by a flow cytometry. (Courtesy of Luminex Corp.)

immunoassay, binding of target analyte brings reporter molecules to the microsphere surface. A green fluorescent dye (phycoerythrin, PE) is pre-conjugated to the reporter molecules and is used to indicate the occurrence of positive binding and quantify the amount of target analytes. The multiplexing detection is performed on a Luminex analyzer, where two lasers are used to quantitate the green, infrared, and red fluorescence of the individual microsphere as they pass through the sample cuvette. The red laser excites the dye molecules inside the microsphere and classifies the microsphere to its unique set (red-infrared fluorochrome ratio measured by FL1, the classifier signal), and the green laser quantifies the immunoassay on the microsphere surface (reporter signal FL2). Only those microspheres with a complete sandwich will fluoresce in the green part of the spectrum, and the signal is proportional to the amount of capture analyte. The reporter signal is measured as the mean or median fluorescence intensity (MFI) for each microsphere set. And quantitation of capture analyte can be achieved with a built in standard curve in the assay. The Luminex xMAP technology has a unique combination of features: high through-put capacity, analyte quantification over a wide range of concentrations, small sample volume, high reproducibility, and high sensitivity. Multiplexed immunoassays have been designed for up to 100-plexed detection (Luminex 100/200™). Recently, Luminex has developed a new instrument (FLEXMAP 3D™) that can perform up to 500 multiplexed immunoassays by using three internal dyes encoded microspheres. More recently, Luminex also introduced the MAGPIX™ system which was based on the principle of fluorescence imaging, where Light Emitting Diodes (LEDs) and a CCD camera were used to replace the lasers and Photo Multiplying Tubes (PMTs) to deliver a cost-effective, compact, and reliable multiplexing platform. The features of these xMAP systems are listed in **Table 3**. The xMAP technology has been demonstrated as a powerful multiplexing method and has found applications in detection of human cytokines[40], single nucleotide polymorphisms (SNPs)[41], allergy testing[42], infectious disease diagnosis[43], and biological warfare agent screening[44].

Instrumentation*	Luminex xMAP (Multi-Analyte Profiling) (www.Luminexcorp.com)	BD™ CBA (Cytometric Bead Arrays) (www.bdbiosciences.com)	Illumina Veracode™/ BeadXpress (www.illumina.com)
Microsphere	5.6 μm Polystyrene/Magnetic	7.5 μm Polystyrene	240 μm (L) X 28 μm (D) Cylindrical silica glass
Bio-conjugation	Covalent: Sulfo-NHS/EDC	Covalent: Sulfo-SMCC	Covalent: Sulfo-NHS/EDC
Fluorescence Detection	Fluorescence signal detector system; PE (phycoerythrin) is normally the reporter molecule	Fluorescence parameters and two size discriminators	Bead identification based on optical "signature" generated by diffraction; four fluorescent dyes can be used for labeling
Multiplexing Capacity	Up to 500	Up to 30	Up to 48 for protein assay
Key Features	Most widely distributed platform; flexible, can test up to 100 analytes simultaneously; commercial kits are available. (New FlexMAP 3D system allows up to 500 multiplexing capability and is compatible with both 96-and 384well plates	Compatible with conventional flow cytometers and capable of cell-based assays	High-purity silica glass beads are used to minimize fluorescence background, two-color laser system, digital coding enables customizable tracking of multiplex assay markers and critical identifiers such as sample ID, laboratory ID, and reagent kits (up to 24 bits)
Applications	Assays for cytokines, hormones, growth factors, proteinases, cancer markers, cardiac markers, metabolic markers, kinases/ phosphorylated proteins are available; can be used for autoimmune disease diagnostics, infectious disease diagnostics etc.	Assays for complement-derived inflammatory mediators, intracellular signaling molecules, and apoptosis have been described. Kits for viral proteins and cytokines are available	Feasible for up to 384-plex genotyping assays. For protein analysis, only a 10-plex cytokine assay is currently available.

*See Ref.6 for more information

Table 2. Overview of commercially encoded-microsphere based multiplexing technologies

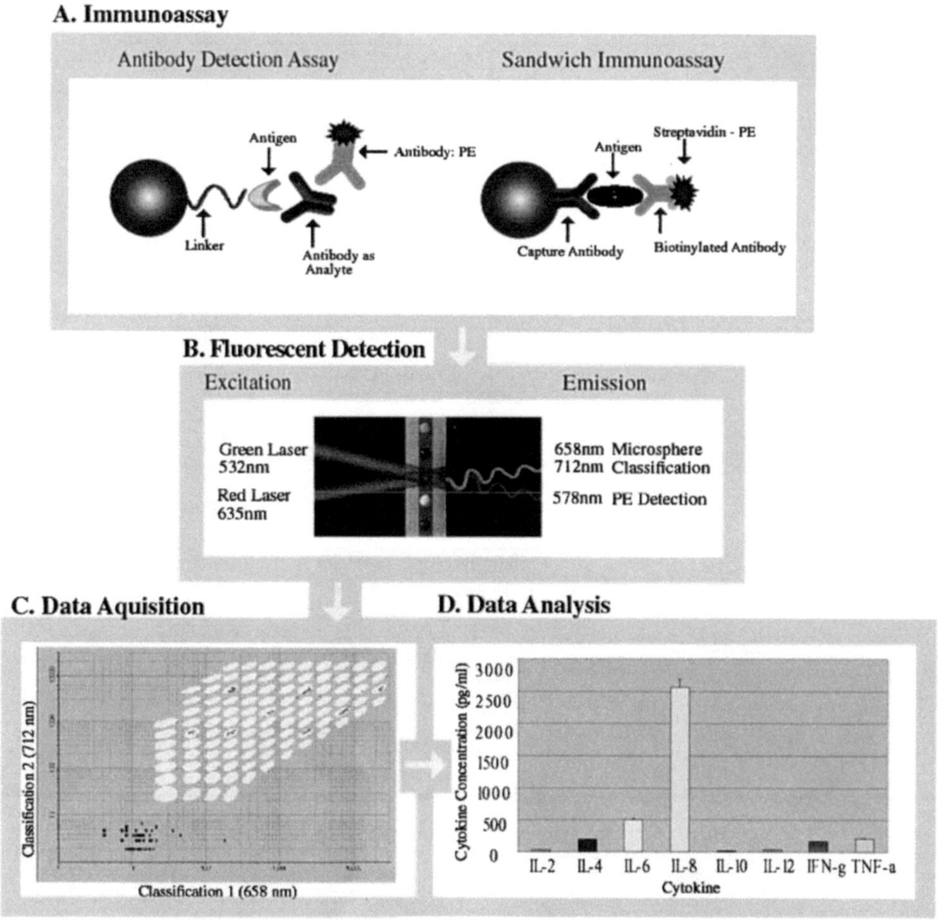

Fig. 3. A schematic illustration of the Luminex xMAP technology: (A) Antibody detection and sandwich immunoassay formats performed on dye encoded microspheres. Any antigen-antibody-based format can be designed with a terminal reporter molecule specific to the laser detection system and distinct from any fluorescence of the microspheres; (B) At the completion of the binding assay, fluorescence intensities associated with each microsphere are measured by flow cytometry (Luminex 100); (C) The dot plot displays 100 distinct regions for each Luminex microsphere population classified on the basis of the intensities of two internal fluorochromes. The instrument was set to acquire at least 100 microspheres each of spectrally distinct populations of microspheres. (D) Multiplexed data from a random sample in an 8-plex assay was calculated. (Reprinted with permission of ref. **44**)

Another similar optically encoded microsphere based multiplexing platform was developed by Becton Dickinson BioSciences, named Cytometric Bead Array system (BD™ CBA). This system uses a series of 7.5 μm microspheres doped with one fluorescent dye at different intensities to simultaneously detect multiple analytes from a single sample.[45, 46] The BD™ CBA combines bead-based immunoassay with sensitivity of amplified fluorescence detection by flow cytometry, creating a powerful multiplexed immunoassay system. The specific capture beads are incubated with tested samples and then mixed with PE conjugated

Features*	Luminex 100/200™	FLEXMAP 3D™	MAGPIX™
Optics	Lasers/APDs/PMTs	Lasers/APDs/PMTs	LED/CCD Camera
Hardware	Flow Cytometry based	Flow Cytometry based	Fluorescent Imager
Beads Compatibility	MagPlex® MicroPlex® SeroPlex® LumAvidin® xTAG®	MagPlex® MicroPlex® SeroPlex® LumAvidin® xTAG®	MagPlex®
Multiplexing Capacity	100 (80 for MagPlex®)	500	50
Read Time	~40 mins/96 well plate	~20 mins/96 well plate	~60 mins/96 well plate
Applications	Protein/Nucleic Acid	Protein/Nucleic Acid	Protein/Nucleic Acid
Dynamic Range	≥ 3.5 logs	≥ 4.5 logs	≥ 3.5 logs
Microtiter Plate	96 well	96 well& 384 well	96 well

* For more detail visit www.luminexcorp.com

Table 3. Technical features of three Luminex XMAP systems

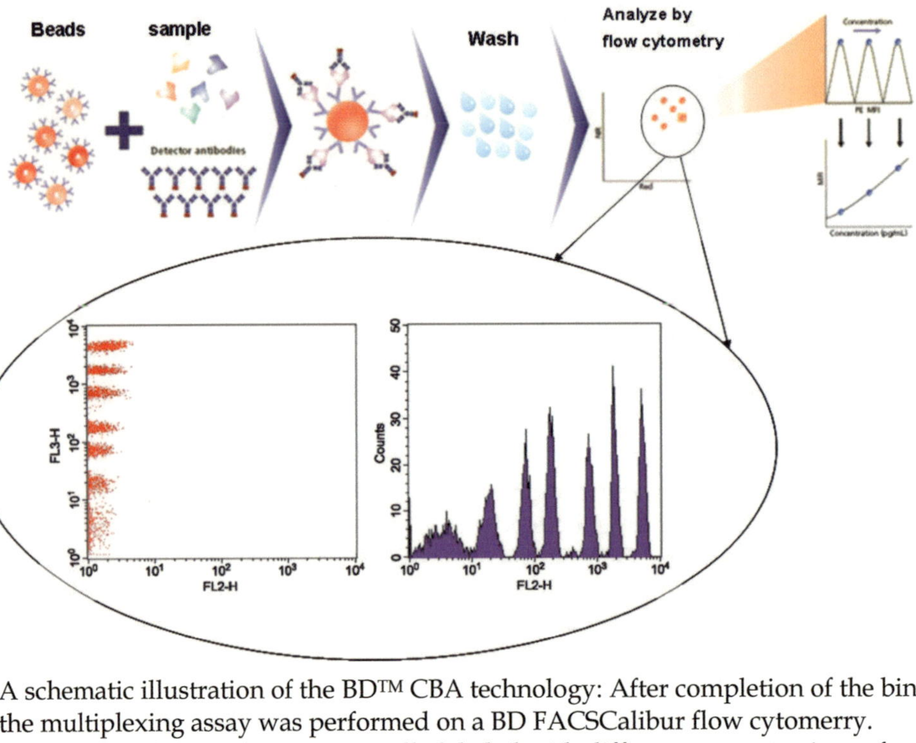

Fig. 4. A schematic illustration of the BD™ CBA technology: After completion of the binding assay, the multiplexing assay was performed on a BD FACSCalibur flow cytomerry. Particles (7.5 µm in diameter) were internally labeled with different concentrations of a dye that emits strong fluorescent signals measured in the FL3 channel while displaying minimal fluorescence measured in the FL2 channel as shown in the two-color analysis dot plot (insert left). The non-overlapping nature of histograms for the bead populations are shown on the inset right. (Courtesy of BD Biosciences).

detection antibodies to form sandwich complexes. Sample data is then obtained using flow cytometry. The CBA analysis is designed to run on FACScan and FACalibur flow cytometers, where microsphere population are gated in the forward and side scatter channel (FSC and SSC) to draw an FL3 (bead channel) histogram (**Figure 4**). Each of the fluorescence intensity peaks identified in the FL3 histogram is first classified as an individual assay (one peak represents each type of analyte-bead complex). The corresponding target analyte concentrations are then measured by their fluorescence intensities in the FL2 reporter channel. While the number of assays that can be performed simultaneously (i.e. multiplexing capacity) is limited due to the use of one fluorescent dye for coding, the CBA assays are compatible with any cytometer that is equipped with a 488 nm laser, and capable of distinguishing emissions at 576 and 670 nm. This advantage enables CBA assays to be performed on widely available commercial benchtop flow cytometry. The BD™ CBA systems have commercialized a larger number of multiplexed immunoassay kits for measurement of a variety of soluble and intracellular proteins, including cytokines, chemokines, growth factors, and phosphorylated cell signaling proteins.

The third commercialized multiplexing platform is VeraCode™ technology from Illumina, which is different from above two platforms that are based on fluorescent dye encoded microspheres. It uses cylindrical glass microbead (240 μm in length and 28 μm in diameter) etched with pre-calculated digital holograms. When illuminated with a red laser beam, the holographic elements diffract the beam to produce a unique image code, where each bright stripe represents '1' and dark strip represents "0" (**Figure 5**). By sequential etching holograms onto microbeads, different patterns of codes can be obtained. The surface of the microbead is functionalized with carboxyl groups for covalent binding of capture ligand. Each set of microbead with a unique digital holographic code is used to attach a specific type of capture ligand for target analyte of interest. Consequently, multiplexed assays can be performed by pooling different microbeads embedded with unique "optical signatures" in the same reaction mixture. And the analytes are labeled with standard fluorescent reporters such as PE, Cy3, Cy5, or AlexaFluor dyes. The multiplexed assays are carried out on the Illumina BeadXpress reader, where the microbeads are deposited into a grooved plate so that they are aligned for reading. During analysis, the fluorescence and code are recorded for each microbead by using a red code-readout laser and a green report laser. The holographic code image in each microbead diffracts the incident read laser beam to make up the optical patterns of the bead code and can be detected with a CCD camera. And the green laser quantifies analyte binding. The company has provided carboxylated microbead sets for custom probe attachment.

3. Applications of multiplexed immunoassays

Multiplexed immunoassays allow simultaneous measurement of multiple analytes in a single biological sample, which enables people to obtain high density of biomolecule information with minimal assay time, cost and sample volume. After overcoming the technical hurdles in encoding, functionalizing, decoding, detecting, and improving the limited number of assays to be performed simultaneously, a great number of multiplexed immunoassay platforms, especially optically encoded microsphere based technologies, have been applied in wide range of fields in the biomedical research and clinical diagnostics.

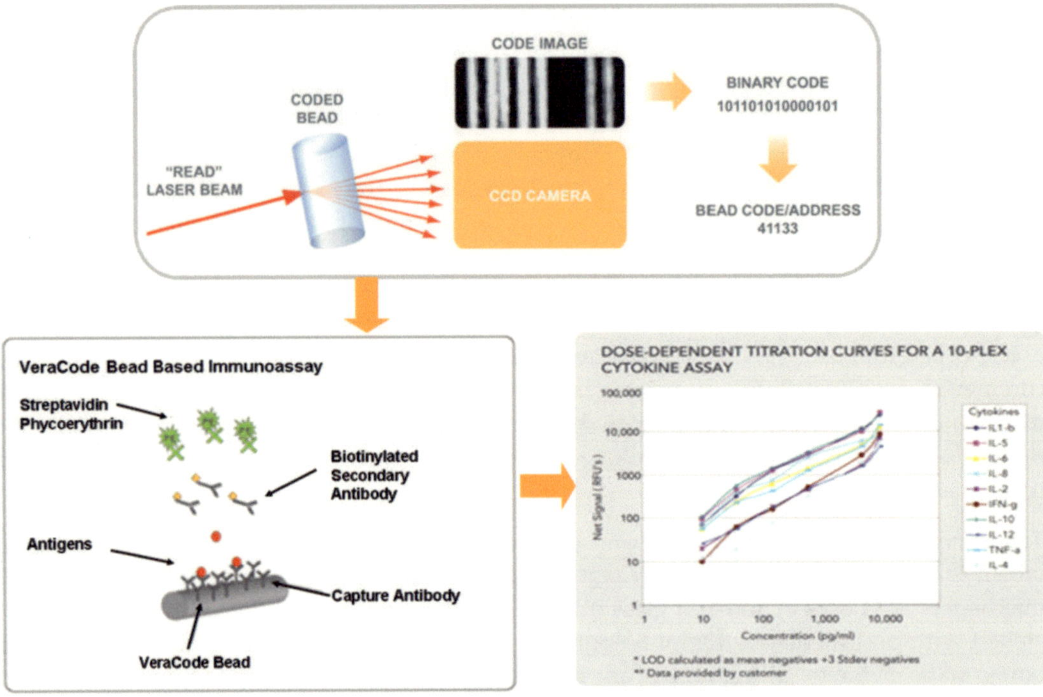

Fig. 5. A schematic illustration of Illumina VeraCode™ techonology: a glass bead containing an etched hologram is illustrated with a laser beam producing a code image. Multiplexed immunoassay can be performed by attached specific capture ligand to individual set of bead. (Courtesy of Illumina, Inc.)

At present, the most successful and robust multiplexing technology is Luminex xMAP platform, which combines advanced fluidics, optics, and digital signal processing with proprietary microsphere technology to deliver multiplexed assay capabilities. Importantly, Luminex is an open technology and numerous companies have marketed the Luminex system, including Bio-Rad, Qiagen, Invitrogen, and Millipore *ect.*. And a steadily growing list of ready-to-use multiplexed immunoassays have also been provided by these companies for applications in biomarker discovery[47-76], autoimmune disease diagnostics[77-80], infectious disease diagnostics[81-93], neurological diseases[94-101], HLA testing[102-104], and drug discovery[105, 106] (**Table 4**).

For example, encoded microsphere based multiplexed immunoassays have been used to analyze the expression of cytokines, chemokines and growth factors in diverse samples (serum, plasma, and tissue culture), and therefore serve as a very straightforward approach for biomarker discovery.[47-63] Cytokines, chemokines, and growth factors are cell signaling proteins that mediate a wide range of physiological responses including immunity, inflammation, and hematopoiesis. Changes in the levels of these biomarkers are associated with a spectrum of diseases ranging from tumor growth, to infections, to Parkinson's disease. One of the many commercially available panels for analysis of cytokines, chemokines and growth factors is a 53-plex by Bio-Rad. This panel can simultaneously measure levels of 53 proteins in biological samples using encoded magnetic microspheres, which allows an investigator to take advantage of flexibility of microsphere arrays to develop a customized

Biomedical Research Partners*	Assays/system	Applications
Affymetrix/Panomics (www.panomics.com)	QuantiGene®, Procarta®	Cardiac Markers; Celluar Signaling; Cytokines, Chemokines and Growth Factors; Endocrine; Gene Expression Profiling; Transcription Factors
Bio-Rad Laboratories (www.bio-rad.com)	X-Plex, Bio-Plex®	Celluar Signaling; Celluar Signaling; Cytokines, Chemokines and Growth Factors; Endocrine; Isotpying
Cayman Chemical Company (www.caymanchem.com)		Apoptosis; Cancer Markers; Cytokines; Endocrine
Charles River Laboratories (www.criver.com)		Accute Phase Inflammation; Autoimmune; Cancer Markers; Cardiac Markers; Cytokines and Chemokines; Endocrines; Infectious Disease
EMD Chemicals (www.emdbiosciences.com)	Novagen Widescreen™	Celluar Signaling; Enzymatic Acitvity
Hitachi/MiraiBio Group		Reagent; Hardware/Software Provider
Indoor Biotechnologies, Inc. (www.inbio.com)	MARIA™	Allergy Testing; Custom Development
Invitrogen (www.invitrogen.com)		Accute Phase Inflammation; Apoptosis; Autoimmune Disease; Cytokines, Chemokines and Growth Factors; Endocrines; Matrix Metalloproteinases; Neuroscience; Signal Transduction
Millipore Corporation (www.millipore.com)	Milliplex™, LINCOplex™, Beadlyte®	Apoptosis; Cancer Markers; Cardiac Markers; Cytokines, Chemokines and Growth Factors; Endocrines; Isotyping; Metabolic Markers
Origene (www.Origen.com)		Genotyping; Transcription Factors
PerkinElmer (www.perkinelmer.com)	Autoplex™	Assay Automation; Hardware/Software Provider
Qiagen, Inc. (www.qiagen.com)		Hardware/Software Provider
R&D Systems (www.rndsystems.com)	Fluoreokine®	Autoimmune Diseases; Cytokines, Chemokines and Growth Factors; Endocrines; Matrix Metalloproteinases
Rules Based Medcine (www.rbmmaps.com)	Human MAPs	Autoimmune Diseases; Cancer Markers; Cardiac Markers; Cytokines, Chemokines and Growth Factors; Endocrines; Infectious Diseases; Isotyping; Metabolic Markers

*Visit www.luminexcorp.com for more information

Table 4.A List of Luminex xMAP biomedical research partners and their application areas

Clinical Diagnostics Partners*	Assays/system	Applications
Abbott Molecular (www.abbottmolecular.com)		Molecular Infectious Disease
Asuragen (www.asuragen.com)	Signature	Human Genetic Testing, Oncology
BMD (www.bmd-net.com)	FIDIS™, CARIS™	Autoimmune Disease
Bio-Rad Diagnostics (www.bio-rad.com)	Bio-Plex®	Autoimmune Disease; Infectious Disease
Eragen Biosciences (www.eragen.com)	MultiCode	Infectious Disease
Celera Diagnostics (www.celeradiagnostics.com)		Human Genetic Testing
Fisher HealthCare (www.fishersci.com)	Prima	Human Genetic Testing; Molecular Infectious Disease
Focus Diagnostics (www.focusdx.com)		Infectious Disease
Innogenetics NV (www.innogenetics.com)		Alzheimer's Disease
INOVA Diagnostics (www.inovadx.com)	QUANTA Plex™	Autoimmune Disease
Inverness Medical Professional Diagnostics (www.invernessmedicalpd.com)	AtheNA Multi-Lyte®	Autoimmune Disease
Microbionix GmbH (www.microbionix.com)		Custom Development
Multimetrix/Progen Biotechnik GmbH (www.multimetrix.com)		Infectious Disease; Custom Development
One Lambda, Inc. (www.onelambda.com)	LABSCreen, LABType	HLA Testing
Qiagen, Inc. (www.qiagen.com)	LiquidChip ™; QIAPlex™	Molecular Infectious Disease
Gen-Probe (www.tepnel.com)	LifeMatch ™	HLA Testing
Zeus Scientific (www.zeusscientific.com)	AtheNA Multi-Lyte®	Autoimmune Disease; Infectious Disease

*Visit www.luminexcorp.com for more information

Table 4.B List of Luminex xMAP clinical research partners and their application areas

multiplex panel for efficient detection of protein of interest. Rules Based Medicine (RBM) also offers a special panel (Human DiscoveryMAP250+) for analysis of up to 250 human biomarkers from human serum sample using minute quantities of sample volume.

Moreover, encoded microsphere based multiplexed immunoassay technology has also been used in cancer biomarker discovery.[64-76] Rapid advance in the genomics and proteomics has generated a plenty of candidate cancer biomarkers that could be useful in early cancer detection and monitoring. However, the capacity to verify and validate these candidate cancer biomarkers is limited, due to the requirement of rigorous testing in a large sample set from many diseases. Recently, Rules Based Medicine has developed a cancer biomarker panel (Human OncologyMAP®) for quantitative measurement of 101 cancer-associated serum proteins. This novel tool is based on encoded microsphere multiplexing technology and offers a powerful tool to aid in the discovery and development of new oncology drugs and diagnostics.

Another example of application of encoded microsphere based multiplexed immunoassay technology is in clinical diagnostics such as autoimmune diseases or infectious diseases. Autoimmune diseases include a wide variety of systemic or organ-specific inflammatory diseases that are characterized by the aberrant activation of immune cells. Many autoimmune diseases are characterized by the presence of specific autoantibody types, which can be used in the diagnosis and classification of autoimmune diseases.[77-80] The BioPlex™ 2200 ANA screen (Bio-Rad) and the AtheNA Multi-Lyte™ ANA test system (Zesus Scientific) have obtained marketing approval from the US FDA. These two tests are used in the diagnostics of autoimmune diseases and based on the simultaneous measurement of multiple auto-antibodies. Moreover, encoded microsphere based multiplexed immunoassay technology could improve diagnostics of infectious diseases by enabling the simultaneous detection of antibodies or antigens to multiple infectious pathogens, such as human immunodeficiency virus (HIV), the Hepatitis A, B, C virus, *Mycobacterium tuberculosis,* as well as a large number of other viral, bacterial and parasitic pathogens.[81-93] FDA-approved assays for infectious diseases (*e.g.* EBV, HSV, MMRV, Syphilis, and ToRC assays on BioPlex™ 2200 or Multi-Lyte™) are already available on market.

Encoded microsphere based multiplexed immunoassays are also effective tools for simultaneously measurement of several biomarkers in Alzheimer's disease (AD).[94, 95] Alzheimer disease is the most common form of age-related neurodegenerative disease, which is a neurodegenerative disorder characterized by accumulation of intracellular neurofibrillary tangles and extracellular amyloid plaques throughout the cortical and limbic brain regions. The development of validated biomarkers for Alzheimer's disease is essential to improve diagnosis and accelerate the development of new therapies. As the list of AD biomarkers is constantly growing, the ability to validate a panel of biomarkers becomes essential. To this end, Innogenetics has offered a multiparameter bead-based immunoassay (**INNO-BIA AlzBio3**) for the simultaneous quantification of 3 key AD markers in human cerebrospinal fluid (CSF): beta-amyloid 1-42, total tau, and tau phosphorylated at threonine 181.

4. Challenges and limitations of current multiplexed immunoassays

Although hundreds of multiplexed immunoassays are introduced to the research market in recent years, only a limited numbers of them have been approved by the FDA for clinical use. The multiplexed immunoassay, as an emerging technology, is not without limitation. Most FDA approved multiplexed immunoassay platforms are based on encoded microsphere arrays by flow cytometry. Development of robust multiplexed immunoassay required rigorous validation of assay configuration and analytical performance to minimized assay imprecision and inaccuracy. Current limitations associated with multiplexed immunoassay technologies include selection of multiple matched antibodies pairs; cross-reactivity between antibodies and analytes and assay diluents; interference from matrix effect; the required compromise of the assay parameters when developing multiple assays; and the requirement for pre-labeling reporter molecules for detection

A major challenge of developing multiplexed immunoassay is the need to obtain a large number of highly specific antibodies for a wide range of analytes. Although there are many monoclonal and polyclonal antibodies commercially available, it is difficult to standardize and screen several hundreds of these antibodies to produce reliable assay in a multiplexed format while fulfilling the required assay sensitivity and specificity. Particularly, antibodies suitable for monoplex immunoassays may display cross-reactivity with other analytes in the multiplexed format. Cross reactivity between antibodies and nonspecific analytes limits the number of antibodies that can be used in a given multiplexed assay. To solve this problem, several attempts have been made to optimize antibodies characterization and selection by using high-throughput methods based on multiplexed immobilized proteins or peptides. For example, Poetz *et al.*[107] reported the use of a protein microarray to simultaneously analyze epitope recognition and binding affinity of antibodies to determine their specificity and affinity.[114] And Schwenk *et al.*[108] also reported the use of Luminex platform to determine antibody specificity towards up to 100 antigens.

Another major problem is that multiplexed immunoassays are prone to interference due to matrix effect, like any other immunoassay.[109] A matrix consists of all the components in the sample other than the analyte. The interference from matrix would limit the performance of multiplexed assays. Potential sources of interference in the multiplexed immunoassay include endogenous plasma/serum proteins, heterophilic antibodies, soluble receptors, complement components, immune complexes, histidine-rich glycolproteins, lysozyme, fibrinogen, lectins, and some acute phase proteins.[110-112] To minimize matrix effect, it is important to select suitable blocker, assay diluents and appropriate dilution factor for the sample matrix that mimics real sample during assay development.[113] However, it is a challenge in the multiplexed format to select assay diluents that interact effectively with all the reagents and proteins, because each protein requires specific conditions to maintain its conformation. Minor changes in buffer pH and ionic strength may change the protein structure, thus impairing assay performance.

Multiplexed immunoassays involve two or more capture molecules and allow the simultaneous measurement of different target analytes. In a monoplex immunoassay (ELISA), the assay parameters such as antibody pairs, sample diluents, and conjugate concentration can be easily optimized for a particular assay. However, in a multiplexed format, those parameters would be different from one analyte to another. They have to be adjusted to suit all the analytes within the multiplexed assay. The required compromise of the assay parameters would limit the assay performance of multiplexed immunoassay. Another major issue that limits the assay performance of multiplexed immunoassay is that an increasing number of detection antibodies results in an increase of background noise, which subsequently decreases assay sensitivity. For example, it has been found that the sensitivity of an 11-plex assay decreased by a factor of 1.75-5.0, compared with monoplex ELISA, due to an increasing in background signal in the multiplexed format.[114]

Current multiplexed immunoassay platforms, based on either planar microarrays or suspended encoding particle arrays, often require an extra labeling step for the detection ligand with reporter molecules (*e.g.* fluorescent dye), which prolongs the assay time and increases the assay cost. Therefore, challenges in simplifying the tagging process and eliminating the need for pre-labeling reporter molecules for detection still remain. The need to overcome such hurdles has motivated research into the development of a label-free multiplexed assay system, where progress has been made in surface plasmon resonance (SPR) and fluorescent conjugated polymers-based optical detection, nanowire-based electrical or electrochemical measurements, and mass spectrometry (MS)-based high-throughput screening.[115-118] Conjugated polymers, especially conjugated polythiophene derivatives, can display remarkable changes of optical properties due to conformational changes of polymer chains when binding to biomolecules, therefore offer a potential opportunity as the optical probe for multiplexed assay in a label-free fashion.[119-121] We have integrated fluorescent conjugated polymers into metallic encoded nanorods for label-free, multiplexed detection of DNA and cancer biomarkers with high specificity and sensitivity.[122, 123]

5. Summary and future prospect of multiplexed immunoassay

Multiplexed immunoassays allow simultaneous measurement of multiple proteins in a single biological sample. They have demonstrated comparable sensitivity to traditional ELISAs, making them great potential for both basic research and clinical diagnostics where assays required multiplexing in small sample volume. Currently, a great numbers of multiplexing technologies have been developed and used in the biomedical research and clinical diagnostics. The optically encoded microsphere-based technology is the most advanced multiplexing technology and has been commercialized on the market. Optically encoded microsphere-based technology offers a robust and efficient approach for setting up multiplexed assays and makes multiplexing assays feasible by flow cytometry. However, there are still a number of challenges to be overcome before encoded microsphere based multiplexing platforms can be fully applied in the field of clinical diagnostics. The need to overcome these challenges motivate people to continue to develop robust, sensitive, specific, rapid, and high-through assays with multiplex capabilities that can fulfill the expectations and demands for basic biomedical research and clinical application. Prospective technology development and research direction of multiplexed immunoassays would focus on the following main areas:

5.1 Miniaturization

Miniaturization has been a driver in assay development for many years. The goal is to obtain increasing amounts of molecular information from ever decreasing volumes of sample. Miniaturized multiplexed immunoassays can be regarded as an ideal solution for applications in which several parameters of a single sample with limited volume needed to be analyzed in parallel.[124] Recent development in the microfluidic system offers great potential in the miniaturized immunoassay.[125] The most common microfluidic platform relies on networks of enclosed micron-dimension channels, where fluids exhibit laminar flow (i.e. fluidic streams) that flow parallel to each other, and mixing occurs only by diffusion.[126] Microfluidic immunoassays have several advantages over conventional methods[127]: (1) increased surface area to volume ratios speeds up molecule binding reactions; (2) smaller dimensions reduce the consumption of expensive reagents and precious samples; and (3) automated fluid handling can improve reproducibility and throughput. These advantages can potentially improve assay performance and reduce the operation cost of conventional immunoassays. Diercks et al. have reported the integration of optically encoded microspheres with microfluidic platform for miniaturized multiplexed immunoassays.[128] In this work, the encoded microspheres were trapped in a microchannel and imaged using a confocal microscope. They detected four different analytes from a 2.7-nL sample.

5.2 Automation

Immunoassay automation promises to be the most rapidly growing area for research and development in the clinical diagnostics industry.[129] In the automated assays, all stages of assays, from sample preparation to instrument operation to data processing are highly compatible with robotics and automation. Therefore, automation can reduce labor requirements and reduce testing costs. Quality testing can be achieved with immunoassay automation due to improved assay performance resulting from improved precision, sensitivity, and wide dynamic ranges, as well as from the elimination of sample handling and processing errors. Bio-Rad has developed a fully automated, random access multiplexed testing platform, Bio-Plex™ 2200. It combines the encoded magnetic microsphere with automated liquid handling workstation. This system addresses the needs for high-throughput analysis of clinical samples, which automatically processes up to 100 samples per hour, for a maximum of 2200 reportable results with eight hours of walk-away capability. First results are available in approximately 20–45 minutes (assay dependent), with subsequent patient samples completed approximately every 30 seconds.

5.3 Improved capture ligands

A key step for development of robust immunoassays is generation and characterization of capture ligands. These systems required high quality of capture ligands with high specificity and sensitivity of recognizing target proteins. Current available antibodies may display cross reactivity with other proteins in the multiplexed assay format. To solve this problem, alternative capture ligands such as engineered protein scaffolds and nucleic acid scaffolds are being evaluated to replace antibodies for the specific protein detection[130-132]. For example, aptamers, highly specific oligonucleic acids or peptide molecules that bind to protein due to their unique three dimensional structure, possess target recognition features as antibodies [133]

5.4 Improved encoding technology

The development of new encoding technology for microparticles may also offer higher and more stable multiplexing capacity. Recent advances in Quantum dots studies have shown a potential for new alternative optical encoding technology. Quantum dots are photoluminescent semiconductor nanocrystals, which typically consist of a core of cadmium selenide (CdSe) surrounded by a shell of zinc sulfide (ZnS).[134, 135] Quantum dots have many advantages over traditional fluorescent dyes as ideal fluorophores for wavelength and intensity multiplxing: (1) their emission spectra are tunable by the size of quantum dots, (2) Quantum dots of different emission profiles can be excited simultaneously at the same excitation wavelength, (3) their emission bands are relatively narrow, which allow more emission bands to be resolved with minimal spectra overlap, and (4) Quantum dots have higher quantum yields than most fluorescent dyes and have better photochemical stability against photo-bleaching. Multicolor optical coding can be achieved by embedding different size of Quantum dots into polymeric microsphere at precisely controlled ratios. [136-138] For example, the use 10 intensity levels and 6 colors can generate up to 10^6 codes, which open up new opportunities for gene profiling, high-throughput screening, and medical diagnostics.

5.5 Improved clinical applications

Early stage detection of many diseases requires distinct pattern recognition of various protein biomarkers to identify at-risk individuals with adequate confidence. Multi-biomarker strategies improve medical diagnostic and prognostic information. Therefore, multiplexed immunoassays are becoming more and more important for clinical diagnostics in the future due to their ability of identifying multiple clinical biomarkers for a wide range of diseases. Multiplexed protein test panels for use in cancer, stroke, diabetes, and cardiovascular diseases would be the interest in the future.

6. References

[1] Wood, C. G. *Clin. Lab.* 2008, *54*, 423-438.
[2] Lequin, R. M. *Clin. Chem.* 2005, *51*, 12-15.
[3] Kitano, H. *Science* 2002, *295*, 1662-1664.
[4] Feinberg, J. G. *Nature* 1961, *192*, 985-986.
[5] Ekins, R. P. *J. Pharm. Biomed. Anal.* 1989, *7*, 155-168.
[6] Nalan, J. P.; Mandy F. *Cytometry A* 2006, *69*, 318-325.
[7] Hsu, H.-Y.; Joos, T. O.; Koga, H. *Electrophoresis* 2009, *30*, 4008-4019.
[8] Krishhan, V. V.; Khan, I. H.; Luciw, P. A. *Ctri. Rev. Biotechnol.* 2009, *29*, 29-43.
[9] Hartmann, M.; Roeraade, J.; Stoll, D.; Templin, M. F.; Joos, T. O. *Anal. Bioanal. Chem.* 2009, *393*, 1407-1416.
[10] Wingren, C.; Borrebaeck, C. A. *Methods Mol. Biol.* 2009, *509*, 57-84.
[11] Wingren, C.; Borrebaeck, C. A. *Drug Discov. Today* 2007, *12*, 813-819.
[12] Li, F.; Guan, Y.; Chen, Z. *Cell. Mol. Life Sci.* 2008, *65*, 1007-1012.
[13] Ramachandran, N.; Anderson, K. S.; Raphael, J. V.; Hainnsworth, E.; Sibani, S.; Montor, W. R.; Pacek, M.; Wong, J.; Eljanne, M.; Sanda, M. G.; Hu, Y.; Logvinenko, T.; LaBaer, J. *Proteomics Clin. Appl.* 2008, *2*, 1518-1527.
[14] Wu, J.; Dyer, W.; Chrisp, J.; Belov, L.; Wang, B.; Saksena, N. *Retrovirlogy* 2008, *5*, 24.
[15] Quintata, F. J.; Farez, M. F.; Viglietta, V.; Iglesias, A. H.; Merbl, Y.; Izquierdo, G.; Lucas, M.; Basso, A. B.; Khoury, S. J.; Lucchinetti, C. F.; Cohen, R. H.; Weiner, H. L. *Proc. Natl. Acad. Sci. U.S.A.* 2008, *105*, 1889.
[16] Leffers, N.; Gooden, M.; de Jong, R.; Hoogeboom, B.; ten Hoor, K.; Hollema, H.; Boezen, H.; van der Zee, A.; Daemen, T.; Nijman, H. *Cancer Immunol. Immunother.* 2009, *58*, 449-459.
[17] Wilson, R.; Cossins, A. R.; Spiller, D. G. *Angew. Chem. Int. Ed.* 2006, *45*, 6104-6117.
[18] Birtwell, S.; Morgan, H. *Integr. Biol.* 2009, *1*, 345-362.
[19] Fulton, R. J.; McDade, R. L.; Smith, P. L.; Kienker, L. J.; Kettman Jr., J. R. *Clin. Chem.* 1997, *43*, 1749-1756.
[20] Battersby, B. J.; Bryant, D.; Meutermans, W.; Matthews, D.; Smythe, M. L.; Trau, M. *J. Am. Chem. Soc.* 2000, *122*, 2138-2139.

[21] Han, M.; Gao, X.; Su, J. Z.; Nie, S. *Nat. Biotechnol.* 2001, *19*, 631-635.
[22] Zhao, X. W.; Liu, Z. B.; Yang, H.; Nagai, K.; Zhao, Y. H.; Gu, Z. Z. *Chem. Mater.* 2006, *18*, 2443-2449.
[23] Dejneka, M. J.; Streltsov, A.; Pal, S.; Frutos, A.; Powell, C.; Yost, K.; Yuen, P.; Muller, U.; Lahiri, J. *Proc. Natl. Acad. Sci. USA* 2003, *2*, 389-393.
[24] Su, X.; Zhang, J.; Sun, L.; Koo, T.; Chan, S.; Sundararajan, N.; Yamakawa, M.; Berlin, A. A. *Nano Lett.* 2005, *5*, 49-54.
[25] Fenniri, H.; Chun, S.; Ding, L.; Zyrianov, Y.; Hallenga, K. *J. Am. Chem. Soc.* 2003, *125*, 10546-10560.
[26] Jin, R.; Cao, Y.; Thaxon, C. S.; Mirkin, C. A. *Small* 2006, *2*, 375-380.
[27] Natan, M. J. *Faraday Discuss.* 2006, *132*, 321-328.
[28] Cunin, F.; Schmedake, T. A.; Link, J. R.; Li, Y. Y., Koh, J.; Bhatia, S. N.; Sailor, M. J. *Nat. Mater.* 2002, *1*, 39-41.
[29] Nicewarner-Peña, S. R.; Freeman, R.G.; Reiss, B. D.; He, L.; Peña, D. J.; Walton, I. D.; Cromer, R.; Keating, C. D.; Natan, M. J. *Science* 2001, *294*, 137-141.
[30] Braeckmans, K.; de Smedt, S.; Roelant, C.; Leblans, M.; Pauwels, R.; Demeester, R. *Nat. Mater.* 2003, *2*, 169-193.
[31] Dames, A.; England, J.; Colby, E. *WO Patent 00/16983*, 2000.
[32] Zhi, Z. L.; Morita, Y.; Hasan, Q.; Tamiya, E. *Anal. Chem.* 2003, *75*, 4125-4131.
[33] Pregibon, D. C.; Toner, M; Doyle, P. S. *Science* 2007, *315*, 1393-1396.
[34] Moran, E. J.; Sarshar, S.; Cargill, J. F.; Shahbaz, M. M.; Lio, A.; Mjalli, A. M.; Armstrong, R. W. *J. Am. Chem. Soc.* 1995, *117*, 10787-10788.
[35] Nicolaou, K. C.; Xiao, X. Y.; Parandoosh, Z.; Senyei, A.; Nova, M. P. *Angew. Chem. Int. Ed.* 1995, *34*, 2289-2291.
[36] Benecky, M. J.; Post, D. R.; Schmitt, S. M.; Kochar, M. S. *Clin. Chem.* 1997, *43*, 1764-1779.
[37] Evans, M.; Sewter, C.; Hill, E. *Assay Drug Dev. Technol.* 2003, *1*, 199-207.
[38] Vignali, D. A. A. *J. Immunol. Methods* 2000,*243*, 243-255.
[39] Kellar, K. L.; Iannone, M. A. *Exp. Hematol.* 2002, *30*, 1227-1237
[40] Kellar, K. L.; Douglass, J. P. *J. Immunol. Methods* 2003, *279*, 277-285.
[41] Hurley, J. D.; Engle, L. J.; Davis, J. T.; Welsh, A. M.; Landers, J. E. *Nucleic Acids Res.* 2004, *32*, e186.
[42] Whitehead, G. S.; Walker, J. K. L.; Berman, K. G.; Foster, W. M.; Schwartz, D. A. *Am. J. Physiol. Lung Cell. Mol. Physiol.* 2003, *285*, L32-L42.
[43] Yan, X.; Zhong, W.; Tang, A.; Schielke, E. G.; Hang, W.; Nolan, J. P. *Anal. Chem.* 2005, *77*, 7673-7678.
[44] McBride, M. T.; Gammon, S.; Pitesky, M.; OKBrien, T. W.; Smith, T.; Aldrich, J.; Langlois, R. G.; Colston, B.; Venkateswaran, K. S. *Anal. Chem.* 2003, *75*, 1924-1930.
[45] Morgan, E.; Varro, R.; Sepulveda, H.; Ember, J. A.; Apgar, J.; Wilson, J.; Lowe, L.; Chen, R.; Shivraj, L.; Agadir, A.; Campos, R.; Ernst, D.; Gaur, A. *Clin. Immunol.* 2004, *110*, 252-266.
[46] Tarnok, A.; Hambsch, J.; Chen, R.; Varro, R. *Clin. Chem.* 2003, *49*, 1000-1002.
[47] Carson, R. T.; Vignali, D. A. *J. Immunol. Methods* 1999, *227*, 41-52.
[48] Prabhakar, U.; Eirikis, E.; Davis, H. M. *J. Immunol. Methods* 2002, *260*, 207-218.
[49] de Jager, W.; te Velthuis, H.; Prakken, B. J.; Kuis, W.; Rijkers, G. T.; *Clin. Diagn. Lab. Immunol.* 2003, *10*, 133-139.

[50] Olsson, A.; Vanderstichele, H.; Andreasen, N.; De Meyer, G.; Wallin, A.; Holmberg, B.; Rosengren, L. *Clin. Chem.* 2005, *51*, 336-345.
[51] de Jager, W.; Rijkers, G. T. *Methods* 2006, *38*, 294-303.
[52] Maier, R.; Weger, M.; Haller-Schober, E. M.; El-Shabrawi, Y.; Theisl, A.; Barth, A.; Aigner, R. *Mol. Vis.* 2006, *12*, 1143-1147.
[53] McDuffie, E.; Obert, L.; Chupka, J.; Sigler, R. *J. Inflamm. (Lond.)* 2006, *3*, 15.
[54] Dunbar, S. A.; Vander Zee, C. A.; Oliver, K. G.; Karem, K. L.; Jacobson, J. W. *J. Microbiol. Methods* 2003, *53*, 245-252.
[55] Chen, R.; Lowe, L.; Wilson, J. D.; Crowther, E.; Tzeggai, K.; Bishop, J. E.; Varro, R. *Clin. Chem.* 1999, *45*, 16931694.
[56] Fulton, R. J.; McDade, R. L.; Smith, P. L.; Kienker, L. J.; Kettman, J. R. Jr. *Clin. Chem.* 1997, *43*, 1749-1756.
[57] Kayal, S.; Jais, J. P.; Aguini, N.; Chaudiere, J.; Labrousse, J. *Am. J. Respir. Crit. Care Med.* 1998, 157, 776-784.
[58] De Freitas, I.; Fernandez-Somoza, M.; Essenfeld-Sekler, E.; Cardier, J. E. *Chest* 2004, *125*, 2238-2246.
[59] Reinhart, K.; Bayer, O.; Brunkhorst, F.; Meisner, M. *Crit. Care Med.* 2002, *30*, S302-S312.
[60] Marshall, J. C. *Intensive Care Med.* 2000, *26*, S75-S83.
[61] Carrigan, S. D.; Scott, G.; Tabrizian, M. *Clin. Chem.* 2004, *50*, 1301-1314.
[62] Bozza, F. A.; Salluh, J. I.; Japiassu, A. M.; Soares, M.; Assis, E. F.; Gomes, R. N.; Bozza, M. T. *Crit. Care* 2007, *11*, R49.
[63] Calvano, S. E.; van der Poll, T.; Coyle, S. M.; Barie, P. S.; Moldawer, L. L.; Lowry, S. F. *Arch. Surg.* 1996, *131*, 434-437.
[64] Bertenshaw, G. P.; Yip, P.; Seshaiah, P.; Zhao, J.; Chen, T. H.; Wiggins, W. S.; Mapes, J. P. *Cancer Epidemiol. Biomarkers Prev.* 2008, *17*, 2872-2881.
[65] Kim, B. K.; Lee, J. W.; Park, P. J.; Shin, Y. S.; Lee, W. Y.; Lee, K. A.; Ye, S. *Breast Cancer Res.* 2009, *11*, R22.
[66] Khan, I. H.; Mendoza, S.; Rhyne, P.; Ziman, M.; Tuscano, J.; Eisinger, D.; Kung, H. J.; Luciw, P. A. *Mol. Cell Proteomics* 2006, *5*, 758-768.
[67] Johnson, T. J.; Wannemuehler, Y. M.; Johnson, S. J.; Logue, C. M.; White, D. G.; Doetkott, C.; Nolan, L. K. *Appl. Environ. Microbiol.* 2007, *73*, 1976-1983.
[68] Allen, C.; Duffy, S.; Teknos, T.; Islam, M.; Chen, Z.; Albert, P. S.; Wolf, G.; VanWaes, C. *Clin. Can. Res.* 2007, *13*, 3182-3190.
[69] Deans, C.; Rose-Zerilli, M.; Wigmore, S.; Ross, J.; Howell, M.; Jackson, A.; Grimble, R.; Fearon, K. *Ann. Surg. Oncol.* 2007, *14*, 329-339.
[70] Shurin, M. R.; Smolkin, Y. S. *Adv. Expl. Med. Biol.* 2007, *601*, 3-12.
[71] Yurkovetsky, Z. R.; Kirkwood, J. M.; Edington, H. D.; Marrangoni, A. M.; Velikokhatnaya, L.; Winans, M. T.; Gorelik, E.; Lokshin A. E. *Clin. Can. Res.* 2007, *13*, 2422-2428.
[72] Ullenhag, G. J.; Spendlove, I.; Watson, N. F.; Indar, A. A.; Dube, M.; Robins, R. A.; Maxwell-Armstrong, C.; Scholefield, J. H.; Durrant, L. G. *Clin. Can. Res.* 2006, *12*, 7389-7396.
[73] Dehqanzada, Z. A.; Storrer, C. E.; Hueman, M. T.; Foley, R.J.; Harris, K. A.; Jama, Y. H.; Shriver, C. D.; Ponniah, S.; Peoples, G. E. *Oncol. Rep.* 2007, *17*, 687-694.
[74] Zhong, H.; Han, B.; Tourkova, I. L.; Lokshin, A.; Rosenbloom, A.; Shurin, M. R.; Shurin, G. V. *Clin. Can. Res.* 2007, *13*, 5455-5462.

[75] Tanaka, M.; Komatsu, N.; Yanagimoto, Y.; Oka, M.; Shichijo, S.; Okuda, S.; Itoh, K. *Kurume Med. J.* 2006, *53*, 63-70.

[76] Keyes, K. A.; Mann, L.; Cox, K.; Treadway, P.; Iversen, P.; Chen, Y. F.; Teicher, B. A. *Can. Chemother. Pharmacol.* 2003, *51*, 321-327.

[77] Gilburd, B.; Abu-Shakra, M.; Shoenfeld, Y.; Giordano, A.; Bocci, E. B.; dell Monache, F.; Gerli, R. *Clin. Dev. Immunol.* 2004, *11*, 53-56.

[78] Shovman, O.; Gilburd, B.; Barzilai, O.; Shinar, E.; Larida, B.; Zandman-Goddard, G.; Binder, S. R. *Ann. NY Acad. Sci.* 2005, *1050*, 380-388.

[79] Barzilai, O.; Ram, M.; Shoenfeld, Y. *Curr. Opin. Rheumatol.* 2007, *19*, 636-643.

[80] Barzilai, O.; Sherer, Y.; Ram, M.; Izhaky, D.; Anaya, J. M.; Shoenfeld, Y. *Ann. NY Acad. Sci.* 2007, *1108*, 567-577.

[81] Clavijo, A.; Hole, K.; Li, M.; Collignon, B. *Vaccine* 2006, *24*, 1693-1704.

[82] Laher, G.; Balmer, P.; Gray, S. J.; Dawson, M.; Kaczmarski, E. B.; Borrow, R. *FEMS Immunol. Med. Microbiol.* 2006, *48*, 34-43.

[83] Morrow, D. A.; de Lemos. J. A.; Sabatine, M. S.; Wiviott, S. D.; Blazing, M. A.; Shui, A.; Rifai, N.; Califf, R. M.; Braunwald, E. *Circulation* 2006, *114*, 281-288.

[84] Khan, I. H.; Mendoza, S.; Yee, J.; Deane, M.; Venkateswaran, K.; Zhou, S. S.; Barry, P. A.; Lerche, N. W.; Luciw, P. A. *Clin. Vac. Immunol.* 2006, *13*, 45-52.

[85] Khan, I. H.; Ravindran, R.; Yee, J.; Ziman, M.; Lewinsohn, D. M.; Gennaro, M. L.; Flynn, J. L.; Goulding, C. W.; DeRiemer, K.; Lerche, N. W.; Luciw, P. A. *Clin. Vac. Immunol.* 2008, *15*, 433-438.

[86] Lukacs, Z.; Dietrich, A.; Ganschow, R.; Kohlschutter, A.; Kruithof, R. *Clin. Chem. Lab. Med.* 2005, *43*, 141-145.

[87] Lal, G.; Balmer, P.; Joseph, H.; Dawson, M.; Borrow, R. *Clin. Diagn. Lab. Immunol.* 2004, *11*, 272-279.

[88] Lal, G.; Balmer, P.; Stanford, E.; Martin, S.; Warrington, R.; Borrow, R. *J. Immunol. Meth.* 2005, *296*, 135-147.

[89] Dias, D.; VanDoren, J.; Schlottmann, S.; Kelly, S.; Puchalski, D.; Ruiz, W.; Boerckel, P.; Kessler, J.; Antonello, J. M.; Green, T.; Brown, M.; Smith, J.; Chirmule, N.; Barr, E.; Jansen, K. U.; Esser, M. T. *Clin. Diagn. Lab. Immuno.* 2005, *12*, 959-969.

[90] Page, B. T.; Kurtzman, C. P. *J. Clin. Microbiol.* 2005, *43*, 4507-4514.

[91] Brunstein, J.; Thomas, E. *Diagn. Mol. Pathol.* 2006, *15*, 169-173.

[92] Mehrpouyan, M.; Bishop, J. E.; Ostrerova, N.; Van Cleve M.; Lohman, K. L. *Mol. Cell Probes* 1997, *11*, 337-347.

[93] Page, B. T.; Shields, C. E.; Merz, W. G.; Kurtzman, C. P. *J. Clin. Microbiol.* 2006, *4*, 3167-3171.

[94] Hansson, O.; Zetterberg, H.; Buchhave, P.; Londos, E.; Blennow, K.; Minthon, L. *Lancet Neurol,* 2006, *5*, 228-234.

[95] Nielsen, H. M.; Minthon, L.; Londos, E.; Blennow, K.; Miranda, E.; Perez, J.; Crowther, D. C.; Lomas, D. A.; Janciauskiene, S. M. *Neurology* 2007, *69*, 1569-1579.

[96] Nelson, P. G.; Kuddo, T.; Song, E. Y.; Dambrosia, J. M.; Kohler, S.; Satyanarayana,G.; Vandunk, C.; Grether, J. K.; Nelson, K. B. *Int. J. Dev. Neurosci.* 2006, *24*, 73-80.

[97] Ichiyama, T.; Siba, P.; Suarkia, D.; Reeder, J.; Takasu, T.; Miki, K.; Maeba, S.; Furukawa, S. *Cytokine* 2006, *33*, 17-20.

[98] Nagafuchi, M.; Nagafuchi, Y.; Sato, R.; Imaizumi, T.; Ayabe, M.; Shoji, H.; Ichiyama,T. *Int. Med,* 2006, *45*, 1209-1212.

[99] Lewczuk, P.; Kornhuber, J.; Vanderstichele, H.; Vanmechelen, E.; Esselmann, H.; Bibl, M.; Wolf, S.; Otto, M.; Reulbach, U.; Kolsch, H.; Jessen, F.; Schroder, J.; Schonknecht, P.; Hampel, H.; Peters, O.; Weimer, E.; Perneczky, R.; Jahn, H.; Luckhaus, C.; Lamla, U.; Supprian, T.; Maler, J. M.; Wiltfang, J. *Neurobiol. Aging* 2008, *29*, 812-818.

[100] Li, G.; Sokal, I.; Quinn, J. F.; Leverenz, J. B.; Brodey, M.; Schellenberg, G. D.; Kaye, J. A.; Raskind, M. A.; Zhang, J.; Peskind, E. R.; Montine, T. J. *Neurology* 2007, *69*, 631-639.

[101] Millward, J. M.; Caruso, M.; Campbell, I. L.; Gauldie, J.; Owens, T. *J. Immunol.* 2007, *178*, 8175-8182.

[102] Colombo, M. B.; Haworth, S. E.; Poli, F.; Nocco, A.; Puglisi, G.; Innocente, A.; Serafini, M.; Messa, P.; Scalamogna, M. *Cytom. B Clin. Cytom.* 2007, *7*, 465-471.

[103] Panigrahi, A.; Gupta, N.; Siddiqui, J. A.; Margoob, A.; Bhowmik, D.; Guleria, S.; Mehra, N. K. *Hum. Immunol.* 2007, *68*, 362-367.

[104] Suarez-Alvarez, B.; Lopez-Vazquez, A.; Gonzalez, M. Z.; Fdez-Morera, J. L.; Diaz-Molina, B.; Blanco-Gelaz, M. A.; Pascual, D.; Martinez-Borra, J.; Muro, M.; Alvarez-Lopez, M. R.; Lopez-Larrea, C. *Am. J. Transplant.* 2007, *7*, 1842-1848.

[105] Zhu, Q.; Ziemssen, F.; Henke-Fahle, S.; Tatar, O.; Szurman, P.; Aisenbrey, S.; Schneiderhan-Marra, N. *Ophthalmology* 2008, *115*, 1750-1755.

[106] Zhang, J. Z.; Ward, K. W. *J. Antimicrob. Chemother.* 2008, *61*, 111-116.

[107] Poetz, O.; Ostendorp, R.; Brocks, B.; Schwenk, J. M.; Stoll, D.; Joos, T. O.; Templin, M. F. *Proteomics* 2005, *5*, 2402-2411.

[108] Schwenk J. M.; Lindberg, J.; Sundberg, M.; Uhlen, M. Nilsson P. *Mol. Cell Proteomics* 2007, *6*, 125-132.

[109] Phillips, D. J.; League, S. C.; Weinstein, P.; Hooper, W. C. *Cytokine* 2006, *36*, 180-188.

[110] deJager, W.; Rijkers, G. T. *Methods* 2006, *38*, 294-303.

[111] Weber, T. H.; Kapyaho, K. I.; Tanner, P. *Scand. J. Clin. Lab. Invest.* 1990, *201*, 77-82.

[112] Selby, C. *Ann. Clin. Biochem.* 1999, *36*, 704-721.

[113] Pfleger, C.; Schloot, N.; Veld, F. T. *J. Immunol. Meth.* 2008, *329*, 214-218.

[114] Kingsmore S. F. *Nat. Rev. Drug Discov.* 2006, 5, 310-320.

[115] Homola, J. *Chem. Rev.* 2008, *108*, 462-493.

[116] Zheng, G.; Patolsky, F.; Cui, Y.; Wang, W. U.; Lieber, C. M. *Nat. Biotenchnol.* 2005, *23*, 1294-1301.

[117] Koehne, J. E.; Chen, H.; Cassell, A. M.; Ye, Q.; Han, J.; Meyyappan, M.; Li, J. *Clin. Chem.* 2004, *50*, 1886-1893.

[118] Higgs, R. E.; Knierman, M. D.; Gelfanova, V.; Butler, J. P.; Hale, J. E. *Methods Mol. Biol.* 2008, *428*, 209-230.

[119] Thomas, S. W.; Joly, G. D.; Swager, T. M. *Chem. Rev.* 2007, *107*, 1339-1386.

[120] Liu, B.; Bazan, G. C. *Chem. Mater.* 2004, *16*, 4467-4476.

[121] Ho, H. A.; Béra-Abérem, M.; Leclerc, M. *Chem. Eur. J.* 2005, *11*, 1718-1724.

[122] Zheng, W.; He, L. *J. Am. Chem. Soc.* 2009, *131*, 3432-3433

[123] Zheng, W.; He, L. *Anal. Bioanal. Chem.* 2010, *397*, 2261.

[124] Joos, T. O.; Stoll, D.; Templin, M. F. *Curr. Opin. Chem. Biol.* 2002, *6*, 76-80.

[125] Uddayasankar, U.; Wheeler, A. R. *Anal. Bioanal. Chem.* 2010, *397*, 991-1007.

[126] Sia, S. K.; Whitesides, G. M. *Electrophoresis* 2003, *24*, 3563-3576.

[127] Bange, A.; Halsall, H. B.; Heineman, W. R. *Biosens. Bioelectron.* 2005, *20*, 2488-2503.

[128] Diercks, A. H.; Ozinsky, A.; Hansen, C. L.; Spotts, J. M.; Rodriguez, D. J.; Aderem, A. *Anal. Biochem.* 2009, *386*, 30-35.
[129] Sokoll, L. J.; Chan, D. W. *Anal. Chem.* 1999, *71*, 356-362.
[130] Nery, A. A.; Wrenger, C.; Ulrich, H. *J. Sep. Sci.* 2009, *32*, 1523-1530.
[131] Hanes, J.; Schaffitzel, C.; Knappik, A.; Pluckthun, A. *Nat. Biotechnol.* 2000, *18*, 1287-1292.
[132] Hallborn, J.; Carlsson, R. *Biotechniques* 2002, *Suppl*, 30-37.
[133] Angenendt, P.; Glokler, J.; Sobek, J.; Lehrach, H.; Cahill, D. J. *J. Chromatogr. A* 2003, *1009*, 97-104.
[134] Sutherland, A. J. *Curr. Opin. Solid State Mater. Sci.* 2002, *6*, 365-370.
[135] Chan, W. C. W.; Maxwell, D. J.; Gao, X. H.; Bailey, R. E.; Han, M. Y.; Nie, S. M. *Curr. Opin. Biotechnol.* 2002, *13*, 40-46.
[136] Xu, H.; Sha, M. Y.; Wong, E. Y.; Uphoff, J.; Xu, Y.; Treadway, J. A.; Truong, A.; O'Brien, E.; Asquith, S.; Stubbins, M.; Spurr, N. K.; Lai, E. H.; Mahoney, W. *Nucleic Acids Res.* 2003, *31*, e43.
[137] Cao, Y. C.; Huang, Z. L.; Liu, T. C.; Wang, H. Q.; Zhu, X. X.; Wang, Z.; Zhao, Y. D.; Liu, M. X.; Lu, Q. M. *Anal. Biochem.* 2006, *351*, 193-200.
[138] Ma, Q.; Wang, X.; Li, Y.; Shi, Y.; Su, X. *Talanta* 2007, *72*, 1446-1452.

9

Multiplexed Bead Immunoassays: Advantages and Limitations in Pediatrics

Emma Burgos-Ramos, Gabriel Ángel Martos-Moreno,
Jesús Argente, Vicente Barrios*
Department of Endocrinology, Hospital Infantil Universitario Niño Jesús,
Instituto de Investigación La Princesa,
Department of Pediatrics, Universidad Autónoma de Madrid, Madrid, and Centro de Investigación Biomédica en Red de Fisiopatología Obesidad y Nutrición (CIBERobn),
Instituto de Salud Carlos III,
Spain

1. Introduction

The development of flow cytometric bead-based technology has afforded new perspectives in basic and clinical investigation, allowing for the simultaneous measurement of multiple analytes in biological samples. In this chapter, we will analyze this innovative technology based upon the use of small fluorescent particles coated with highly specific antibodies.

When performing an immunoassay, a specific antibody is used to identify and quantify the concentration of target molecules or analytes in complex samples, such as serum or urine. The use of monoclonal antibodies, highly specific, was a great improvement in these assays. Currently, the combination of these specific antibodies with different fluorophores and novel detection technologies has allowed the achievement of higher sensitivity and several improvements in this technique.

This review will be focused on the multiplexed bead immunoassay (MBIA), which has emerged as a powerful tool to simultaneously quantify several analytes in limited sample volumes. This is of great interest in Pediatrics, given the difficulty to obtain biological samples, particularly in newborns and the clinical interest of this specific type of analysis has increased in recent years (Lee et al., 2008). In fact, MBIA presents several advantages over the classically used immunoassays in pediatric samples, showing better reliability and consistency in the measurements, what is of great interest in longitudinal studies and clinical trials (Bomert et al., 2011).

This multi-analyte analysis method is a solid-phase immunoassay sandwich that uses a capture monoclonal antibody for every molecule aimed to study, that are joined to a specific microsphere with unique features. This microsphere combines two fluorescent compounds that allow for the discrimination from other particles in the assay. A second antibody recognizes another epitope, and detects each analyte bound to the complex, by using several

* Corresponding Author

detection methods, such as secondary or tertiary antibodies with fluorescent probes or the use of phycoerytrin-streptavidin, among others (Chandra et al., 2011). A flow cytometer, based in X-map technology, recognizes and integrates the emission of the last signal discriminating it according to the specific emission of each microsphere (Vignali et al., 2000). Currently, the color-coded microspheres allow the simultaneous performance of up to 100 determinations.

However, the development of assays focused on the diagnosis in pediatric disorders is still sparse, with new antibody detection panels needed, especially in growth and pubertal disorders. The acceptance of MBIA depends on the acquisition of comparable results to those achieved by using classical techniques, such as radioimmunoanalysis (RIA) or enzyme-linked immunosorbent assay (ELISA), accepted as "gold standards" to date. Although some studies have comparatively quantified the measurement of some hormones by using classical inmunoassays and MBIA (Liu et al., 2006), further comparisons are needed, especially for analytes present at low concentrations, that show significant differences in their values according to the methodology used. Therefore, the establishment of reference values for the pediatric population and the improvement in the detection of those parameters present in a low concentration in samples constitute new challenges for both, the investigators and the MBIA manufacturers.

2. Multiplexed bead immunoassays: principles and technology development

The limited sample volume and time-saving gains of the MBIA have made it an election technique for studies involving multiple factors, such as cytokines and pituitary hormones, among others (Djoba-Siawaya et al., 2008). In fact, these complex profiles require an arduous procedure and high volume samples when numerous analytes were analyzed by classical methods. Nevertheless, this laborious process has been improved by the introduction of fluorescent bead assays.

2.1 General considerations

The analytes measured by the immunoassays are extensive, including proteins and low molecular weight molecules, and have been widely utilized in the diagnosis for over forty years (Tetin & Stroupe, 2004). Immunoassays were applied initially to the determination of hormones and the antibodies used were polyclonal (Yalow & Berson, 1959). Its routine use led to a revolution in the field of endocrinology, as well as to the introduction of new tests for the diagnosis and management of endocrine disorders. Subsequently, the use of this technique was extended to other areas, such as biochemical disorders and oncology, by the determination of enzymes, vitamins and tumor markers.

Nevertheless, these classical assays show several limitations. Probably the most important, is that they only measure the levels of one analyte as a time. Proteins are a part of a complex system and clinical diagnosis requires the determination of multiple factors to interpret the pathophysiology of a single health problem. Thus, these requirements increase the cost, due to the number of assays, with the subsequent economic pressures for the Health Systems. In addition, the time spend in their performance is increased and this must be optimized in a diagnostic setting. Besides, the determination of several analytes included into an endocrine system may lead to different error degrees in each individual determination that may avoid a desirable interpretation of the illness. In addition, there is a minimal risk of radiation and the problems of stability of radioisotopes may interfere in the quality of radioimmunoassay.

All these concerns have been minimized in the past decades. As previously reported, one of the greatest advances has been the use of monoclonal antibodies, which represents a continuous source of identical molecules with high affinity and specificity (Hoogenboom, 2005). Also, the development of software for data processing and the incorporation of non-isotopic reporters, such as enzymes that generate chromogenic, fluorescent and chemiluminescent products have improved these classical assays. The development of amplification methods (Figure 1) together with the use of above mentioned products has improved the sensitivity of these assays, allowing for the progressive use of smaller sample size, making it possible their application to pediatric samples (Barrios et al., 2007).

2.2 Basic principles

The discovery of new fluorescent compounds has improved the sensitivity of classical immunoassays. In recent years, protein microarrays have emerged as a powerful tool to provide quantitative data of proteins in biological samples. In traditional protein microarrays, capture reagents are immobilized in defined locations and in the presence of substrates, microspots are generated. After that, the deconvolution of the multiplexed measurements, allows for the identification and quantification of the set of selected proteins (Mirzabekov & Kolchinsky, 2002).

A key advance in multiplexed measurements has been the spatial segregation of the mentioned immobilized protein, encoded beads yield so-called MBIA. Multiplexed bead immunoassay kits contain microspheres, that are highly uniform with the same size (around 3-6 µm, depending of the manufacturer) and are polystyrene beads cross-linked during polymerization for physical and thermal stability. These microspheres are grouped into sets; each one is subsequently embedded with specific quantities of red and orange fluorescent dyes. The different proportion of these dyes gives each specific set of microspheres a unique spectral signature. Each specific set of microspheres is used as the solid support for the conjugation with a distinct reactant for each particular analyte. Among the reactants, there are enzyme substrates, antigens, receptors and antibodies.

In the MBIA, the capture antibody of each immunosorbent assay is coupled to one of 100 different microsphere bead sets, a 10 x 10 matrix with capacity and the combination of red and orange florescent dyes. After the capture of the analyte, the complexes are washed applying vacuum separation. The vacuum is applied to a 96-well plate, in order to separate the liquid, whereas the microspheres are retained in the filter. Afterwards, the addition of a solution with a second biotinylated antibody followed by resuspension allows for the creation of a "sandwich". After a new washing, a complex of streptavidin conjugated to phycoerythrin is added. The amount of the analyte binded to the beads is then quantified through the use of phycoerythrin, a green-fluorochrome reported dye, excited by the array reader at a wavelength of 532 nm, whereas the emission is detected around 575 nm (Figure 2). Thus, in each immunosorbent assay, the intensity of this green fluorochrome measured by the reader is directly proportional to the amount of analyte bound to the surface of each microsphere (Thrailkill et al., 2005; Van der Heyde & Gramaglia, 2011).

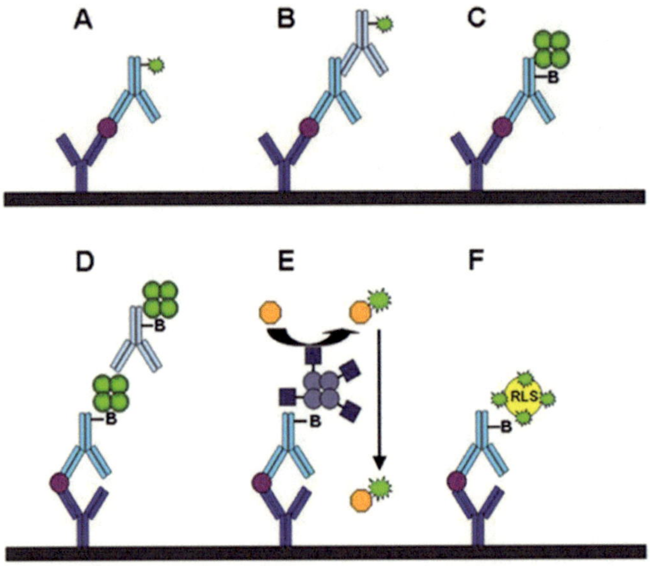

A, fluorescent bound detection antibodies. B, fluorescent labeled compounds-tertiary antibodies. C, biotinylated detection antibodies with streptavidin-phycoerythrin conjugate. D, streptavidin-phycoerythrin conjugate staining amplified with biotinylated anti-streptavidin-phycoerythrin antibodies. E, streptavidin-linked horseradish peroxisade linked to a species-specific tertiary antibody activates chemiluminiscent substrates or generates different flourophores. F, resonance light-scattering colloid gold particles coated with an antibiotin antibody. Modified from Nielsen & Geierstanger. J Immunol Methods 2004; 290: 107-120.

Fig. 1. Signal generation and amplification methods.

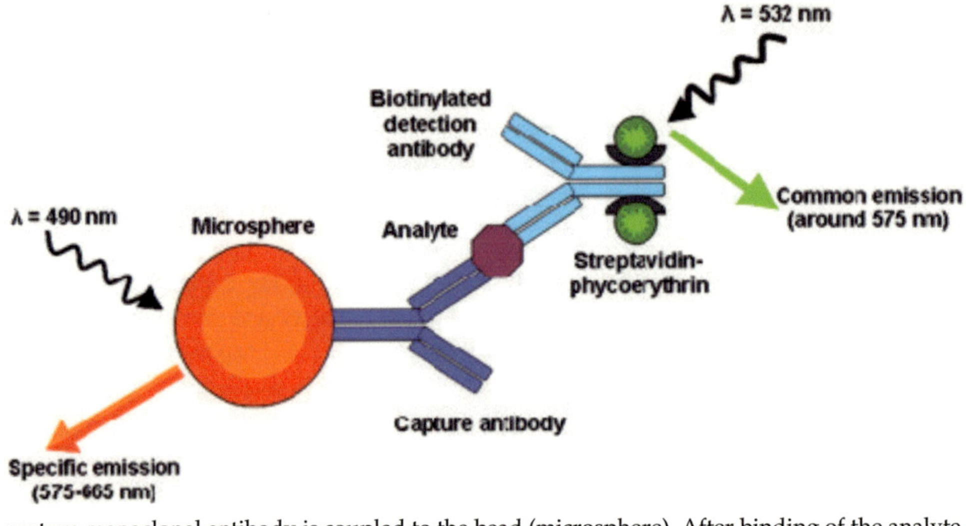

The capture monoclonal antibody is coupled to the bead (microsphere). After binding of the analyte a second biotinylated antibody is added. After addition of a streptavidin-phycoerythrin conjugate, dyes embedded in the beads and phycoerythrin are excited (wavy lines) and both compounds give two types of light emission. Modified from Barrios et al., Rev Esp Pediatr 2007; 63: 157-161.

Fig. 2. Schematic representation of an isolated reaction of a MBIA with the reagents used in this technique.

There are two lasers in the adapter array reader for MBIA, the first laser classifies each microsphere and its bound analyte and the second quantifies the amount of analyte bound to each microsphere. The first laser, known as red laser, excites the dyes of each microsphere and the fluorescent signal of each microsphere is separated with selective filters and converted in intensity units by the combination of fluorescent detectors and a digital processor, being the microsphere arranged. The second laser, named green laser, stimulates the fluorochromes bound to the analytes (in our case, phycoerythrin) and the signal is distinguished with emission filters and translated to intensity units by specific detectors and a signal processor, and the amount of analyte is measured. This data are acquired by different adapted flow cytometers attached to computers with special software (Figure 3).

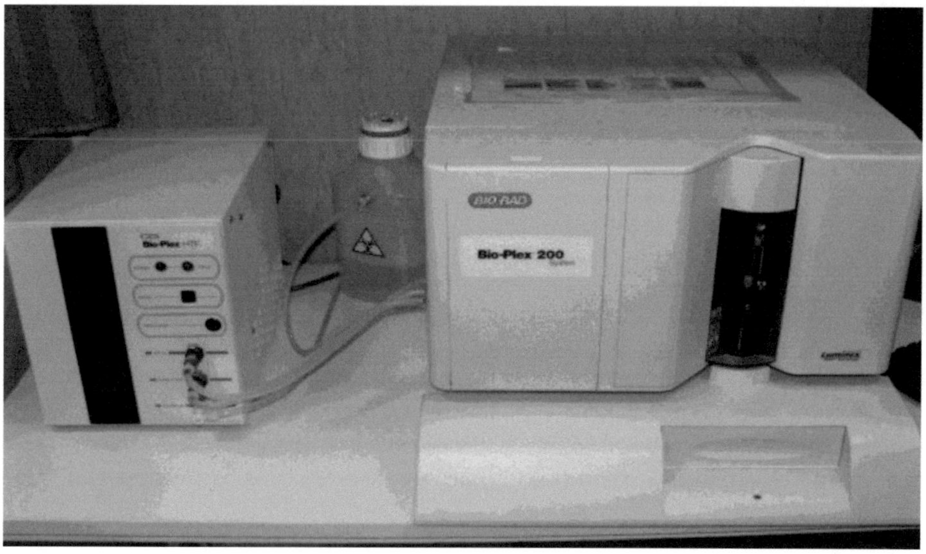

Fig. 3. Suspension array system with high throughout put fluidics system.

This special cytometer is a dual-laser, flow-based microplate reader system. The content of each well is drawn up into the reader. The laser and associated optics detect the fluorescence of the individual beads and the fluorescence signal on the bead surface. This identifies each assay and reports the levels of target protein in the well. The detected intensity of fluorescence on the beads indicates the quantity of analytes. Thus, the system calculates the green fluorescence and the combination of red and orange fluorescence of each microsphere by using three detectors. The software separates the pool of microspheres using the orange and red fluorescence data and integrates these data with the average amount of green fluorescence for each bead set (Figure 4). A high-speed digital processor manages the data output, analyzed as fluorescence intensity on the software.

2.3 Assay guidelines and technical considerations

One of the main focuses of this review is to analyze the assay procedure in order to obtain reliable results with this technique. The current literature contains many examples of user and manufacturer product evaluations; however, some recommendations that will improve the performance of MBIA must be taken into account.

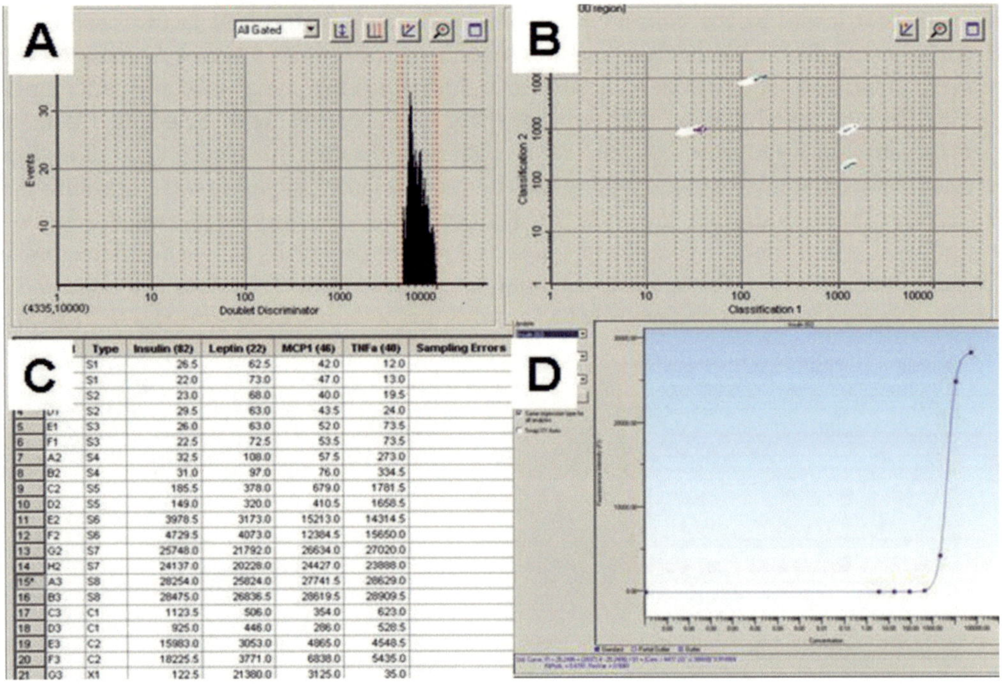

Each set of microbeads is quantitated in the histogram (A) and separated by the Luminex© system in a two-dimensional bead map (B), permitting the simultaneous quantitation of different analytes in the same sample. Results are given as fluorescence mean intensity (C) and the concentration of the analyte in the problem sample is obtained by extrapolation from a standard curve (D).

Fig. 4. Separation and quantification of the analyte concentrations by the suspension array reader system.

As the microspheres have different fluorescent dyes that are light sensitive, we must protect the beads from direct light by covering the tubes with aluminium foil. Sometimes, this procedure is not necessary, because the manufacturer provides the MBIA kits with dark tubes, thus avoiding light exposition. We also must keep the microspheres at 4°C, avoiding freezing.

Another problem is the eventual aggregation of the microspheres. Sonication during 15-60 seconds keeping the tubes on ice is a procedure to separate aggregated microspheres, but it may cause hurt in the microsphere suspension. We usually used gentle vortexing during 5-10 minutes to obtain a homogeneous mixture. Thus, we may avoid not only a potential harmful effect on the sample, but also the possible loss of a part of the liquid phase during sonication. Another common alternative process is the use of a bath sonicator, by placing the probe sonicator tip in a bath of water and inserting the tube with microspheres near the tip, avoiding touching it.

Multiplexed bead immunoassays require washing during the assay period to separate the analyte of second antibody bound to the microsphere surface from the unbound reactants. The most common procedure is the vacuum separation. The reactions are performed in microtiter filter-bottom 96-well plates and vacuum is applied to the plate allowing the liquid to filter through while retaining the microbeads on the filter (Figure 5A). A new procedure is the use of magnetic microbeads and conventional 96 well plates. In this situation, a microplate washer with a magnetic platform is used to separate these microspheres of unbound fraction (Figure 5B).

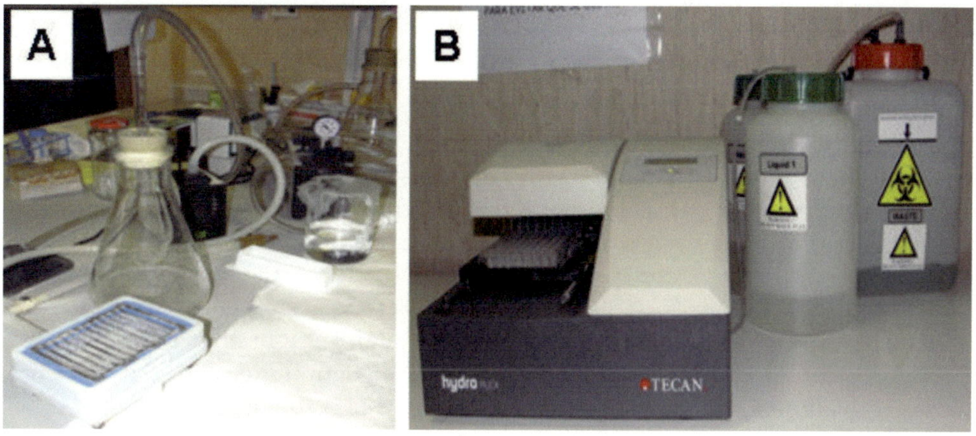

A, vacuum manifold system. The microtiter filter-bottom 96-plate is on a support and vacuum is applied with a conventional pump. Liquid is collected into a manifold. B, Microplate washer with magnetic platform. Conventional ELISA 96-plate and magnetic microbeads are used to separate liquid of microbeads.

Fig. 5. Separation of microbeads and liquid containing unbound fraction.

We may also develop new MBIAs, coupling the capture antibodies to the microspheres. First, we must choose a set of microbeads with significant diverse proportion of dyes fluorescence compounds (red and orange) in order to maintain sufficiently separated the reading areas obtained in the two-dimensional diagram by the suspension array reader system (see figure 5B). In this way, we will avoid potential overlapping among different bead readings.

Microspheres with fluorescent dyes are supplied at standard concentrations, but during the coupling process may diminish due to loss during washing. This loss is not uniform and it may change for multiple causes, such as pressure of vacuum manifold, and reactant employed in coupling, among others (Bio-Plex Manager Software, User Guide). It is difficult the optimization of the assay because we must take into consideration the different proportions of reactants (antibodies, analytes, fluorophore conjugates, assay buffers, etc.), temperatures and times of incubation and perhaps the most critical variable, the total surface area (total number of microbeads). To obtain reliable results, it is necessary to know the number of microspheres by counting them in a hemocytometer. These are also crucial aspects in the new MBIA using small quantity of sample, the microfluidic bead-based immunoassay that it was be developed to perform a multiplexed assay in a capillary, requiring only 1 µl assay volume (Yu et al., 2010).

Monoclonal capture antibodies must be bound to a specific each set of microspheres. There are some kits to perform this procedure; however is difficult to establish not only the adequate number of beads and concentration of the capture antibody, but also the quantity of secondary antibody to obtain a good assay performance (Djoba-Siawaya et al., 2008). Assay performance of new developed MBIAs must be compared with classical methods, such as radioimmunoassay o ultra-sensitive enzyme-linked immunosorbent assay, considered as "gold standards" in the laboratory (Krouwer et al., 2002; Elshal & McCoy, 2006). The development of new panels using MBIA requires testing the effect of the biological matrix. Serum or plasma specimens are complex samples that are frequently diluted before addition in the well. The diluent has to imitate the sample matrix in order to obtain the same fluorescent background. There are many commercially available diluents and it is also necessary to analyze the effect of dilution and its addition to interpolate unknown concentrations (Pfleger et al., 2008).

Another aspect is the optimization of the parameters of the acquisition of data and analysis of results in the reader, by using the associated software. We must start by adjusting the needle according the manual instructions. The height of the array reader sample needle must be adjusted when the style of microtiter plate has been modified, to optimize the sample acquisition. The next step is the calibration of the array reader, necessary for optimal performance and reproducibility of results (Bio-Plex Manager Software, User Guide). Commercial manufacturers provide some kits containing calibration microspheres with stable fluorescent intensities in the emission wavelength ranges of the classification channels. The calibration process employs these microbeads to regulate voltage settings for optimal microsphere classification and reporter readings over time.

After preparation of the protocol, we need to define additional characteristics, as the number of bead counts, sample size and bead map selection to obtain an adequate histogram and bead map (Figures 4A & 4B). These graphs are updated during the reading (Figure 4C). Results are extrapolated from each standard curve for each analyte (Figure 4D). At the end of the reading process, the software generates a results file, containing the data, protocol parameters used and analysis tools for interpreting the data. Thus, we can reanalyze raw data by testing the effect of dilution or the regression method used. We are also able to change the double discriminator gate range and to recalculate the data based in the new range. During the reading, this discriminator of the array reader determines the amount of light scatter of the beads detected by the red laser. Particle size is proportional to light scatter and an internal discriminator gate identifies particles smaller o larger than single microbeads, including aggregates that may interfere in the results.

In addition to these studies, development of a new MBIA or the inclusion of a new analyte to a pre-existent multiplexed panel also requires the analysis of classical assay characteristics, as sensitivity, specificity, precision, recovery and linearity, among others (Krouwer et al., 2002; Liu et al., 2005; Dossus et al., 2008; Martos-Moreno et al., 2010).

3. Interest of MBIA in pediatrics

The study of growth hormone axis, pituitary hormone panel or cytokine expression profiling, among other examples, have become as established guidelines for the identification and characterization of several diseases. However, the determination of multiple parameters by classical immunoassays is a laborious process requiring a big amount sample volume, a problematic aspect for patients, especially when these subjects are newborns or children.

Multiplexed immunoassays based on protein microarray platforms have been used in the detection and confirmation of biomarkers associated with several diseases (Hsu et al., 2008; Sauer et al., 2008; Paczesny et al., 2009). Nevertheless, most of these studies have been performed in adults and it is necessary to carry out these determinations in children. Among studies in children, most of them have been conducted to analyze serum cytokine profiling (Pranzatelli et al., 2011). In addition, most of the parameters determined in boys and girls during pubertal development show variations in their concentrations, due to anthropometric and biochemical changes influencing some of these variables. Thus, MBIA is a good method, because it allows for the simultaneous determination of multiple parameters in a single assay, avoiding inter-assay variations. This property offers reliable data and could help in the diagnosis and or follow up of pediatric patients. Thus, different studies, clinical trials or monitoring of pediatric patients during disease treatment require the determination of multiple parameters during extended periods of time (Martos-Moreno et al., 2011a). As an example, in the Table 1, we show the effect of weight loss on several adipokines in obese children after dietary intervention.

This technique also facilitates in obtaining a "pool" of reference values during childhood and puberty and may improve the knowledge of the physiology of any given endocrine axis. As it is mentioned above, the determination of several analytes at the same time, avoid the variability among them and allows a better interpretation of the physiology of the studied axis. In addition, the obtaining of reference data in children involves the recruitment of boys and girls in different Tanner stages, due to the effect of sex and biochemical changes through pubertal development. MBIA could be a choice method, as not only integrates all parameters in one determination, but also allows analyzing longitudinal changes in all of them. Here we show reference data of different adipokines in boys and girls through childhood and adolescence (Table 2).

Group	Adiponectin	Leptin	Resistin	TNF-α	IL-6
Control	15.8 ± 6.3	4.3 ± 3.1	13.8 ± 6.2	4.6 ± 2.2	2.2 ± 2.0
Obese B	16.3 ± 7.4	36.9 ± 13.6**	14.7 ± 6.5	6.1 ± 2.0	2.5 ± 2.0
Obese -1	19.1 ± 7.2	16.4 ± 13.3**##	12.2 ± 5.5	5.4 ± 3.2	2.1 ± 1.5
Obese -2	25.7 ± 11.4*#	16.1 ± 11.3**##	15.7 ± 8.4	4.8 ± 2.4	2.0 ± 1.3

Adiponectin, leptin, resistin, tumoral necrosis factor-α (TNF-α) and interleukin-6 (IL-6) levels were measured by MBIA in healthy children (control) and prupubertal obese subjects at baseline (Obese B) and after reduction of their body mass index by 1 SDS (Obese -1) and 2 SDS (Obese -2). Data expressed as mean ± standard deviation. *p<0.01, **p<0.001 vs. control; #p<0.01, ##p<0.001 vs. obese B. Modified from Martos-Moreno et al. Clin Chem Lab Med 2010; 48: 1439-1446.

Table 1. Serum concentrations of adipokines in control and obese children

Another aspect of special interest in Pediatrics is the sensitivity of the MBIAs. Serum samples of children and newborns have low levels of some analytes and sensitivity is crucial to determine them. The fluorescent readout if MBIA is more sensitive than the colorimetric signal of ELISA, where it is required a step of enzyme amplification. Moreover, the sensitivity can be augmented by reducing the number of bead in each assay, increasing in this manner the ratio of analyte to capture antibody without reducing the number of capture antibodies per bead. In addition, MBIA may be more reproducible than ELISA. Thus, the replicates usually show little variation in fluorescence, whereas ELISA significant variations between experiments and between plates within assays (Leng et al., 2008). Multiplexed bead assays are more accurate because the data are calculated from the mean of 50-100 beads, each of which functions as an individual replicate. This is an additional advantage in longitudinal studies, very frequents in pediatric population.

The MBIAs may be adapted to carry out immunoassays for identifying antibodies. It is necessary to introduce variations in the assay design (Morgan et al., 2004). Here, purified antigens are conjugated to the beads and incubated with any sample of interest, followed with species-specific anti-immunoglobulin reagent, labelled with a fluorochrome. The mean fluorescence intensity is directly proportional to the amount of antibody bound to the antigen on the bead. These adapted assays have been employed to detect antibodies in diagnosis of celiac disease (Yiannaki et al., 2004), autoimmune thyroid disease (Tozzoli et al., 2006) and meningitis (Shoma et al., 2011) during childhood.

Multiplex applications are not restricted to the detection of proteins and antibodies, as this technique has also been used during a decade for the simultaneous detection of different DNA sequences. Among the specific applications include genotyping of single nucleotide polymorphisms, screening of genetic diseases, genotyping of the major histocompatibility complex and molecular analysis of infectious organisms (Ye et al.., 2001; Cesbron-Gautier et al., 2004; Dunbar et al., 2003). The main use of MBIA in this field has been the detection of mutations associated with disease; so, one of the first applications of genotyping was the analysis of multiple variants of β-globin in capillary blood of neonates (Colinas et al., 2000). Also this technology has been used for genotyping in samples from patients with a predisposition to thrombophilia (Musher et al., 2002) and detection of fusion transcripts of chromosomal translocations in children with acute lymphoblastic leukemia (Wallace et al., 2003).

Tanner stage	Adiponectin	Leptin	Resistin	TNF-α	IL-6
I					
Female	15.6 ± 4.2	4.8 ± 3.6	13.5 ± 5.0	4.2 ± 1.6	2.6 ± 2.2
Male	16.2 ± 5.6	3.9 ± 2.7	12.6 ± 6.3	4.2 ± 2.0	1.9 ± 1.8
II					
Female	16.7 ± 12.2	5.7 ± 2.7	15.9 ± 4.3	4.0 ± 1.6	2.6 ± 2.2
Male	17.0 ± 5.0	4.1 ± 2.8	16.9 ± 7.1	4.0 ± 1.3	2.4 ± 1.8
III + IV					
Female	18.0 ± 6.2	11.4 ± 4.2	16.5 ± 3.8	4.6 ± 1.7	1.3 ± 0.4
Male	13.4 ± 6.8	6.4 ± 2.7	16.8 ± 7.0	4.4 ± 1.3	1.5 ± 0.6
V					
Female	12.1 ± 4.9	12.1 ± 4.3	29.4 ± 8.9	4.9 ± 1.1	1.5 ± 1.2
Male	18.3 ± 5.2	6.2 ± 3.1	22.8 ± 8.5	4.6 ± 1.6	1.0 ± 0.5

Adiponectin, leptin, resistin, tumoral necrosis factor-α (TNF-α) and interleukin-6 (IL-6) levels were measured by MBIA in healthy girls and boys in the different pubertal stages (Tanner stage). Data expressed as mean ± standard deviation. Modified from Martos-Moreno et al. An Pediatr (Barc.) 2011b; 74: 356-362.

Table 2. Reference values of adipokines in children throughout development

4. Limitations

In spite of the advantages of this technology, it is important to keep in mind the scarce development of assays in the field of pediatric disorders. Therefore, the development of new multiplexed panels is needed, especially in those pediatric pathologies related to endocrinology of growth and pubertal disorders.

Special attention should be paid when reporting absolute values with MBIA. The acceptance of this technique depends on the acquisition of comparable results to those achieved by using classical techniques, accepted as the "gold standards" in the laboratory. To date, we and others have compared these methodologies for some hormones (Martos-Moreno et al., 2010; Liu et al., 2005), but further comparisons are needed, especially for analytes that are present at very low concentrations in pediatric samples, since the concentrations obtained with MBIA and classical ultra-sensitive immunoassays are distinct for some analytes and also show that the differences between the methods are composed of both constant and proportional components, preventing a direct comparability between both assays.

A limitation in some MBIAs is the interpretation and reporting of analyte values at extremely low concentrations. One of the possible advantages of this assay is that the dynamic range seems to be much broader than classical ELISAs. However, many sensitivity issues in the very low range of concentrations remain unresolved (Liu et al., 2005; Leng et al., 2008), especially for several cytokines.

Therefore, the establishment of reference values for the pediatric population and the improvement in the detection of determined parameters that are present at low levels in serum is a challenge for the investigators and the MBIA manufacturers, respectively.

5. Future research

These methods have an excellent accuracy and reliability, together with an excellent sensitivity for most analytes. However, some analytes are currently determined by ultra-sensitive immunoassays. A challenge of this technology is to improve the sensitivity of some analytes present at very low concentrations in biological fluids, as well as in tissues, in order to its applicability in new areas of routine diagnosis.

Another important aspect is the improvement of specificity for some parameters, which is essentially limited by the quality of antibodies employed in the MBIA (Vignali, 2000). Thus, the use of some monoclonal antibodies in classical immunoassays, such as enzimoimmunoassay or radioimmunoassay, does not affect in a significant manner the results, but it may be a big issue for MBIA. The near future will show whether MBIA exhibit a greater applicability in diagnostics in Pediatrics.

Another objective is the development of commercial kits that allow the simultaneous analysis of factors that require extractive procedures or alternative processes for assessment, such as growth factors, together with other molecules in which it is not necessary this preliminary stage. It is also required the improvement of MBIAs to evaluate the molecular heterogeneity of certain hormones that have several isoforms (Popii & Baumann, 2004). In this sense, the development of immunology allows characterizing new monoclonal antibodies against different epitopes, solving some problems of inadequate sensitivity or cross-reactivity with classical antibodies (Feldhaus et al., 2003).

These assays will improve the throughput by greatly enhancing the quantity of information achieved from a single experiment. Moreover, the development of new microfluidic bead-based immunoassays will allow diminishing the expenditures of reagents and reducing the requirements of biological sample, very important in pediatric patients. Based upon their capabilities, MBIA will be proposed for use in disease screening and probably will open up new possibilities in the follow up of patients during therapy.

6. Conclusion

Multiplexed bead immunoassays could result more cost-effective for the measurements of selected analytes, diminishing inter-assay variations and reducing the volume of sample needed, what would be particularly interesting in Pediatrics, especially when limited amounts of samples are available, which is usually the case of young children. The current advantages in time, ability to simultaneously measure analyte concentrations in the same conditions and high performance of multiplex analysis will allow MBIA to be a more useful tool in evaluating the pediatric diseases.

7. Acknowledgments

The authors wish to thank Dr. Julie Ann Chowen for English revision and critical review of the manuscript. This work was supported by grants of Fondo de Investigación Sanitaria (CD07/00256 to E.B.R.), CIBERobn and Fundación Endocrinología y Nutrición.

8. References

Barrios, V.; Martos-Moreno, G.A. & Argente, J. (2007). Aspectos metodológicos y utilidad diagnóstica de los inmunoensayos múltiples en suspensión en Pediatría. *Revista Española de Pediatría*, Vol.63, No.2, pp. 157-161, ISSN 0034-947X

Bio-Plex Manager Software 4.1. User Guide. (2005) Bio-Rad Laboratories, Inc. 2000 Alfred Nobel Drive. Hercules, CA, USA, P/N 10003414.

Bomert, M.; Köllisch, G.; Roponen, M.; Lauener, R.; Renz, H.; Pfefferle, P.I. & Al-Fakhri, N. (2011) Analytical performance of a multiplexed, bead-based cytokine detection system in small volume samples. *Clinical Chemistry and Laboratory Medicine*, (DOI: 10.1515/CCLM.2011.631), ISSN 1434-6621

Cesbron-Gautier, A.; Simon, P.; Achard, L.; Cury, S.; Follea, G. & Bignon J.D. (2004). Luminex technology for HLA typing by PCR-SSO and identification of HLA antibody specificities. *Annales de Biologie Clinique (Paris)*, Vol.62, No.1, pp. 93-98, ISSN 0003-3898

Chandra, H.; Reddy, P.J. & Srivastava S. (2011). Protein microarrays and novel detection platforms. *Expert Review of Proteomics*, Vol.8, pp. 61-79, ISSN 1478-9450

Colinas, R.J.; Bellisario, R. & Pass, K.A. (2000). Multiplexed genotyping of beta-globin variants from PCR-amplified newborn blood spot DNA by hybridization with allele-specific oligodeoxynucleotides coupled to an array of fluorescent microspheres. *Clinical Chemistry,* Vol.46, No.7, pp. 996-998, ISSN 0009-9147

Djoba Siawaya JF, Roberts T, Babb C, Black G, Golakai HJ, Stanley K, Bapela NB, Hoal E, Parida, S.; van Helden, P. & Walzl G. (2008). An evaluation of commercial fluorescent bead-based luminex cytokine assays. *PLoS One,* Vol.3:e2535, ISSN 1932-6203

Dossus, L.; Becker, S.; Achaintre, D.; Kaaks, R. & Rinaldi, S. (2009) Validity of multiplex-based assays for cytokine measurements in serum and plasma from "non-diseased" subjects: comparison with ELISA. *Journal of Immunological Methods,* Vol. 350, pp. 125-132, ISSN 0022-1759

Dunbar, S.A.; Vander Zee, C.A.; Oliver, K.G.; Karem, K.L. & Jacobson, J.W. (2003). Quantitative, multiplexed detection of bacterial pathogens: DNA and protein applications of the Luminex LabMAP system. *Journal of Microbiological Methods,* Vol.53, No.2, pp. 245-252, ISSN 0167-7012

Elsshal, M.F. & McCoy, J.P. (2006). Multiplex bead array assays: performance evaluation and comparison of sensitivity to ELISA. *Methods,* Vol.38, No.4, pp. 317-323, ISSN 1046-2023

Feldhaus, M.J.; Siegel, R.W.; Opresko, L.K; Coleman, J.R.; Feldhaus, J.M.; Yeung, Y.A.; Cochran, J.R.; Heinzelman, P.; Colby, D.; Swers, J.; Graff, C.; Wiley, H.S. & Wittrup. KD. (2003). Flow-cytometric isolation of human antibodies from a nonimmune Saccharomyces cerevisiae surface display library. *Nature Biotechnology,* Vol.21, No.2, pp. 163-170, ISSN 1087-0156

Hoogenboom, H.R. (2005). Selecting and screening recombinant antibody libraries. *Nature Biotechnology,* Vol.23, pp. 1105-1116, ISSN 1087-0156

Hsu, H.Y.; Wittemann, S.; Schneider, E.M.; Weiss, M. & Joos T.O. (2008) Suspension microarrays for the identification of the response paterns in hyperinflammatory diseases. *Medical Engineering & Physics,* Vol.30, No.8 , pp. 976-983, ISSN 1350-4533

Krouwer, J.S.; Tholen, D.W.; Garber, C.C.; Goldschmidt, H.M.J.; Harris-Kroll, M.; Linnet, K.; Meier, K.; Robinowitz, M. & Kennedy, J.W. (2002) Method comparison and bias estimation using patient samples; approved guideline. 2nd edition (EP9-A2). *Clinical and Laboratory Standards Institute;* Vol.22, No.19, pp. 1-53, ISSN 0273-3099.

Lee SA; Tsai HT; Ou HC; Han CP; Tee YT; Chen YC; Wu, M.T.; Chou, M.C.; Wang, P.H. & Yang, S.F. (2008). Plasma interleukin-1beta, -6, -8 and tumor necrosis factor-alpha as highly informative markers of pelvic inflammatory disease. *Clinical Chemistry and Laboratory Medicine,* Vol.46, No.7, pp. 997-1003, ISSN 1434-6621

Leng, S.X.; McElhaney, J.E.; Walston, J.D.; Xie, D.; Fedarko, N.S. & Kuchel, G.A. (2008) ELISA and multiplex technologies for cytokine measurement in inflammation and aging research. *Journal of Gerontology Series A Biological Sciences and Medical Sciences,* Vol.63, No.8, pp. 879-884, ISSN 1079-5006

Liu, M.Y.; Xydakis, A.M.; Hoogeveen, R.C.; Jones, P.H.; Smith, E.O.; Nelson, K.W. & Ballantyne, C.M. (2005). Multiplexed analysis of biomarkers related to obesity and the metabolic syndrome in human plasma, using the Luminex-100 system. *Clinical Chemistry,* Vol.51, No.7, pp. 1102-1109, ISSN 0009-9147

Martos-Moreno, G.A.; Burgos-Ramos, E.; Canelles, S.; Argente, J. & Barrios, V. (2010) Evaluation of a multiplex assay for adipokine concentrations in obese children. *Clinical Chemistry and Laboratory Medicine,* Vol.48, No.10, pp. 1439-1446, ISSN 1434-6621

Martos-Moreno, G.A.; Kratzsch, J.; Körner, A.; Barrios, V.; Hawkins, F.; Kiess, W. & Argente J. (2011a) Serum visfatin and vaspin levels in prepubertal children: effect of obesity and weight loss after behavior modifications on their secretion and relationship with glucose metabolism. *International Journal of Obesity (London),* (DOI: 10.1038/ijo.2010.280), ISSN 0307-0565

Martos-Moreno, G.A.; Burgos-Ramos, E.; Canelles, S.; Argente, J. & Barrios, V. (2011b). Analysis of insulin and cytokines during development using a multiplexed immunoassay: implications in pediatrics. *Anales de Pediatría (Barcelona),* Vol.74, No.6, pp. 356-362, ISSN 1695- 4033

Mirzabekov, A. & Kolchinsky, A. (2002). Emerging array-based technologies in proteomics. *Current Opinion in Chemical Biology,* Vol.6, No.1, pp. 70-75, ISSN 1367-5931

Morgan, E.; Varro, R.; Sepulveda, H.; Ember, J.A.; Apgar, J.; Wilson, J.; Lowe, L.; Chen, R.; Shivraj, L.; Agadir, A.; Campos, R.; Ernst, D. & Gaur, A. (2004). Cytometric bead array: a multiplexed assay platform with applications in various areas of biology. *Clinical Immunology,* Vol.110, No.3, pp. 252-266, ISSN 1521-6616

Musher, D.; Goldsmith, E.; Dunbar, S.; Tilney, G.; Darouiche, R.; Yu Q.; López, J.A. & Dong, J.F. (2002). Association of hypercoagulable states and increased platelet adhesion and aggregation with bacterial colonization of intravenous catheters. *The Journal of Infectious Diseases,* Vol.186, No.6, pp. 769-773, ISSN 0022-1899

Nielsen, U.B. & Geierstanger, B.H. (2004) Multiplexed sandwich assays in microarray format. *Journal of Immunological Methods,* Vol.290, pp.107-120, ISSN 0022-1759

Paczesny, S.; Krijanovski, OI; Braun, TM; Choi, SW; Clouthier, SG; Kuick, R; Misek, DE; Cooke, KR; Kitko, CL; Weyand, A; Bickley, D; Jones, D.; Whitfield, J.; Reddy, P.; Levine, J.E.; Hanash S.M. & Ferrara J.L. (2009). A biomarker panel for acute graft-versus-host disease. *Blood,* Vol.113, No. 2, pp. 273-278, ISSN 0006-4971

Pfleger, C.; Schloot, N. & ter Veld, F. (2008). Effect of serum content and diluent selection on assay sensitivity and signal intensity in multiplex bead-based immunoassays. *Journal of Immunological Methods,* Vol.329, No.1-2, pp. 214-218, ISSN 0022-1759

Popii, V. & Baumann, G. Laboratory measurement of growth hormone. *Clinica Chimica Acta,* 2004; Vol.350, No.1-2, pp. 1-16, ISSN 0009-8981

Pranzatelli, M.R.; Tate, E.D.; Travelstead, A.L. & Verhulst, S.J. (2011) Chemokine/cytokine profiling after rituximab: reciprocal expression of BCA-1/CXCL13 and BAFF in childhood OMS. *Cytokine,* Vol.53, No.3, pp. 384-389, ISSN 1043-4666

Sauer, G.; Schneiderhan-Marra, N.; Kazmaier, C.; Hutzel, K.; Koretz, K.; Muche, R.; Kreienberg, R.; Joos, T. & Deissler, H. (2008). Prediction of nodal involvement in breast cancer based on multiparametric protein analyses from preoperative core needle biopsies of the primary lesion. *Clinical Cancer Research,* Vol.14, No.11, pp. 3345-3353, ISSN 1078-0432

Shoma, S.; Verkaik, N.J.; de Vogel, C.P.; Hermans, P.W.; van Selm, S.; Mitchell, T.J.; van Roosmalen, M.; Hossain, S.; Rahman, M.; Endtz, H.P.; van Wamel, W.J. & van Belkum, A. (2011). Develpoment of a multiplexed bead-based immunoassay for the simultaneous detection of antibodies to 17 pneumococcal proteins. *European Journal of Clinical Microbiology & Infectious Diseases,* Vol.30, No.4, pp. 521-526, ISSN 0934-9723

Tanner, J.M. (1962). Growth and Adolescence, 2nd edition. Oxford: Blackwell Scientific Publications.

Tetin, S.Y. & Stroupe, S.D. (2004). Antibodies in diagnostic applications. *Current Pharmaceutical Biotechnology,* Vol.5, pp. 9-16, ISSN 1389-2010

Thrailkill, K.M.; Moreau, C.S.; Cockrell, G.; Simpson, P.; Goel, R.; North, P.; Fowlkes, J.L. & Bunn, R.C. (2005). Physiological matrix metalloproteinase concentrations in serum during childhood and adolescence, using Luminex Multiplex technology. *Clinical Chemistry and Laboratory Medicine,* Vol.43, No.1, pp. 1392-1399, ISSN 1434-6621

Tozzoli, R.; Villalta, D.; Kodermaz, G.; Bagnasco, M.; Tonutti, E. & Bizzaro, N. (2006). Autoantibody profiling of patients with autoimmune thyroid disease using a new multiplexed immunoassay method. *Clinical Chemistry and Laboratory Medicine,* Vol.44, No.7, pp. 837-842, ISSN 1434-6621

Van der Heyde, H.C. & Gramaglia, I. (2011) Bead-based multiplexed analysis of analytes by flow cytometry. *Methods in Molecular Biology,* Vol.699, pp. 85-95, ISSN 1064-3745

Vignali, DAA. (2000). Multiplexed particle-based flow cytometric assays. *Journal of Immunological Methods,* Vol. 243, pp. 243-255, ISSN 0022-1759

Wallace, J.; Zhou, Y.; Usmani, G.N.; Reardon, M.; Newburger, P.; Woda, B. & Pihan, G. (2003). BARCODE-ALL: accelerated and cost-effective genetic risk stratification in acute leukemia using spectrally addressable liquid bead microarrays. *Leukemia,* Vol.17, No.7, pp. 1404-1410, ISSN 0887-6924

Yalow, R.S & Berson, S.A. (1959). Assay of plasma insulin in human subjects by immunological methods. *Nature,* Vol. 184, pp. 1648-1649, ISSN 0028-0836

Ye, F.; Li, M.S.; Taylor, J.D.; Nguyen, Q.; Colton, H.M.; Casey, W.M.; Wagner, M.; Weiner, M.P. & Chen, J. Fluorescent microsphere-based readout technology for multiplexed human single nucleotide polymorphism analysis and bacterial identification. *Human Mutation,* 2001; Vol.17, No.4, pp. 305-316, ISSN 1059-7794

Yiannaki, E.E.; Zintzaras, E.; Analatos, A.; Theodoridou, C.; Dalekos, G.N. & Germenis, A.E. (2004). Evaluation of a microsphere-based flow cytometric assay for diagnosis of celiac disease. *Journal of Immunoassay and Immunochemistry,* Vol.25, No.4, pp. 345-357, ISSN 1532-1819

Yu, X.; Hartmann, M.; Wang, Q.; Poetz, O.; Schneiderhan-Marra, N.; Stoll, D.; Kazmaier, C. & Joos, T.O. (2011) μFBI: a microfluidic bead-based immunoassay for multiplexed detection of proteins from a μl sample volume. *PLos one*, Vol.5, No.10, e13125, ISSN 1932-6203